Veterinary Lactation Physiology

Joydip Mukherjee • Pradip Kumar Das
Dipak Banerjee • Kalyan De

Veterinary Lactation Physiology

A Textbook

Springer

Joydip Mukherjee
Department of Veterinary Physiology
West Bengal University of Animal
and Fishery Sciences
Kolkata, West Bengal, India

Pradip Kumar Das
Department of Veterinary Physiology
West Bengal University of Animal
and Fishery Sciences
Kolkata, West Bengal, India

Dipak Banerjee
Department of Veterinary Physiology
West Bengal University of Animal
and Fishery Sciences
Kolkata, West Bengal, India

Kalyan De
ICAR - National Research Centre on Pig
Rani, Assam, India

ISBN 978-3-032-21122-4 ISBN 978-3-032-21123-1 (eBook)
https://doi.org/10.1007/978-3-032-21123-1

This Springer imprint is published by the registered company Springer Nature Switzerland AG
The registered company address is: Gewerbestrasse 11, 6330 Cham, Switzerland

This book is dedicated to dairy farmers, veterinarians, and livestock professionals whose daily efforts translate scientific knowledge into productive and sustainable dairying.

Foreword

Over the past several decades, global milk production from dairy cows has increased substantially. This growth has been supported by extensive research in lactation physiology aimed at enhancing milk yield, composition, quality, and production efficiency while safeguarding the health and welfare of dairy animals. A solid understanding of the physiological, nutritional, and molecular mechanisms governing lactation is essential for developing effective management strategies that benefit both farmers and the dairy industry at large.

Veterinary Lactation Physiology serves as a comprehensive and insightful resource for students, teachers, researchers, and professionals engaged in the study of lactation biology. This book covers both fundamental and advanced aspects of mammary gland development and function, including mammogenesis, lactogenesis, and galactopoiesis across various farm animal species. Special emphasis is placed on elucidating the mechanisms underlying key physiological processes, integrating molecular insights with clinical perspectives to bridge the gap between basic science and practical application.

The text is carefully organized into concise sections with clear headings and subheadings, facilitating easy navigation for readers with diverse academic backgrounds. Each topic is discussed in depth, connecting physiological events with their clinical, production, and management implications. Notably, the book includes several unique chapters not commonly found in traditional lactation physiology textbooks—such as species-specific molecular and endocrine regulation of mammary gland development, mechanisms of milk secretion and lactation persistency, mammary gland metabolism, and the nutraceutical significance of milk.

In essence, this volume stands out as a distinctive and comprehensive textbook that brings together the full breadth of lactation biology under one cover. Its balanced and integrative approach makes it an invaluable reference not only for veterinary and animal science students but also for faculty members, researchers, and professionals in related disciplines who seek to deepen their understanding of the fascinating science of lactation.

Research Scientist, American Institute for Goat Research
Langston University
Langston, OK, USA

Amlan Patra

Preface

The book *Veterinary Lactation Physiology* is an earnest attempt to provide comprehensive and accessible learning material for students, teachers, researchers, and professionals associated with the subject. It encompasses the fundamental and advanced aspects of lactation physiology in various farm animal species. Recognizing the diverse background of potential readers, the content is presented in concise, well-organized paragraphs with relevant headings and subheadings to facilitate easy navigation and understanding.

Special emphasis has been placed on elucidating the mechanisms underlying physiological and molecular events of lactation, bridging general concepts with in-depth explanations. The text further explores the clinical and field implications of physiological processes, linking them with allied basic, clinical, and production-related disciplines.

Distinct from conventional textbooks, this volume introduces several unique sections such as the species-specific molecular and endocrine basis of mammary gland development, initiation and maintenance of lactation, mammary gland metabolism, and nutrient dynamics. The inclusion of these advanced topics, coupled with detailed mechanistic insights and species-wise variations, makes this book a singular reference source that caters to diverse learners. Its comprehensive scope is expected to serve not only undergraduate students but also postgraduate and doctoral scholars as a lifelong academic companion.

The book is organized into 12 chapters, each structured with a detailed table of contents, an abstract, keywords, graphical abstract, learning objectives, exercises, glossary, and suggested readings. Complex physiological processes are clarified through illustrations and tables, accompanied by descriptive footnotes to strengthen the understanding of cause-and-effect relationships among various systems. Numerical data and key information are presented in tables for ease of memorization and review. "Knowledge corner" in each chapters provide interesting facts about the topics.

Each chapter begins with an engaging abstract to capture the reader's interest and concludes with learning outcomes to reinforce comprehension of major concepts. The exercises comprising both objective and subjective formats enable self-assessment and examination readiness. A concise glossary supports clear conceptual understanding, while comprehensive references in the suggested reading section guide further exploration of the subject.

In essence, this book represents a unique and inclusive endeavor to present the entire field of lactation physiology within a single volume. It aims to serve as a reliable academic resource and ready reference for students, faculty members, and researchers across the core and allied disciplines of animal physiology.

Kolkata, West Bengal, India Joydip Mukherjee
Kolkata, West Bengal, India Pradip Kumar Das
Kolkata, West Bengal, India Dipak Banerjee
Rani, Assam, India Kalyan De

Competing Interests The authors have no competing interests to declare that are relevant to the content of this manuscript.

Contents

About the Authors

Joydip Mukherjee MVSc, PhD is an Associate Professor in the Department of Veterinary Physiology at the West Bengal University of Animal & Fishery Sciences, Kolkata, India. His research has focused extensively on lactation physiology, with particular emphasis on the innate immune mechanisms of the mammary gland in crossbred cattle and buffaloes. His notable contributions include the standardization of protocols to assess mammary gland immune competence, especially through in vitro evaluation of milk leukocyte activity, and their validation under different physiological conditions. He has also elucidated the molecular and endocrine regulation of milk leukocyte function and demonstrated the modulation of in vitro immune responses through micronutrient supplementation. Currently, he is engaged in research on electrocardiography in companion animals and diagnostic imaging. He serves as an editor and contributing author of multiple chapters in the *Textbook of Veterinary Physiology* (ISBN: 978-981-19-9410-4; Print ISBN: 978-981-19-9409-8) and is also a coauthor of the book *Techniques in Veterinary Physiology* (ISBN: 978-81-929,561-0-7). His scholarly output includes more than 70 research and review articles published in peer-reviewed journals. He has supervised and mentored numerous postgraduate and doctoral students. In recognition of his research achievements, he has received several prestigious fellowships and honors, including the Junior Research Fellowship, Senior Research Fellowship, DST-INSPIRE Fellowship, and the Young Scientist Award from the Society of Animal Physiologists of India. He is an active member of various professional bodies, such as the Indian Science Congress Association, the Society of Animal Physiologists of India, the Society of Domestic Animal Biodiversity, and the Association of Public Health Veterinarians. Presently, he is the section editor (Physiology and Anatomy) of the *Indian Journal of Animal Health*.

Pradip Kumar Das MSc, PhD is a Professor in the Department of Veterinary Physiology at West Bengal University of Animal & Fishery Sciences, Kolkata, West Bengal, India, with specialization in reproductive, lactational, cardiovascular, environmental, and poultry physiology. He has made substantial research contributions in the areas of repeat breeding, use of phytochemicals as antimicrobial agents, development of poultry husbandry databases, and studies on the transmission of environmental pollutants through the food chain. He has led several research projects and pioneered a sustainable backyard poultry farming model. He has supervised and mentored numerous postgraduate and doctoral students. His academic output includes 5 books, 30 book chapters, and 10 practical manuals for students, along with more than 170 research and review articles published in reputed peer-reviewed journals. In addition, he has authored 20 books aimed at entrepreneurs and produced 7 feature films to promote scientific awareness among the public. He has been actively associated with various scientific societies and served as the General Secretary of the Society of Animal Physiologists of India. He has coordinated over 100 capacity-building programs and organized approximately 20 national and 5 international scientific symposia. He has also served as an advisor to the District Planning Committee of the Animal Resources Development Department, Government of West Bengal, and as Secretary of the Education, Research, Training, and Extension Subcommittee of the State Agriculture Commission. In recognition of his scientific and academic contributions, he was awarded the SAPI Fellowship and the A. Roy Award by the Society of Animal Physiologists of India. Currently, he serves as the Editor-in-Chief of the *Indian Journal of Animal Health*.

Dipak Banerjee MVSc, PhD is an Associate Professor in the Department of Veterinary Physiology at the West Bengal University of Animal & Fishery Sciences, Kolkata, West Bengal, India. He has more than 14 years of teaching and research experience in Veterinary and Animal Physiology. He received his PhD in Animal Physiology from the National Dairy Research Institute (NDRI), Karnal, India. Before joining his present institution, he worked as an Assistant Professor at Anand Agricultural University, Anand, Gujarat, India. His research focuses on how animals adapt to different environmental conditions. His main areas of interest include stress physiology, environmental physiology, reproductive neuroendocrinology, and lactation physiology. His work uses molecular, endocrine, and physiological methods to study how stress and environmental factors affect reproduction and milk production. He has handled research projects funded by different funding agencies. He has guided several master's and PhD students. He also acts as a reviewer and editorial board member of scientific journals. He is an editor and contributing author of several chapters in the *Textbook of Veterinary Physiology* (ISBN: 978-981-19-9410-4; Print ISBN: 978-981-19-9409-8) and a coauthor of the book *Techniques in Veterinary Physiology* (ISBN: 978-81-929,561-0-7). He has published more than 56 research and review articles in peer-reviewed journals. He has delivered around 25 invited and lead presentations at national and international conferences. He has received several awards for his research, including the Young Scientist Award from the Society of Animal Physiologists of India.

Kalyan De MVSc, PhD is a scientist at the ICAR–National Research Centre on Pig, Rani, Guwahati, India. He earned his PhD in Livestock Production and Management from the National Dairy Research Institute (NDRI), Karnal, where he developed strong expertise in applied dairy animal production and management. An animal scientist by training, he has conducted extensive research on animal behavior, welfare, and thermal adaptability in the context of changing environmental conditions. His work has significantly advanced the understanding of physiological and behavioral responses of livestock to environmental stress, thereby contributing to improved livestock production and management practices. His research emphasizes the use of scientific interventions and management strategies to enhance both animal welfare and productivity. Currently, he is engaged in studies on colostrum production and intake, along with research on pig behavior and welfare, with a particular focus on their behavioral responses to evolving environmental cues. He has authored 3 books, contributed to 15 book chapters, and prepared 4 practical manuals for students. His academic contributions also include over 50 research and review articles published in peer-reviewed journals. In recognition of his scientific contributions, he was awarded the Young Scientist Award by the Indian Society for Sheep and Goat Production and Utilization (ISSGPU).

Abbreviations

ACAT	Acetyl-CoA acetyltransferase
ACC	Acetyl CoA carboxylase
ACP	Acyl-carrier protein
ACSL	Acyl-coA synthetase
ALDH2	Aldehyde dehydrogenase 2
AMP	Adenosine monophosphate
AMPK	Adenosine 5′-monophosphate-activated protein kinase
ANGPTL4	Angiopoietin-like 4
APase	Acid phosphatase
AQP	Aquaporin
AREG	Amphiregulin
ASase	Aryl sulfatase
ASCT	Alanine, serine, cysteine amino acid transport protein
ATGL	Adipose triglyceride lipase
B4GALT1	β-1,4-Galactosyltransferase-1
BALT	Bronchus-associated lymphoid tissue
BCAA	Branched chain amino acids
BCAT	BCAA transaminase
BCKA	Branched-chain α-ketoacids
BLG	Beta-lactoglobulin
BM	Basement membrane
BMP4	Bone morphogenetic protein 4
BoHV-2	Bovine herpesvirus-2
C/EBP	CCAAT/enhancer-binding proteins
CAD	Caspase-activated DNase
CavME	Caveolae-mediated endocytosis
CCK	Cholecystokinin
CD	Cluster of differentiation 24
CFU	Colony-Forming Unit
CIDR	Controlled Internal Drug Release
CK	Cytokeratins
CLD	Cytoplasmic lipid droplets
CMKLR1	Chemokine receptor-like 1

CMT	California mastitis test
c-Myc	Myelocytomatosis oncogene
CNH	Casein hydrolysates
CNN1	Calponin 1
COX-2	Cyclooxygenase-2
CREB	cAMP-response element binding protein
CRISPR/Cas9	Clustered Regularly Interspaced Short Palindromic Repeats
CRL	Crown-Rump length
CTX-I	C-terminal cross linking telopeptide of type I collagen
DCT	Dry cow therapy
DGAT	Diacylglycerol acyltransferase
DH	β-Hydroxyacyl dehydratase
DISC	Death-inducing signaling complex
dL	Deciliter (a unit of fluid measure equal to 10^{-1} L)
DMI	Dry matter intake
DNA	Deoxyribonucleic acid
Dsc	Desmocollin
Dsg	Desmoglein
e.g.	Exempli gratia, the Latin phrase meaning “for example”
EAAT	Excitatory amino acid transporter
eCG	Equine Chorionic Gonadotropin
ECM	Extracellular matrix
EEF1A1	Eukaryotic translation elongation factor 1 alpha 1
eIF	Eukaryotic initiation factors
ELISA	Enzyme-Linked Immunosorbent Assay
ER	Endoplasmic reticulum
ERGIC	Endoplasmic reticulum-Golgi intermediate compartment
et al.	“Et alia” meaning “and others.” It is used in academic citations
ETT	Embryo Transfer Technology
FAK	Focal adhesion kinase
FALT	Furstenberg’s rosette associated lymphoid tissue
FAS	Fatty acid synthetase
FASN	Fatty acid synthase
FATP	Fatty acid transport proteins
FCM	Fat corrected milk
FGF	Fibroblast growth factor
FIL	Feedback inhibitor of lactation
FN	Fibronectin
FPP	Farnesyl pyrophosphate
FSP1	Fibroblast specific protein 1
fT3	Free T3
FTAI	Fixed-time artificial insemination
g	Gram (a metric unit of mass equal to 1/1000 (one-thousandth) of a kilogram)
G3PD	Glyceraldehyde-3-phosphate dehydrogenase

G6P	Glucose-6-phosphate
GALT	Gut-associated lymphoid tissue
GEBV	Genomic Estimated Breeding Value
GH	Growth hormone
GHR	GH receptor
GLUT	Glucose transporters
GLYCAM1	Glycosylation-dependent cell adhesion molecule 1
GM-CSF	Granulocyte macrophage colony-stimulating factor
GnRH	Gonadotropin-releasing hormone
GPAM	Glycerol-3-phosphate acyltransferase
GPAT	Glycerol-3-phosphate acyltransferases
GPCR	G protein-coupled receptor
GPP	Geranyl pyrophosphate
GT	Galactosyl transferase
H^+	Hydrogen ion
HARP	Heparin affin regulatory peptide
HGF	Hepatocyte growth factor
HK	Hexokinase
HMG CoA	β-Hydroxy β-methylglutaryl CoA
hnRNA	Heterogeneous nuclear RNA
HSL	Hormone sensitive lipase
i.e.	"Id est," a Latin term means "that is" or "in other words"
IFN-γ	Interferon- γ
Ig	Immunoglobulin
IGF-1	Insulin-like growth factor-1
IGF-1	Insulin-like Growth Factor-1
IGFBP	IGF-binding proteins
IL	Interleukin
IM	Intramuscular
INF	Inflammation-associated fibroblasts
IoT	Internet of Things
IP3	Inositol 1,4,5-trisphosphate
IRP	Inflammation-related proteins
IRS	Insulin receptor substrates
IVF	In vitro fertilization
JAK2-STAT5	Janus kinase 2-signal transducer and activator of transcription 5
kg	Kilograms (a unit of length equal to one thousand grams)
KR	β-Ketoacyl reductase
KS	β-Ketoacyl synthase
L	Liter
LALBA	α-Lactalbumin
LAMP	Loop-mediated isothermal amplification
LAT	L-type amino acid transporter
LCFA	Long-chain fatty acids
LDH	Lactate dehydrogenase

LDPP	Long-day photoperiods
Lef	Lymphoid enhancer-binding factor
LEF1	Lymphoid enhancer-binding factor 1
LM	Laminin
LOX	Lysyl oxidase
LPA	Lysophosphatidic acid
LPC	Laboratory pasteurized count
LPL	Lipoprotein lipase
LPS	Lipopolysaccharide
LS	Lactose synthase
LTA	Lipoteichoic acid
LTBP	TGFβ binding protein
LVDd	Left ventricular diameter in diastole
LVVd	Left ventricular volume in diastole
m	Meter, the fundamental unit of length in the International System of Units (SI)
MAF	Musculoaponeurotic fibrosarcoma
MAS	Marker-assisted selection
MaSC	Mammary stem cell
MAT	Acetyl/malonyl-CoA transferase
MCP-1	Monocyte chemoattractant protein 1
MEC	Mammary epithelial cells
MEPI	Myoepithelium-derived serine proteinase inhibitor
mEq/L	Milliequivalents per liter
mg	Milligram (a unit of mass equal to 1/1000 (one-thousandth) of a gram)
MGL	Monoglyceride lipase
MIC	Minimum inhibitory concentration
miRNA	microRNA
mL	Milliliter (a unit of capacity equal to 1/1000 (one-thousandth) of a liter)
MLD	Microlipid droplet
mm	Millimeter (a unit of length equal to 1/1000 (one-thousandth) of a meter)
mM	Millimolar
MMA syndrome	Mastitis, metritis and agalactia syndrome
mmHg	Millimeter mercury
mmol/L	Millimole per liter
MMP	Matrix metalloproteinase
MMUT	Methylmalonyl-CoA mutase
mRNA	Messenger ribonucleic acid
mTOR	Mammalian target of rapamycin
MUN	Milk urea nitrogen
Mvb	Multivesicular bodies
NADP	Nicotinamide adenine dinucleotide phosphate

NAGase	N-acetyl-β-D-glucosaminidase
NEB	Negative energy balance
NEFA	Nonesterified fatty acids
NF1	Nuclear factor 1
NF-κB	Nuclear factor-κB
ng	Nanogram (a unit of mass equal to 10^{-9} g)
NIRD	National Institute for Research in Dairying
NIS	Sodium/iodide symporter
nm	Nanometer (a unit of mass equal to 10^{-9} m)
NMR	Nuclear magnetic resonance
NO	Nitric oxide
NOS	Nitric oxide synthase
NRG	Neuregulins
Nrg3	Neuregulin 3
NSF	N-ethylmaleimide–sensitive fusion
OAT	Ornithine aminotransferase
ODC	Ornithine decarboxylase
P5CD	Δ^1-l-pyrroline-5-carboxylate dehydrogenase
P5CR	Δ^1-l pyrroline-5-carboxylate reductase
PA	Plasminogen activators
PABP	Poly(A)-binding protein
PAI-1	Plasminogen activator inhibitor-1
PAX	Phosphorylates adapter protein paxillin
PBAA	Peptide bound amino acids
PCoAC	Propionyl-CoA carboxylase
PCR	Polymerase chain reaction
PDGFRα	Platelet derived growth factor receptor α
PDGFRα	Platelet-derived growth factor receptor α
PDK1	Phophoinositide dependent kinase1
PEP	Phosphoenolpyruvate
PEPCK	Phosphoenolpyruvate carboxykinase
pg	Picogram (one-trillionth of a gram, a unit of mass equal to 0.000000000001 g)
$PGF_2α$	Prostaglandin $F_2α$
p-glu-ase	P-glucuronidase
PI3K	Phosphatidylinositol 3′kinase
PKA	Protein kinase A
PKB	Protein kinase B
PLA2	Phospholipase A2
PLC	Phospholipase C
PMCA2	Plasma membrane calcium ATPase isoform 2
PMN	Polymorphonuclear neutrophil
PPARγ	Peroxisome proliferator-activated receptor γ
PRL	Prolactin
PtdSer	Phosphatidylserine

PTHrP	Parathyroid hormone-related protein
PTN	Pleiotrophin
QTL	Quantitative trait loci
RANKL	Receptor activator of NFKB1 ligand
RAR	Retinoids
RARRES2	Retinoic acid receptor responder protein 2
RBP4	Retinol-binding protein 4
rBST	Recombinant bovine somatotropin
RER	Rough endoplasmic reticulum
RFI	Lower residual feed intake
RNA	Ribonucleic acid
RNA-Seq	RNA sequencing
ROS	Reactive oxygen species
rRNA	Ribosomal RNA
RT-PCR	Reverse transcription polymerase chain reaction
RXR	Retinoid X receptor
SAA	Serum amyloid A
SARS	Seryl-tRNA synthetase
SCC	Somatic cell count
SCD	Stearoyl-CoA desaturase
SCNT	Somatic Cell Nuclear Transfer
SDF-1	Stroma cell-derived factor-1
SDPP	Short day photoperiod
SGLT	Na^+/glucose cotransporters
SNAP	Synaptosomal-associated protein
SNARE	Soluble N-ethylmaleimide–sensitive fusion (NSF) attachment protein receptor
SNAT	Sodium-coupled neutral amino acid transporter
SNP	Single nucleotide polymorphism
SOCS	Suppressors of cytokine 1Signaling
SPC	Standard plate count
SREBP	Aterol-regulatory element binding protein
ST	Somatotropin
Stat5	Signal transducer and activator of transcription 5
T1MP-1	Tissue inhibitor of metalloproteinases
T3	Triiodothyronine
T4	Thyroxine
TCA cycle	Tricarboxylic acid cycle
Tcf	T-cell factor
TDLU	Terminal ductal-lobular unit
TDU	Terminal ductal unit
TE I	Thioesterase I
TEB	Terminal end bud
TEER	Trans-epithelial electrical resistance
Tf	Transferrin

TGF	Transforming growth factor
TGF-β	Transforming growth factor-β
TGN	Trans-Golgi network
TIMP	Inhibitors of metalloproteinases
TLN	Talin
TNFSF11	Tumor necrosis factor ligand superfamily, member 11
TNF-α	Tumor necrosis factor- α
tPA	Tissue-type plasminogen activator
TPH1	Tryptophan hydroxylase 1
TPM2	Tropomyosin 2
tRNA	Transfer RNA
TRPV5	Transient receptor potential vanilloid type 5
TSH	Thyroid-stimulating hormone
TUNEL	Terminal deoxynucleotidyl transferase dUTP Nick End Labeling
UDP	Uridine diphosphate glucose
UGPA	UTP-glucose-1-phosphate uridylyltransferase
uPA	Urokinase-type plasminogen activator
USG	Ultrasonography
UTP	Uridine triphosphate
VCL	Vinculin
VCP	Valosin-containing protein
VDMI	Voluntary dry matter intake
VEGF	Vascular endothelial growth factor
VFA	Volatile fatty acids
VLDL	Low-density lipoproteins
WAP	Whey acidic protein
Zo	Zonula occluden
±	Both plus and minus
°C	Degree Centigrade
°F	Degree Fahrenheit
2D-GE	Two-dimensional gel electrophoresis
αSMA	Alpha smooth muscle actin
β-TrCP	Beta-transducing repeat-containing protein
μg	Microgram (a unit of length equaling 1×10^{-6} g)
μm	Micrometer (a unit of length equaling 1×10^{-6} m)

Landscape of World Milk Production: Prospects and Challenges

1

Contents

Abstract

The global milk production continues to grow and is now approximately 982 million tonnes. Worldwide, milk is among the most produced and valuable agricultural commodities. Asia has emerged as the highest contributor to the global milk production, and currently India is the largest milk producer in the world. The average per capita milk consumption is approximately 322 grams per day globally in 2023. Cow milk represents 81% of global milk production, followed by milk from buffaloes (15%), goats (2%), sheep (1%), and camels (0.4%). Other minor dairy species like yak, horse, donkey, reindeer, llama, and alpaca contribute less than 1% of global milk production, mostly in diverse climatic zones. The per-animal productivity varies by species and region. More than 150 million farmers raise dairy animals, and the dairy sector supports almost one billion

J. Mukherjee et al., *Veterinary Lactation Physiology*,
https://doi.org/10.1007/978-3-032-21123-1_1

people in their livelihoods. However, only 3% of the dairy farms have more than 10 cows. The average dairy herd size is approximately 2.4 cows per farm. Milk is mainly consumed domestically; only around 9% of total milk production is traded globally. Milk and dairy products (butter, cheese, skim milk powder, and whole milk powder) contribute approximately 14% to global agricultural trade. The major opportunities in the dairy sector are in the continuous production and demand of milk and dairy products, constant innovation, and adoption of modern technologies, despite the region-specific constraints broadly due to climate change, environmental regulations, feed and labor shortages, price volatility, disease outbreaks, antimicrobial resistance, infrastructure gaps, etc. A holistic region-specific, climate-smart practice and regulation, supportive labor and trade policies, and stronger disease forecast and control with judicial antimicrobial use can make the milk production sustainable.

Graphical Abstract

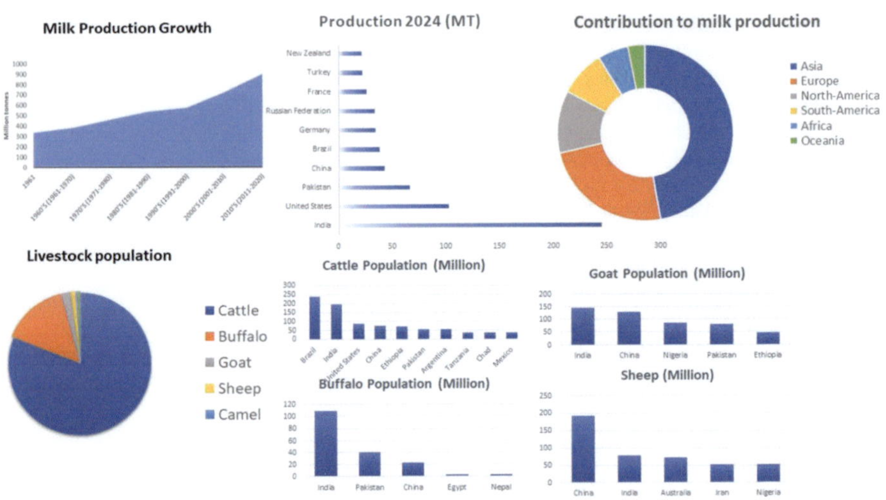

Description of the graphic: Global milk production is ~982 million tonnes, led by Asia, with India as the largest producer and per capita consumption of ~322 g/day. Cow milk accounts for 81% of output, followed by buffalo (15%), with minor species contributing <1%. The sector supports nearly one billion livelihoods through mostly smallholder farms, trades only ~9% of milk globally, and contributes ~14% to agricultural trade. Sustainable growth depends on climate-smart, region-specific practices, supportive policies, technological innovation, and effective disease and antimicrobial management

Keywords

Milk production · Per capita availability · Livestock · Dairy

Inside the Chapter
- Current status of milk production
- Decade-wise growth in milk production
- Leading milk-producing continents and countries
- Worldwide per capita milk availability
- Milk-producing species and breeds, their population and contribution
- Dairy products production status
- Imports and exports in the dairy sector
- Challenges and prospects of dairy

Learning Objectives
- Contemporary milk production status and its growth
- Contribution of continents, countries, species, and breeds in global milk production
- Worldwide availability of milk and production of milk products
- Diary trading nations, imports and exports, emerging challenges, and prospects of the dairy sector

1.1 Introduction

Milk is nature's perfect food. It provides essential nutrients to billions of people. For generations, milk and dairy foods have consistently served as dependable sources of nutrition. The global human population is expected to reach ten billion by 2050. For such a booming global population, nutritional security is going to be a greater challenge. Hence, the global dairy sector is in continuous growth despite different challenges. Approximately 6.50 billion people, that is, more than 80% of the global population consume milk or dairy products, reflecting its nutritional importance and universal acceptance. More than 80% of the global population, approximately 6.50 billion people, regularly consume milk or dairy products, showing its universal appeal and nutritional value. Milk and dairy foods are rich in essential nutrients, offering energy, high-quality protein, and important micronutrients such as calcium, magnesium, selenium, riboflavin, and vitamins B_5 and B_{12}. Milk provides approximately 5% of energy, 10% of protein, and 9% of fat globally. Around the world, people receive roughly 134 kcal of energy, 8.3 g of protein, and 7.6 g of fat per day from milk.

Milk production is an energy-demanding complex physiological process involving hormonal regulation, nutrient metabolism, and cellular secretion mechanisms. The milk production scenario of the present world is continuously transforming, which requires understanding and managing lactation through better management, adequate precision nutrition, and genetic improvement. Since the 1970s, South East Asia emerged as a major contributing region for increased milk production. The global milk production was about 982 million tonnes in 2024, showing a 1.4% rise from 2023. A major portion of the milk production comes from small and marginal farmers in rural households. Smallholder dairy plays a crucial role in advancing women's empowerment in developing countries. Approximately 22% of women of working age globally are engaged in agricultural activities, with nearly one-quarter of farms maintaining dairy animals. Globally, more than 150 million maintain at least one milk-producing animal, including cattle, buffalo, goats, or sheep. Milk production remains a foundational pillar of global food security and rural livelihoods, providing essential nutrition and income to millions of smallholder farmers and commercial producers worldwide.

The fast growth of the dairy sector is facing sustainability challenges. The major challenges appear from climate change, heat stress, heat waves, environmental regulations, feed and fodder shortages, animal health issues, political tension, trade disruptions, infrastructure, and market limitations. However, more sustainability can be achieved with the use of modern technologies like robotics, artificial intelligence (AI), big data (BD), and blockchain. Precision management and feeding, development of climate-resilient breeds, real-time disease detection, and use of energy-efficient technologies are going to be key to the success of the dairy industry. This chapter highlights some key aspects of the landscape of milk production to recognize the importance and implications of lactation physiology for humanity in ensuring nutritional security, employment generation, and poverty alleviation.

1.2 Dynamic Growth

The global milk production was approximately 982 million tonnes in 2024. Over the last six decades, the global milk production dynamic has changed immensely (Table 1.1). The world milk production has increased almost three times since 1960 over the last six decades. The highest growth was recorded during the last two decades, that is, 2001–2010 and 2011–2020, whereas the lowest was during the 1990s, that is, 1991–2000.

Table 1.1 Milk production across decades and corresponding growth

Decades	Approximate milk production (million tonnes)	Increase from previous decades (%)
1961	344.00	
1960s (1961–1970)	391.95	13.94
1970s (1971–1980)	465.82	15.86
1980s (1981–1990)	542.45	14.12
1990s (1991–2000)	579.31	6.36
2000s (2001–2010)	724.45	20.03
2010s (2011–2020)	906.00	20.04

Data compiled from FAO, FAOSTAT, and NDDB databases

Table 1.2 Continent-wise milk production

Rank	Continent	Approximate milk production (million tonnes)	Contribution to milk production (%)
1	Asia	459	47
2	Europe	235	24
3	North America	111	11.4
4	South America	82	8.4
5	Africa	54	5.6
6	Oceania	30	3.1

FAO (2025a)

1.3 Continent Contribution

Currently, almost half (47%) of the total milk production comes from Asia, with nearly 460 million tonnes of milk production (Table 1.2). Europe accounts for almost 24% of the world's milk production, with approximately 236 million tonnes of milk production. North America produced almost 112.5 million tonnes, contributing 11.4% of global output. South America produces about 69 million tonnes, contributing almost 7% of the world's milk production. Africa produces approximately 54 million tonnes of milk, contributing 5.5% of output. Oceania contributes 30 million tonnes, representing 3.1% of world milk production.

The Food and Agriculture Organization (FAO) projects that world milk production reached 982 million tonnes in 2024, representing a 1.4% increase from 2023.

The milk production of Asia increased several fold in the 1970s to 459 million tonnes in 2024, making it the world's largest milk-producing region. In Asia, India, Pakistan, and China are the major milk-producing countries. In Europe, the European Union collectively produces the majority of the milk, which includes Germany, France, the Netherlands, and Ireland. In North America, the United States is the major milk-producing region. In South America, Brazil is a major contributor to milk production, followed by Argentina. In Africa, Egypt, Kenya, Algeria, Ethiopia, South Africa, and Tanzania were the continent's primary producing nations. In Oceania, New Zealand produces approximately 21.5–22 million tonnes, and Australia produces 8.3–8.5 million tonnes of milk.

1.4 Milk-Producing Countries

Presently, India is the largest milk producer in the world, with a total milk production of 239–245 million tonnes during 2023–2024, which contributes almost 25% of the global total milk production (Table 1.3). India has been the leading milk producer since 1998. India's large milk production is due to a huge cattle and buffalo population and the effective cooperative networks of small-scale dairy producers. The United States is the second-largest milk producer in the world with 102.5 MT

Table 1.3 Leading countries in milk and dairy product production (milk equivalent basis)

Rank	Country	Approximate production 2024 (MT)
1	India	245.0
2	The United States	102.5
3	Pakistan	66.3
4	China	43.2
5	Brazil	38.2
6	Germany	34.4
7	Russian Federation	34.1
8	France	26.2
9	Turkey	22.0
10	New Zealand	21.5

Data source: FAO/Development Aid/Wikipedia/USDA FAS

milk production. Pakistan is the third-largest milk-producing nation, producing nearly 66.3 MT of milk annually. China is holding the fourth rank in milk-producing countries with 43.2 MT milk production. Brazil is the fifth-largest milk producer with 38.2 MT milk production. The other major milk-producing countries are Germany (34.4 MT), Russian Federation (34.1 MT), France (26.2 MT), Turkey (22.0 MT), New Zealand (21.5 MT), the United Kingdom (15.5 MT), Poland (15.1 MT), the Netherlands (14.9 MT), Italy (14.3 MT), Mexico (13.2 MT), Argentina (11.9 MT), Canada (10.1 MT), Australia (9.2 MT), Ireland (9.1 MT), and Belgium (8.6 MT).

1.5 Per Capita Availability

Approximately 80% of the global population (6.5 billion people) consumes milk or milk products. The per capita availability of milk is approximately 119.1 kg per year or 322 grams per day globally in 2023. It has increased from 97 kg in the 1990s. The per capita availability of milk is diversely distributed in different regions of the world. Europe, North America, Argentina, Armenia, Australia, Costa Rica, Israel, Kyrgyzstan, and Mongolia are among the high milk-consuming regions with more than 150 kg/capita/year milk (or milk equivalent) consumption. Mostly the Islamic Republic of Iran, Senegal, Thailand, most of Central Africa, and most of East and Southeast Asia are the low-consumption regions, with less than 30 kg/capita/year milk (or milk equivalent) consumption. In 2023, per capita milk availability in Asia surpassed 100 kg. Most of the European countries have per capita milk consumption between 150 and 200 liters, which is more than three times higher than the world average. Currently, India's per capita availability of milk is 485 grams per day or 176.9 kg per year, despite India's huge population. In India, Punjab has the highest milk per capita availability of 1245 grams per day in 2023–24, followed by Rajasthan at 1171 grams and Haryana at 1105 grams per day.

1.6 Distribution of Milk Production Among Different Species

The majority of milk is produced from cattle. Approximately 783 million tonnes of milk, that is, 81% of total global milk production is produced from cattle. Buffalo is the second-largest contributor to total global milk production. Approximately 145 million tonnes of milk, which contribute almost 15% of the total milk production, comes from buffalo. Goat produces approximately 19 million tonnes of milk, which contributes almost 2% of the global milk production. Sheep milk contributes 1% of the global milk production, with 10.00 million tonnes of milk. Camel also produces almost *four* million tonnes of milk, which contributes approximately 0.4% of total global milk production. The rest of the milk is produced by yaks, donkeys, Mithun, etc. (approximately five million tonnes; 0.6%).

In India, crossbred cow contributes approximately 29.81%, exotic cow 1.86%, indigenous cow 10.73%, nondescriptive cow 9.51%, indigenous buffalo 31.94%, and nondescriptive buffalo12.87%, and goat 3.3% of the country's total milk production.

1.6.1 Major Milk-Producing Species

Dairy Cattle

Currently, the world cattle population is approximately 1.57 billion. Depending on the land availability, climate conditions, agricultural policies, and market demand, the dairy cattle population is concentrated on a relatively small number of countries (Table 1.4). Currently, Brazil has the highest cattle population. India ranks second in the total cattle population, but has the highest dairy cattle population. The United States is in third position in cattle population.

Table 1.4 Ten leading countries in cattle population

Rank	Country	Approximate cattle population (million)
1	Brazil	238.6
2	India	194.5
3	The United States	88.8
4	China	73.6
5	Ethiopia	70.9
6	Pakistan	55.5
7	Argentina	54.2
8	Tanzania	37.9
9	Chad	37.6
10	Mexico	37.6

Source: World Population Review. (2025). Cattle Population by Country 2025

Table 1.5 Leading dairy cattle breeds

Breed name	Origin	Approximate average lactation yield
Holstein-Friesian	The Netherlands	10,000–10,500 kg
Jersey	The United Kingdom (Isle of Jersey)	4000–6100 kg
Guernsey	The United Kingdom (Isle of Guernsey)	6000–7700 kg
Brown Swiss	Switzerland (Alps)	7000–8000 kg
Ayrshire	Scotland	9000–10,000 kg

Table 1.6 Five leading countries in buffalo population

Rank	Country	Approximate population (million)
1	India	109.85
2	Pakistan	41.19
3	China	23.27
4	Egypt	3.68
5	Nepal	3.50

Source: FAO (Food and Agriculture Organization), FAOSTAT database 22–23; Livestock Census (2019)

For milk production, based on environmental conditions, the developed countries have developed different cattle breeds through selective breeding for many years (Table 1.5).

Globally, the Holstein-Friesian is the most widely distributed dairy breed, originating from the Netherlands. Holstein cows can produce between 7000 and 10,000 liters of milk per lactation. Jersey cattle are also a well-known dairy breed that originated from the Isle of Jersey. Being a smaller-sized breed compared to the Holstein, its feed requirement is less and it can adapt to various climatic conditions. Guernsey cattle are also a leading dairy breed in the world, originating from the Island of Guernsey in the English Channel. Due to high beta-carotene content in the milk, Guernsey milk is of a golden color. It is also a medium-sized breed and an efficient converter of feed and well adapted to diverse climatic conditions. Brown Swiss cattle and Ayrshire cattle are also among the world's leading milk-producing breeds.

In India, Sahiwal, Gir, Red Sindhi, and Rathi are the major milch breeds. Tharparkar, Kankrej, Deoni, Hariana, and Krishna Valley are dual-purpose breeds. Karan Swiss is a high-yielding crossbred. India's 31.11% milk is produced from cross-bred cattle, 11.36% milk is produced from indigenous cattle, and 10.11% milk from nondescript cattle.

Dairy Buffalo

Buffalo is the major contributor to global milk production after cattle. The global buffalo population is presently estimated at around 205 million. The vast majority of the global buffalo population (98%) is concentrated in Asia, mainly in India (53%), Pakistan (20.1%), and China (11%) (Tables 1.6 and 1.7). Nepal, Indonesia, Vietnam,

Table 1.7 Leading dairy buffalo breeds

Breed	Origin	Approximate lactation yield
Murrah	Haryana/Punjab, India	2200–2500 kg
Nili-Ravi	Punjab (Indo-Pak)	1850–1929 kg
Jaffarabadi	Gujarat, India	2000–2500 kg
Mehsana	Gujarat, India	1600–2000 kg
Surti	Gujarat, India	1500–1800 kg
Bhadawari	Madhya Pradesh, India	1500–2000 kg
Mediterranean	Italy	1600–2000 kg
Khuzestan	Iran and Iraq	1950 kg

Table 1.8 Five leading countries in goat population

Rank	Country	Approximate population (millions)
1	India	148.88
2	China	132.4
3	Nigeria	88.0
4	Pakistan	82.5
5	Ethiopia	49.3

Source: India's 20th Livestock Census (2019)

Table 1.9 Leading dairy goat breeds

Breed	Origin	Approximate lactation yield
Saanen	Switzerland	1285 kg
Alpine	France	950 kg
Toggenburg	Switzerland	740 kg
Nubian	Africa/Sudan	690 kg
British Alpine	The United Kingdom	1200 kg
Oberhasli	Switzerland	748 kg
Jamunapari	India	540 kg

the Philippines, Myanmar, Bangladesh, Brazil, and Egypt also have a good number of buffalo populations. About 0.8% of the world's buffalo population is found in Africa (mainly Egypt), 0.9% in South America, and 0.2% in Europe. India's indigenous buffalo contributes approximately 31.49% of the national milk production (Table 1.7).

Dairy Goat

Dairy goats also contribute approximately 2% of world milk production with their 1.1 billion population. Although out of 1.1 billion, approximately 20–25% is dairy breed. Goat is mostly distributed in Asia and Africa. India has the highest goat population (appoximately14%) in the world and is among the world's top goat milk producers (Table 1.8). However, dairy goats are mainly concentrated in Europe (France, Spain, Greece, Italy) (Table 1.9).

Table 1.10 Five leading countries in sheep population

Rank	Country	Approximate population (millions)
1	China	193
2	India	77.4
3	Australia	72.1
4	Iran	52.0
5	Nigeria	51.4

Source: FAOSTAT 23–24

Table 1.11 Leading dairy sheep breeds

Breed	Origin	Lactation yield
East Friesian	Germany	500–700 kg
Lacaune	France	180–320 kg
Awassi	Syria and Jordon	300–350 kg
Assaf	Israel [cross of Awassi (5/8) with the German East Friesian (3/8)]	260–500 kg
Sarda	Italy	200–400 kg
Chios	Greece	200–250 kg
British Milk	The United Kingdom	650–750 kg

Dairy Sheep

Globally, sheep contribute approximately 1.0% of the milk production, with approximately 1.3 billion, out of which approximately 15–20% is only dairy sheep. Sheep are mostly distributed in Africa and Asia. China has the highest sheep population, followed by India and Australia (Table 1.10); however, notable dairy sheep breeds are found in Germany, France, Syria, and Jordon (Table 1.11).

Dairy Camel

The global camel population totals approximately 37.5 million head, distributed mainly in Africa (87%) and Asia (12%). Chad (nine million) has the maximum population of camels, followed by Sudan (4.9 million), Somalia (7.24 million), Kenya (4.7 million), Ethiopia (1.28 million), and Mali (1.24 million). India has 1.20 million camel population. Approximately 40–50% of global camels are dairy breeds, and Kenya is the world's largest camel milk producer. Kohi (Pakistan), Barela (Pakistan), Marecha (Pakistan), Kachhi (India), Hoor (Somalia), Sifdaar (Somalia), Majaheim (Saudi Arabia), and Arvana (Afghanistan) are the leading milk-producing breeds of camel. In India, Kachchhi, Bikaneri, Jalori, Jaisalmeri, Mewari, and Khimari (Sindhi) are used for milk production.

1.6.2 Other Dairy Species

Cattle, buffalo, sheep, goat, and camel are the major dairy species. Yak (approximately 15–17 million), horse (approximately 58.4–60 million), donkey (approximately 50 million), reindeer (approximately 2–3 million), llama (approximately 3 million), and alpaca (approximately 3.72 million) contribute less than 1% of global milk production. But they have a unique importance because of their production distributed across diverse climatic zones from Arctic regions to high mountains to arid deserts. China is the leader in milk production from minor dairy species. China has approximately 90% of the world's yak population and is the leading yak milk producer, followed by Mongolia, Nepal, and India. India's main milk-producing minor species is the yak (population 76,000). The average daily milk yield of a yak is around 1.0–2.5 kg/day. The countries with the largest horse populations include the United States, Mexico, China, Brazil, Argentina, Mongolia, Kazakhstan, and Romania. The top horse milk-producing countries are Mongolia, Kazakhstan, and Russia. Ethiopia, Sudan, Pakistan, and Chad are the leading countries with the highest donkey populatios. The major reindeer milk-producing countries are Sweden, Russia, Finland, and Norway. The average daily milk yield of a reindeer is approximately 0.72–0.98 kg/day. Peru, Bolivia, and Chile are the top llama/alpaca milk-producing countries. The daily average milk production of llama/alpaca is around 0.4–1.2 liters/day. India, China, and Myanmar have Mithun populations. The average milk yield of a Mithun is approximately 0.87–1.62 kg/day.

1.6.3 Per Animal Milk Productivity

Per animal productivity varies as per species and country. Currently, Israel has the maximum per animal productivity, that is, approximately 32.9/kg/cow/day or 12,025 kg/cow/year. The leading countries with higher per animal productivity are Estonia, the United States, Denmark, the Netherlands, Belgium, Canada, Spain, Germany, etc.

India is in the top position in terms of per buffalo annual milk productivity, with 2440 kg/year (6.63–7.0 kg/day). The other leading countries with higher per buffalo productivity are Pakistan, Egypt, and Italy.

Among the goat milk-producing countries, the leading countries with higher per goat milk productivity are the Netherlands, Switzerland, France, Norway, Ukraine, etc.

Switzerland, Austria, Spain, France, and Kuwait are the leading countries with higher per sheep milk productivity.

1.7 Utilization of Milk

Globally, approximately 23.8–26 million metric tons of cheese were produced in 2024. The majority of production is concentrated in developed countries. The United States (6.3–6.6 million tonnes), Germany, France, Italy, and the Netherlands are the leading cheese-producing countries. Butter production was approximately 11.75–11.98 million Metric tonns in 2024–25, globally. India is the largest butter-producing country, with 6.95 million metric tons (58% of global production), followed by the European Union, with 2.08 million metric tons (17% of global production), and the United States, with 1.02 million metric tons (8% of global production). Milk powder has mainly two categories: skimmed milk powder (SMP) comprises milk with a maximum fat content of 1.5% by weight, while whole milk powder (WMP) contains 26–42% of milk fat content. Globally, skim milk powder (SMP) production was 5.1 million tonnes and whole milk production was 4.7 million tonnes in 2023.

1.8 Milk Export and Import

Milk is mainly consumed domestically because of its perishability and volume-to-value ratio; hence, global dairy trade is only approximately 9% of the total milk production, which accounts for approximately 86 million tonnes (milk equivalent). New Zealand, Germany, the Netherlands, France, and the United States are the major milk product-exporting countries. China and the European Union countries are the largest milk importers. The European Union (EU), the United States, and New Zealand are major cheese exporters, and the United Kingdom, Russia, and Japan are major export destinations. New Zealand, the EU, and Belarus are the major exporters of butter and butter oil to China, Russia, and the United States. New Zealand, the EU, and the United Arab Emirates (UAE) are the major whole milk powder (WMP) exporters, and the top destinations of export are China, Algeria, and Brazil. The SMP top three exporters are the United States, the EU, and New Zealand, and Mexico, China, and Indonesia are the export destinations.

1.9 Employment Generation and Farm Structure

Worldwide, almost 150 million dairy farms exist and involve approximately 150 million households. Approximately one billion people globally depend on the dairy sector for their livelihoods and engaged communities in all corners of the world. Approximately 600 million people are directly involved in milk production and sales. Another 400 million are employed in activities, including feed supply, milk handling, processing, and distribution. Globally, around 80 million women are involved in the dairy sector, and around 37 million women are heading their own farms. In India, almost 80 million people are involved in the dairy sector. In India, 70% of the dairy workforce is women.

The average dairy herd size is approximately 2.4 cows per farm globally, as per the FAO & International Farm Comparison Network (2007). The majority of countries' hard size is less than 10 cows. As per the IFCN (2025) world dairy map, only 3% of the world's dairy farms have more than 10 cows, yet they house a third of all dairy animals and produce nearly 60% of the world's milk. Argentina, Australia, the Czech Republic, New Zealand, South Africa, and the United States have an average hard size of more than 100.

1.10 Challenges of the Dairy Sector

The challenges of the dairy sector destabilize the nutritional security, threaten farmers' profitability, and disrupt production performance. Although the challenges are not similar throughout the world, they vary according to the region and country. However, the dairy industry, as well as farmers of developing countries, is more vulnerable due to a lack of capital and a regulatory framework.

Currently, the major challenges in the dairy sector come from climate and the environment. Climate change and heat stress reduce the productivity of dairy animals. The climate-oriented natural disasters like drought, flood, and storm destroy the feed, fodder land, and infrastructure. Water stress causes depletion and destruction of grazing land as well as natural grazing land. The dairy sector emits almost 4% of the anthropogenic greenhouse gas. The regulations for reduction in methane emission and climate policies of New Zealand, as well as the European Union countries, threatens the less efficient farms. The regulations are compelling to innovation for sustainable production, which simultaneously increases the capital cost.

The global dairy sector consumes huge amounts of dry matter feed annually. Shortage of quality feed and fodder in Southeast Asia and Africa is causing production loss and increasing the production cost. The increased feed cost poses serious challenges to small holding farms. Labor shortage in different regions causes disruption of the supply chain and closure of dairy farms. Another challenge is that persistent milk price fluctuation risks the profitability and sustainability of dairy farms. Disease outbreaks like lumpy skin disease in India and other endemic diseases like foot-and-mouth disease, brucellosis, hemorrhagic septicemia, and climate change-oriented vector-borne diseases are leading to decreased per animal productivity that hinders the sustainability of dairy farms, especially in developing countries. In the dairy sector, antimicrobial resistance is a public health concern as well as a sustainability threat in low- to middle-income countries, where antimicrobials are used extensively for disease treatment and regulatory infrastructure and disease surveillance are not strong. They may develop antimicrobial resistance. In some areas, infrastructure shortage in the cold chain and processing reduces the return and increases waste in the dairy sector.

1.11 Prospects in the Dairy Sector

The major opportunity in the dairy sector is the constant demand for milk and dairy products, which supports the constant growth and market expansion throughout the world, especially in the developing countries due to increasing population, urbanization, and improvement of incomes. Along with that the per capita consumption of dairy products is also in an increasing trend. Constant innovation, like present-day utilization of artificial intelligence, robotics, genetic improvement in the high-yielding animals, precision management and feeding, development of climate-resilient breeds, real-time disease detection, and use of energy-efficient technologies, may reduce the production cost and reduce the environmental impact. The growth in demand for dairy products like cheese, butter, and fermented dairy products as well as organic dairy product increases the profitability of the sector, and consumers are ready to pay for the value-added products. Blockchain and advanced tracking technologies, cold chain improvement, processing modernization, and logistic upgrade are building the trust of consumers and ensuring premium quality product supply that strengthens the sustainability of the dairy sector.

Addressing the challenges of the dairy sector requires a holistic approach combining the adoption of climate-smart technology and management; better policy for solving labor immigration, import export and transportation issues; strengthening disease surveillance and prevention infrastructure; incentivization for activities toward antimicrobial resistance prevention; and promoting sustainable production according to the region and countries' needs.

Exercises

Objective Questions

1. Which continent is the largest milk producer ____________________ with _____________ of milk production?
2. ______________________ is the largest milk producing country in the world.
3. ______________________ is the highest milk-consuming country with per capita availability of ______________________ kg/capita/year milk.
4. ___________________ animal is the second-largest contributor to total global milk production.
5. Most widely distributed dairy cattle breed is _________________________.
6. Which country has highest goat population in the world ___________________.
7. World's largest camel milk-producing country is ___________________.
8. ______________________ country has maximum per animal productivity of 32.9/kg/cow/day.
9. The dairy sector emits almost ____________________ of the anthropogenic greenhouse gas.
10. __________________ country is the leading in milk-producing country from minor dairy species.

Subjective Questions

1. Highlight the prospects and challenges of the global dairy industry.
2. Give a brief account of the milk from minor dairy species.
3. Write a short note on the role of the dairy industry in livelihood generation.
4. Write in brief about the contribution of buffaloes in global milk production.

Answers to Objective Questions

1. Asia, 460 million tonnes
2. India
3. Mongolia, 150
4. Buffalo
5. Holstein-Friesian
6. India
7. Kenya
8. Israel
9. 4%
10. China

References

Research Articles

Abdullah HM, Sheikh A (2024) History of a dairy camel (NAQA) and machine milking in Saudi Arabia: challenges and prospective. Trop Anim Health Prod 56(8):352. https://doi.org/10.1007/s11250-024-04211-8

Antunović Z, Mioč B, Klir Šalavardić Ž, Širić I, Držaić V, Mikulec N, Krivohlavek A, Novoselec J (2024) Physical and chemical properties, hygienic quality and fatty acid profile in milk of lactating Lacaune dairy sheep. Arch Anim Breed 67:37–49

Bhat R, Di Pasquale J, Bánkuti FI, Siqueira TT, Shine P, Murphy MD (2022) Global dairy sector: trends, prospects, and challenges. Sustainability 14(7):4193. https://doi.org/10.3390/su14074193

Chen X, Li C, Fang T, Yao J, Gu X (2024) Effects of heat stress on endocrine, thermoregulatory, and lactation capacity in heat-tolerant and -sensitive dry cows. Front Vet Sci 11:1405263. https://doi.org/10.3389/fvets.2024.1405263

Dobson H, Smith R, Royal M, Knight C, Sheldon I (2007) The high-producing dairy cow and its reproductive performance. Reprod Domest Anim 42(Suppl 2):17–23. https://doi.org/10.1111/j.1439-0531.2007.00906.x

Dong S, Long R, Kang M (2007) Milking performance of China yak (Bos grunniens): a preliminary report. Afr J Agric Res 2(3):52–57

Faraz A, Waheed A, Mirza RH, Nabeel MS, Ishaq HM (2020) Milk yield and composition of Barela dromedary camel in Thal Desert, Punjab, Pakistan. Pak J Zool 52(3):1221–1224

Faraz A, Waheed A, Mustafa AB, Tauqir NA, Mirza RH, Ishaq HM, Bilal RM, Nabeel MS (2021) Milk production potential of Marecha camel (Camelus dromedarius) in extensive and semi-intensive management systems. Pak J Zool 53(1):273–280

Faye B (2020) How many large camelids in the world? A synthetic analysis of the world camel demographic changes. Pastoralism 10:25. https://doi.org/10.1186/s13570-020-00176-z

Gauly M, Ammer S (2020) Review: challenges for dairy cow production systems arising from climate changes. Animal 14(S1):s196–s203. https://doi.org/10.1017/S1751731119003239

Gjøstein H, Holand Ø, Weladji RB (2004) Milk production and composition in reindeer (Rangifer tarandus): effect of lactational stage. Comp Biochem Physiol A Mol Integr Physiol 137(4): 649–656. https://doi.org/10.1016/j.cbpb.2004.01.002

Gross JJ (2022) Limiting factors for milk production in dairy cows: perspectives from physiology and nutrition. J Anim Sci 100(3):skac044. https://doi.org/10.1093/jas/skac044

Hamid M, Siddiky M, Rahman M, Hossain K (2017) Scopes and opportunities of buffalo farming in Bangladesh: a review. SAARC J Agric 14(2):63–77. https://doi.org/10.3329/sja.v14i2.31246
Hassoun A, Garcia-Garcia G, Trollman H, Jagtap S, Parra-López C, Cropotova J, Bhat Z, Centobelli P, Aït-Kaddour A (2023) Birth of dairy 4.0: Opportunities and challenges in adoption of fourth industrial revolution technologies in the production of milk and its derivatives. Curr Res Food Sci 7:100535. https://doi.org/10.1016/j.crfs.2023.100535
Li A, Liu C, Han X, Zheng J, Zhang G, Qi X, Du P, Liu L (2023) Tibetan Plateau yak milk: a comprehensive review of nutritional values, health benefits, and processing technology. Food Chem X 20:100919. https://doi.org/10.1016/j.fochx.2023.100919
Nagy PP, Skidmore JA, Juhasz J (2022) Intensification of camel farming and milk production with special emphasis on animal health, welfare, and the biotechnology of reproduction. Anim Front 12(4):35–45. https://doi.org/10.1093/af/vfac043
Oselu S, Ebere R, Arimi JM (2022) Camels, camel milk, and camel milk product situation in Kenya in relation to the world. Int J Food Sci 2022:1237423. https://doi.org/10.1155/2022/1237423
Riek A, Gerken M (2006) Changes in llama (Lama glama) milk composition during lactation. J Dairy Sci 89(9):3484–3493. https://doi.org/10.3168/jds.S0022-0302(06)72387-6
Talafha AQ, Ababneh MM (2011) Awassi sheep reproduction and milk production: review. Trop Anim Health Prod 43(7):1319–1326. https://doi.org/10.1007/s11250-011-9858-5

Reports and Database

Animal Husbandry Statistics Division, Department of Animal Husbandry and Dairying, Ministry of Fisheries, Animal Husbandry and Dairying, Government of India (2019) 20th livestock census 2019: All India report. https://ruralindiaonline.org/en/library/resource/20th-livestock-census-2019-all-india-report/
APEDA (2025) Monthly dashboard Dairy-Oct-2025. Agricultural and Processed Food Products Export Development Authority, Government of India
Basic Animal Husbandry Statistics-2025 (2025) Govt. of India, Ministry of Fisheries, Animal Husbandry & Dairying, Department of Animal Husbandry & Dairying, Krishi Bhawan, New Delhi
Department of Animal Husbandry and Dairying, Ministry of Fisheries, Animal Husbandry and Dairying, Government of India (2025) Basic animal husbandry statistics 2025. https://dahd.gov.in/sites/default/files/2025-12/BasicAnimalHusbandryStatistics2025.pdf
FAO (2025) Milk production – Gateway to dairy production and products. Food and Agriculture Organization of the United Nations, Rome
FAO & International Farm Comparison Network (IFCN) (2007) The global dairy sector: Status and trends, farm structure and herd size. FAO Animal Production and Health Division, Rome
Food and Agriculture Organization of the United Nations (2016) World milk production dataset (Elaborated from FAOSTAT and the World Bank Development Indicators Database), Rome
Food and Agriculture Organization of the United Nations (2022) Agricultural production statistics, 2000–2021 (FAOSTAT Analytical Brief Series No. 60). Rome. https://doi.org/10.4060/cc3751en
Food and Agriculture Organization of the United Nations (2023) Dairy market review: Emerging trends and outlook in 2023. Rome
Food and Agriculture Organization of the United Nations (2024a) Agricultural production statistics 2010–2023 (FAOSTAT Analytical Briefs No. 96). Rome. https://openknowledge.fao.org/handle/20.500.14283/cd3755en
Food and Agriculture Organization of the United Nations (2024b) World food and agriculture: statistical yearbook 2024. Rome. https://doi.org/10.4060/cd2971en
Food and Agriculture Organization of the United Nations (2025a) Dairy market review: overview of global market developments in 2024. Rome

Food and Agriculture Organization of the United Nations (2025b) History of camelids. In: Camelids: heroes of deserts and highlands, nourishing people and culture, vol 1, Rome. https://doi.org/10.4060/cd5819en

International Farm Comparison Network (IFCN) (2024a) IFCN dairy report 2023. International Farm Comparison Network (IFCN), Kiel

International Farm Comparison Network (IFCN) (2024b) IFCN Dairy Report 2024: Improved global milk production growth and recovery in demand in 2023. International Farm Comparison Network, Kiel

International Farm Comparison Network (IFCN) (2025) World dairy map 2025: Dairy's path forward—Insights for a profitable tomorrow [Map]. International Farm Comparison Network, Kiel

National Dairy Development Board (2024) Annual report 2023–24. National Dairy Development Board

OECD & FAO (2023) OECD-FAO agricultural outlook 2023–2032. OECD Publishing. https://doi.org/10.1787/08801ab7-en

OECD & FAO (2024) OECD-FAO agricultural outlook 2024–2033, Paris/Rome. https://doi.org/10.1787/4c5d2cfb-en

OECD & FAO (2025) OECD-FAO agricultural outlook 2025–2034, Paris/Rome. https://doi.org/10.1787/601276cd-en

Press Information Bureau, Government of India (2025, November 26) Release of Basic Animal Husbandry Statistics 2025. PIB, New Delhi

United States Department of Agriculture, National Agricultural Statistics Service (2025, July 25) Cattle inventory report. USDA NASS

Evolutionary Aspects of the Mammary Gland

2

Contents

Abstract

The mammary gland and the capacity for lactation emerged through a gradual and prolonged evolutionary trajectory, shaped by slow, incremental adaptations over time rather than by rapid or abrupt changes. Because soft tissues rarely fossilize, direct evidence is limited; therefore, several hypotheses have been proposed to explain the evolutionary transition of glands from their ancestral precursors. It is believed that the mammary gland evolved from the synapsid lineage, the last common ancestor of present mammals. The skin gland of the amniotes produced watery antimicrobial secretion to moisturize and protect their eggs. The basic structure of the present mammalian mammary gland is envisaged to originate from the skin's apocrine glands, sebaceous glands, and hair developing an apo-pilo-sebaceous unit in their successors, viz. monotremes and eutherians. Evidence from a range of genetic molecules associated with different nutritional components supports the view that the mammary gland and its secretory products

J. Mukherjee et al., *Veterinary Lactation Physiology*,
https://doi.org/10.1007/978-3-032-21123-1_2

have an ancient evolutionary origin, dating back to approximately 340 million years ago. The mammary gland evolutionary process demonstrated the theory of the survivability of the fittest as explained by Charles Darwin. The structure and composition of milk constituents in mammals were altered with the emergence of placentation followed by domestication.

Graphical Abstract

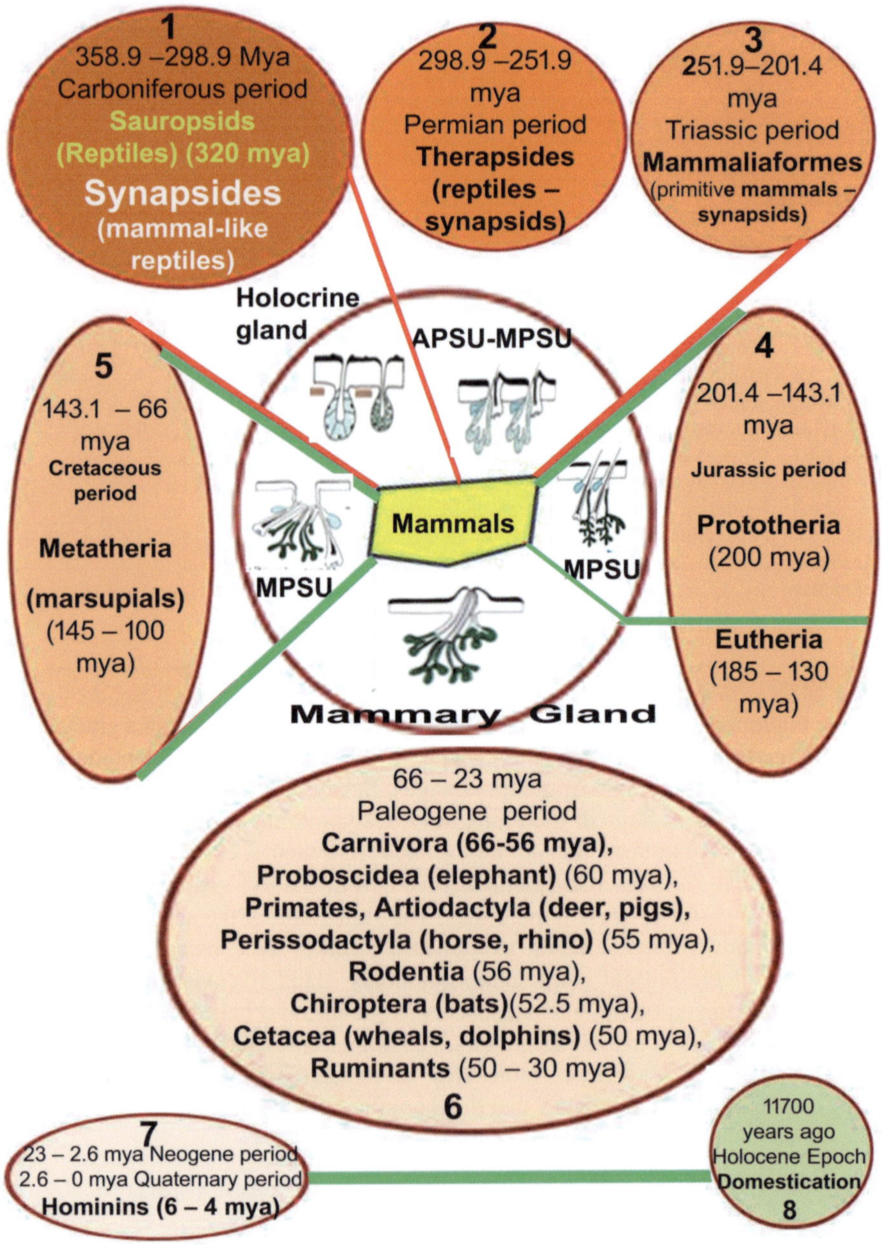

Description of the graphic: The evolutionary process of the mammalian mammary gland commenced during the Carboniferous period (358.9–298.9 million years ago, mya), with the origin of Synapsida (mammal-like reptiles) (**1**) having a holocrine milk-secreting gland. The existence of the apo-pilo-sebaceous unit–mammolobular-pilo-sebaceous unit (APSU-MPSU) persisted in the pre-mammalian Synapsida during the Permian period (**2**) and the Triassic period (**3**). Only the MPSU prototype milk-secreting gland was evaluated with the appearance of mammalian classes, in Prototheria and Metatheria, during the Jurassic period (**4**) and the Cretaceous period (**5**), respectively. The distinctive mammary gland appeared in the placenta-bearing Eutheria at the late Jurassic period (**4**). The evaluation of the mammary gland was continued till then in all the mammals, in the Paleogene period (**6**) and also in humans in the Neogene period and Quaternary period (**7**). The milk yield and composition were altered rapidly with domestication in Holocene Epoch (**8**)

Keywords

Adaptation of milk composition · Egg yolk into the milk · Eutherian milk · Mammo-pilo-sebaceous unit · Placentation · Synapsids lineage

Inside the Chapter

- *Origin of the mammary glands and lactation*
  - Amniotes to Synapsids
  - Appearance of nipples
  - Conversion of egg yolk into the milk
  - Mammary gland and placentation
- *Morphological evolution of the mammary gland*
- *Evolution of milk constituents*
  - Protective and nutritive role of milk
  - Diversity of fat molecules in milk
  - Evolution of protein spectrum in milk
  - Adaptation of milk composition in domestic mammals

Learning Objectives

- Evolution of the mammary gland from amniotes and synapsids during the Carboniferous and Pennsylvanian periods
- Transformation of apocrine skin gland secretions into milk for nourishment and protection of the young
- Structural and compositional changes following the emergence of nipples
- Adaptive evolution of the mammary gland and milk constituents driven by natural selection and survival of the fittest

2.1 Introduction

The mammary gland is a unique characteristic of the class Mammalia in the animal kingdom for the terrestrial quadrupeds with dolphins and whales, competence to produce milk for their young, coined by *Carl Linnaeus* in 1758. Mammalia was derived from the Latin word Mamma, meaning breast, that is, mammary gland. Animals having mammary glands are known as mammals. About 6000 species belong to the Mammalia class, having three subclasses: *Prototheria,* including Monotremes, the egg-laying mammals, *Metatheria,* distinguished by the mother's pouch, and *Eutheria,* comprising placenta. Hence, Prototheria, Metatheria, and Eutheria are the common ancestors of present mammals. The gland is present in both males and females of the same mammalian species, but remains nonfunctional and rudimentary in all males, with some exceptions. Androgens suppress the growth and development of the gland in males. Male marsupials, like kangaroos, koalas, and opossums, lack mammary glands, whereas male monotremes, viz. platypus and echidna, can excrete milk through the skin from the abdomen, but do not have nipples. Male mice and horses lack nipples. The white-colored secretory product of the mammary gland is milk, the source of major nutrients for the young. Considering the functional nature of milk, the product secreted from the crop of the birds to provide nutrients to the young is called crop milk, found in pigeons, flamingos, doves, and penguins. The tsetse flies and some types of jumping spiders secrete some nutritious substances for their larva and spiderlings, respectively, also termed milk. The word uterine milk denotes the secretory substances of the uterus that provide nutrients to the fetus. Often, white-colored plant-origin juices like coconut milk, rice milk, and soy milk are termed milk. The composition and nature of milk of the mammals diverged from species to species and are keenly related to their evolutionary aspect.

Knowledge Corner. . .

The mammary gland did not evolve originally to produce milk, but likely from skin glands that secreted moisture and antimicrobial substances to protect eggs.

2.2 Origin of the Mammary Glands and Lactation

2.2.1 Amniotes to Synapsids

The evolutionary process of the mammalian mammary gland is linked with the appearance of *amniotes* from the amphibians, approximately 340 million years ago (mya) during the *Carboniferous* period (360–300 mya). The amniotes vertebrates adapted with amnion in their body and are either able to lay eggs on land or keep the fertilized egg within the body. In a short period, at about 320 mya, the *synapsids* and *sauropsids* originated from amniotes, presently extinct. Synapsids are mammal-like reptiles and are believed to be the ancestors of Prototheria, Metatheria, Eutheria, and modern mammals. Sauropsids are the ancestors of reptiles, birds, and dinosaurs. The mammary glands are not fossilized well. It is believed that all the amniotes and their descendants moisten their eggs or hatched young, keep them free from any infection, and provide nutrition by their secretory glands. Considering the abundant watery secretion of the glands, the mammalian mammary gland is supposed to have originated from the eccrine sweat glands of amniotes. However, the mammary gland resembles the apocrine and sebaceous glands rather than eccrine glands based on their anatomical, physiological, developmental, and topographical distribution. Hence, the mammalian mammary gland is supposed to have originated with the adaptation and evolution of cutaneous sebaceous, eccrine, and apocrine glands of amniotes. The secretions of the glands have a major role in providing nutrition and protection to the young.

2.2.2 Appearance of Nipples

During the Pennsylvanian period, approximately 323.2–298.9 mya (a part of the Carboniferous period), the reptiles emerged in the terrestrial life, having prominent glandular rather than scaled integument. Mammals originated after this period, having some evolutionary features in the mammary gland. The hair follicles were associated with the reptiles' apocrine-like glands. The hairy mammary patch is the salient feature of the oviparous ancestor of early mammals. These glands were gradually restructured and void of hair follicles due to the cytotoxic effect of the tedious radiation. The vestigial mammary hair in the marsupials (about 145–100 mya) substantiated this conception. The glands progressively intensified and clustered as evidenced during early ontogenetic development in the *earlier mammals*. The pilosebaceous units open onto a nipple-less mammary patch to provide moisture and other nutrients to permeable eggs and hatchlings that demonstrated monotremes (around 115–108 mya). The appearance of nipples was highly correlated with the emergence of secondary hard-palate and jaw structures that support sucking milk from the newborn of the viviparous. Manifestation of nipples was also linked with the smaller egg mass due to the incompatibility of spreading the fluid (milk) over the egg. Thus, lactation must have developed before the appearance of viviparous at least 200 mya in oviparous.

2.2.3 Conversion of Egg Yolk into Milk

In the late *Triassic* period (approximately 201.4 mya), the advanced Triassic *therapsids*, like cynodonts and therocephalians, and early mammalian forms or mammal-like reptiles are considered close relatives of mammals. These animals are believed to have been *endotherms*. Hence, they required more body fluids to restore incubatory water losses of eggs, resulting in small-sized eggs. The altered dental pattern of the newborn was associated with faster growth. The adaptation process supported the commencement of feeding, indicating more dependency on the mother's milk. Thus, animals secrete a mixture of antimicrobial and nutrient-rich milk that provides nutrition to the neonates and immature young. Steadily, the egg yolk contents were gradually replaced in the milk to supplement nutrients to the young. The gene for *vitellogenin*, precursor to the egg yolk protein, was progressively lost from the synapsids, as evidenced by about 170 mya (*Jurassic* period).

2.2.4 Mammary Gland and Placentation

Placentation developed around 150–200 mya in a few fish, reptiles, amphibians, invertebrates, and mammals. *True placenta* evolved in eutherian mammals between 163 and 157 mya during the Jurassic period. However, ancient mammary glands emerged before placentation in some primitive mammals through the process of natural selection at about 190 mya. The ventral epidermal glands of the thorax and abdomen were favored to provide the secretory nutrients efficiently to the newborns. These features were documented in primitive mammals or mammalian-like reptiles, like monotremes (Prototheria), the echidna (*Tachyglossus aculeatus*), and the duck-billed platypus (*Ornithorhynchus anatinus*). Another evolutionary trend confirmed the mammary gland development in mammals with the rise of nipples from the hairless mammary patch and the concurrent presence of placental structures that allowed milk-like secretion in the eutherians, at about 120–140 mya. The full emergence of the mammary gland is supposed to have evolved from the ventral thoracic-abdominal epidermal glands of synapsid reptiles, first in the *Multituberculates* or *Rodentia* at around 100–120 mya (mid Jurassic period).

Differentiation and control of the copious alveolar secretory cells in the mammary gland radically changed during gestation and parturition in eutherians. In eutherians, the functional ability of the secretory cells to secrete profuse milk synthesis is controlled by the endocrines, viz. glucocorticoids, insulin, growth hormone, prolactin, and estrogens, superseding the negative role of progesterone. This adaptation supports them in developing an extended gestation period and short lactation. Early to eutherian, the marsupials were incompetent to inhibit the progesterone; hence, they have an extended lactation period and short gestation. It supported that the survivability of the neonate was the principle of lactation, as explained by *Charles Darwin*—the *survivability of the fittest*. Thus, lactation evolved through a very slow process. Presently, bovine genomes, concerning milk and mammary glands, have close similarities to eutherians—mouse, rat, dog, and human, marsupial—opossum, and monotreme—platypus.

2.3 Morphological Evolution of the Mammary Gland

The appearance of mammo-pilo-sebaceous unit (MPSU), a typical structure of hair follicles and sebaceous glands that open into the infundibulum of the hair follicle, has been recognized in the mammary patch of monotremes. In monotremes, about 100–200 MPSUs fused in a nipple-less small oval mammary patch resemble the galactophores of the mature and lobular mammalian mammary gland. Thus, the advanced mammary gland of mammals is likely to be analogous to the apocrine gland of its ancestors. In marsupials, the oval primary primordium separates the rudimentary structures (*nipple primordial*), considered nipples in higher mammals. It extends into knobs and buds that originate from the hair follicles (*primary sprout*). The branching structures developed from the primary sprouts in marsupials, called *secondary sprouts,* regarded as the mammary glands when elongated and canalized, and in due course formed the lactiferous ducts with their branches. In marsupials, the sebaceous glands were considered *tertiary sprouts*, which are assumed to be a complex ductal structure developed by the progesterone, prolactin, and other biomolecules, and differentiated into a milk-secreting cell, the alveoli, in higher mammals. About 100 MPSUs form nearly a dozen nipples in marsupials, where hair follicles gradually fall off, leaving galactophores that evidenced the evolutionary origin of mammary glands in higher mammals. The emergence of myoepithelial cells associated with the mammalian mammary gland for ejecting milk was documented in the early synapsids.

In the early synapsids, the oviparous transfers the heat through the mammary patch. It supported the animal in thermoregulation. The appearance of nipples may be considered the origin of marsupials, which developed the suckling behavior in the young. The emergence of simultaneous vomeronasal organs probably supported the young receiving the pheromone signaling released through milk. Thus, young–mother affection developed with the manifestation of nipples in mammals. Nipples control the milk seepage, caused milk to be yielded more than in early mammals. Downward movement of the posterior tongue of the calf caused vacuum and simultaneous compression of the teat caused it to secrete more milk in a given period to the cows than other mammals, viz. sows, rabbits, etc.

2.4 Evolution of Milk Constituents

Milk composition and energy concentration are greatly variable between species. The common macronutrients are water, sugars, lipids, and proteins in diverse concentrations. The sugars and lipids are the major sources of energy. Various proteins and amino acids have principally contributed to protective functions. Considering the unusual nutritional and pathogens confronted during the survivability of existence in various evolutionary periods, several lactation genomes evolved. Evolutionary history supported diversity. Some of the milk constituents, viz. α-lactalbumin, β-lactoglobulin, whey acidic protein, α-, β-, and κ caseins, lactose, membrane enveloped lipid droplets, and some oligosaccharides exceptionally originate in the mammary tissue, not elsewhere in nature.

2.4.1 Protective and Nutritive Role of Milk

The evolutionary process of the mammary gland from the apocrine-like gland confirmed the emergence of the primary mammalian milk constituents from their ancestors, like amniotes. Calcium-binding *phosphoproteins* of the apocrine-like gland's secretion implied its role in calcium delivery to eggs to protect the parchment-like shell of the early mammals. Later, calcium secretion supported the development of the hard eggshell. The complex *casein* micelles appeared later, during the Pennsylvanian period, around 310 mya. The casein proteins facilitate conveying the amino acids, calcium, and phosphorus to their eggs. The presence of three primary type caseins, α-, β-, and κ-casein, had been identified before the origin of monotremes, marsupials, and eutherians. The occurrence of immune proteins, viz. *butyrophilin* and *xanthine oxidoreductase* (XOR), has been identified in the apocrine-like gland's secretion during the same period. These proteins are associated with the milk fat globule membrane (MFGM) and were involved mostly in energy transfer. The ancestral c-lysozyme, an antimicrobial enzyme, gradually transforms into α-lactalbumin, a heat-stable whey protein in milk, supporting the synthesizing of the novel milk sugars, the lactose in the mammalian milk. Evidence suggested that the precursors of some whey proteins of mammalian milk, viz. *β-lactoglobulin* and whey acidic proteins, are ancestral *lipocalin* and whey acidic protein four-disulphide core (WFDC) protein. The role of transportation and antimicrobial functions of lipocalin and WFDC proteins are gradually limited to providing sulfur amino acids to the young. It indicates that the primary function of milk is protection for the young and the secondary is to provide nutrition, at least up to the Jurassic period. The occurrence of the Monotreme Lactation Protein (MLP) gene in the monotremes is an instance of this concept.

MLP is an antimicrobial protein, typically identified in the milk of monotremes and considered an ancient constituent of milk-mediated innate immunity, absent in other mammals. The MLP gene is profusely expressed in the milk cells of platypus and short-beaked echidna. This amphipathic, α-helical, N-linked glycosylated protein acted against opportunistic pathogens, like *Staphylococcus aureus* and commensal *Enterococcus faecalis*. The MLP played a critical protective role in monotremes, where milk secreted from the abdomen's nipple-less mammary patches to support the eggs and hatched young for a long pre-weaning period.

The natural selection process favored the accretion of certain innate immune factors, like immunoglobulin, iron-binding proteins, lysozyme, oligosaccharides, and leukocytes in the milk of protheria and eutheria. These substances are considered the precursors of various anti-inflammatory and immunomodulating factors in mammalian milk. The immune factors continued to be secreted in the milk up to their postnatal development. Their concentrations depend upon the placentation type, lactation pattern, and atmosphere. For example, marsupials require more nutrients in milk as they have no placenta than the eutherian milk. Hence, the composition of milk constituents was greatly altered with the evolution of the placenta in eutherians.

2.4.2 Diversity of Fat Molecules in Milk

The mammalian milk constituents and compositions have been widely altered according to *natural selection*. The milk fats are present as *milk fat globules* (MFG), the unique characteristics of mammalian milk. To conserve energy, the milk lipids are structured multilayered, consecutively with a phospholipid mono- and bilayer and a glycosylated surface having an inner protein coat. So many lipids have been demonstrated in the ancestors of the eutherians. However, MFG was not found in any pre-mammalian species and was also not secreted in any gland other than the mammary gland of the mammals. It is the major energy source of some mammals living in colder climates. Thus, wide variation in milk fat exists among the mammalian species, viz. less than 1% in rhinoceros and nearly 60% in *seals* and wheals. The mammals that have a low milk fat comprise more lactose to keep a steady energy source through milk to the young, like ruminants and humans. It is mostly related to natural selection and the ability of digestion and assimilation of the young of various food items. For example, the gene for *α-lactalbumin* has been mutated and changed in transcription rates in fur seals and sea lions (family Otariidae). Hence, lactose or lactose-based oligosaccharides are absent in these seals and have a high milk fat. About 200 genes for milk proteins and over 6000 other analogous genes were identified in the cow's mammary gland and apocrine glands of its ancestors, from amniotes.

2.4.3 Evolution of Protein Spectrum in Milk

Various caseins have a nutritive role providing calcium, phosphate, and amino acids to the young. Whey proteins have innate and adaptive immune functions. Some metalloproteins, like lactoferrin and transferrin, are bactericidal and bacteriostatic. Diversified bioavailability of whey proteins in different mammalian milk is the cause of evolutionary adaptation for their young. Considering the necessity of easily digestible lactose, more essential amino acids and immunoprotective proteins with balanced fat and carbohydrates, the fundamentals for an infant's brain development, ample α-lactalbumin is available in human milk. Conversely, β-lactalbumin is the chief whey protein in the ruminant's milk due to its diversified role in nutrition and immunity, including the transportation of various proteins and intestinal uptake of vitamin A, vitamin D, fatty acids, minerals, and various essential lipophilic compounds that are prerequisites for their rapid growing young compared to humans. The presence of β-lactalbumin has been recognized in the milk of monotremes, some marsupials, and a few eutherians during the Jurassic period. Interestingly, β-lactalbumin is lacking in the milk of guinea pigs, some mice and rats, domestic rabbits, one-humped camels (dromedary camels), llamas, and humans. Hence, the functional characteristic of β-lactalbumin is still indistinct. A cysteine-rich acidic protein, the whey acidic protein (WAP), is abundantly present in the milk of pig, camel, rabbit, mouse, rat, echidna, platypus, tammar wallaby, and brushtail possum. The WAPs regulate the growth and development of mammary epithelial cells and, consequently, milk production, reducing the degradation of laminin by serine proteases. It is absent in ruminants, where the mammary gland development is controlled by prolactin. WAPs are also good sources of essential amino acids, necessary for muscle growth and the overall health of the young.

2.4.4 Adaptation of Milk Composition in Domestic Mammals

The composition of milk constituents in mammals, particularly in domestic lactating animals, was fundamentally altered during the inception of human civilization. The transition of wild mammals to domestication was possibly considered about 11,000 years ago. Some animals were recognized as dairy animals, viz. cattle, buffaloes, sheep, goats, camels, yaks, etc. The composition of their milk is distinguished from the ancestor eutherian milk and wild mammals, with a reduced quantity of fats, caseins, and whey proteins and moderately higher levels of lactose. The major adaptation was targeted to maximize the total yield. This evolutionary alteration in the domesticated mammalian milk composition with its diluted nature of major milk constituents supported to accumulate the milk for a long period in their extensive storage cisterns. The less concentrated propped up the young of dairy animals and suitable for human consumption.

The morphology of the mammary glands, milk yield, and milk components is highly adapted to the mammals' physiology, behavior, and feeding characteristics (Table 2.1). The nipples' number is associated with the litter size. The fast-growing animals took less time to gain more weight with short lactation length. The immunological substances are highly related to the placentation pattern of mammals. Milk yield and components are linked with the physiological variations, including diurnal rhythm, and suckling patterns of the neonates associated with the milk removal and intramammary pressure. Feeding behavior involves feeding frequency and fermentation. The physiological and feeding adaptation processes eventually affect the hormonal and metabolic status of mammals related to lactation.

Table 2.1 Variation in the lactation characteristics of some wild and domestic animals

Attributes/species	Wild	Domesticate	Domesticate
	Rabbits (*Oryctolagus cuniculus* L.)	Cows (*Bos taurus*)	Pigs (*Sus scrofa*)
Litter size (average)	6	1	10
Nipples (no.)	8–10	4	12–16
Birth weight (kg)	0.050–0.090	22.00–38.00	1.20–1.70
Time to double the birth weight (d)	6–7	36	8
Weaning weight vs. birth weight (times)	4–6	4–6	4–6
Lactation length (d)	28–35	180–240	56
Average daily milk yield (kg)	0.14–0.32	5–10	4.50–5.70
Feeding interval (h)	24	5	1
Immunoglobulin transfer during pregnancy	IgG	None	None
Immunoglobulin in colostrum	IgA > IgG > IgM	IgG > IgA, IgM	IgG > IgA > IgM
Total immunoglobulin (mg/mL)	7.1	58	72
Total fat (g/L)	22	48	55
Major fatty acids	Short-chain fatty acids	Long-chain fatty acids	Medium- and long-chain fatty acids
Total protein (g/L)	103	32	56
β-Lactoglobulin	No	Present	Present
Major carbohydrate	Lactose	Lactose	Lactose
Lactose concentration (g/L)	22	48	55

Compiled from McClellan et al. (2008), Perumal et al. (2019), Szendrő et al. (2019), and Jankowiak et al. (2020)

Exercises

Objective Questions

1. The word *Mammalia* was coined by ______________________ .
2. Synapsids and sauropsids are originated from _______________ .
3. Mammary hairs were gradually voided due to the cytotoxic effect of __________ .
4. During _______________ period, the egg yolk contents were gradually replaced in the milk.
5. Placentation evolved at around ___________ million years ago.
6. The full form of MPSU is ________________________________ .

7. Lactose or lactose-based oligosaccharides are absent in fur seals due to mutation of ____________ gene.
8. The diluted nature of major milk constituents was prominently noticed during ___________ phase of the evolution of the mammals.
9. The whey acidic proteins regulate the growth and development of mammary epithelial cells by protecting the _______________ .
10. Three primary type caseins are _______________________________ .

Subjective Questions

1. The anatomical, physiological, developmental, and topographical distribution of the mammalian mammary gland resembles which glands? Write some evidence in support of your justification.
2. What are the evolutionary alterations that occurred with the development of nipples in the mammary gland?
3. Write in brief about the evolutionary changes in the mammary gland with the placentation.
4. Describe the evolutionary features of the nutritive role of milk.
5. How were fat molecules diversified in the evolutionary process?
6. Write about the protein spectrum concerned with the evolution of milk.
7. Describe the adaptation of milk composition in domestic mammals.
8. How did physiology, behavior, and feeding characteristics have evolutionary influences on mammalian milk composition?
9. Describe the evolutionary aspects of the protective function of milk.
10. Write in brief about the evolution of nipples.

Answers to Objective Questions

1. Carl Linnaeus
2. Amniotes
3. Radiation
4. Jurassic period
5. 150–200
6. Mammo-pilo-sebaceous unit
7. α-lactalbumin
8. Domestication
9. Laminin
10. α-, β-, and κ-casein

References

Articles

Biswas SK, Banerjee S, Baker GW, Kuo C-Y, Chowdhury I (2022) The mammary gland: basic structure and molecular signaling during development. Int J Mol Sci 23:3883. https://doi.org/10.3390/ijms23073883

Capuco AV, Akers RM (2009) The origin and evolution of lactation. J Biol 8:37. https://doi.org/10.1186/jbiol139

Cattaneo L, Piccioli-Cappelli F, Minuti A, Trevisi E (2023) Metabolic and physiological adaptations to first and second lactation in Holstein dairy cows: postprandial patterns. J Dairy Sci 106(5):3576–3585. https://doi.org/10.3168/jds.2022-22685

Enjapoori AK, Grant TR, Nicol SC, Lefe'vre CM, Nicholas KR, Sharp JA (2014) Monotreme lactation protein is highly expressed in Monotreme milk and provides antimicrobial protection. Genome Biol Evol 6(10):2754–2773. https://doi.org/10.1093/gbe/evu209

Freund J (2015) The evolution of the mammary gland. Master's Dissertation, Ghent University, Faculty of Veterinary Medicine, Academic year 2014–2015

Jankowiak H, Balogh P, Cebulska A, Weisbauerová E, Bocian M, Reszka P (2020) Impact of piglet birth weight on later rearing performance. Vet Med 65(11):473–479. https://doi.org/10.17221/117/2020-VETMED

McClellan HL, Miller SJ, Hartmann PE (2008) Evolution of lactation: nutrition v. protection with special reference to five mammalian species. Nutr Res Rev 21:97–116. https://doi.org/10.1017/S0954422408100749

Oftedal OT (2012) The evolution of milk secretion and its ancient origins. Animal 6(3):355–368. https://doi.org/10.1017/S1751731111001935

Perumal P, De AK, Bhattacharya D, Kundu A, Sunder J, Ravi SK, Bala PA, Alyethodi RR, Zamir Ahmed SK (2019) Birth rate and birth weight of crossbred calves in Andaman and Nicobar Islands. Int J Bioresour Stress Manage 10(3):323–328. https://doi.org/10.23910/IJBSM/2019.10.3.2000

Szendrő Z, Cullere M, Atkári T, Zotte AD (2019) The birth weight of rabbits: influencing factors and effect on behavioural, productive and reproductive traits: a review. Livest Sci 230(Suppl.1):103841. https://doi.org/10.1016/j.livsci.2019.103841

Anatomy and Histology of the Mammary Gland

3

Contents

J. Mukherjee et al., *Veterinary Lactation Physiology*,
https://doi.org/10.1007/978-3-032-21123-1_3

Abstract

Mammary gland is a modified sweat gland evolved exclusively to nourish the young. In cows, four mammary glands are joined together to form an udder from which the milk is drained through teat. Internally the mammary gland is lobuloalveolar in nature composed of secretory tissues, connective tissues and ductular system. The secretory tissue produces the milk and drains through the ductular system. Connective tissues act as a supporting system to the udder. The primary secretory unit of the mammary gland is the alveoli lined by luminal epithelial cells and myoepithelial cells. Luminal epithelial cells produce the milk, and contractile myoepithelial cells support the gland and help in milk secretion. These secretory tissue components are embedded within the stromal tissue comprising fibroblasts, adipocytes, extracellular matrix proteins, blood vessels, and lymphatics. The contact between epithelial cells and myoepithelial cells is facilitated by tight junctions, adherens junctions, desmosomes, and gap junctions, and the cellular interactions are mediated by junctional proteins such as zonula occluden, occludin, cingulin, cadherin, catenin, desmoglein, desmocollin, and connexin. The interaction between mammary epithelial cells and ECM is crucial for the development and survival of mammary epithelial cells. These interactions are facilitated by transmembrane receptors (integrins) in the mammary epithelial cells and their ligands (collagen, laminin, fibronectin, vitronectin) in the ECM components.

Graphical Abstract

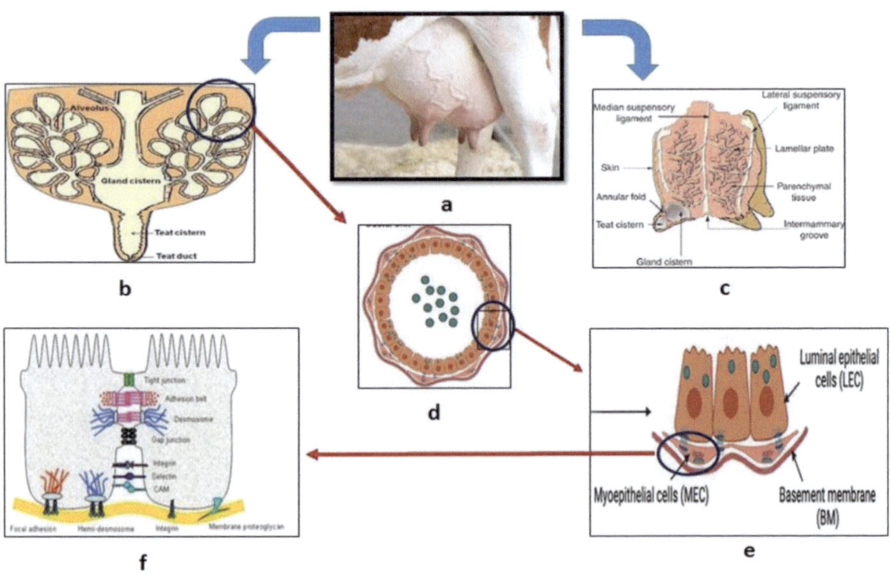

Description of the graphic: Mammary gland (**a**) is made of secretory components (**b**) and supporting structure (**c**). The primary secretory unit is called alveoli (**d**) composed of luminal epithelial cells and myoepithelial cells embedded within the stromal tissue and extracellular matrix (**e**). The contact between epithelial cells and myoepithelial cells is facilitated by tight junctions, adherens junctions, desmosomes, and gap junctions (**f**), which are crucial for cell–cell interactions that controls the functions of the mammary gland

Keywords

Alveoli · Epithelial cells · Stroma · Cell–cell interaction · Junctional proteins · Myoepithelial cells · Mammary artery · Milk vein

Inside the Chapter

- *External anatomy of the mammary gland*
- *Supporting structure of the mammary gland*
- *Functional histo-morphology of mammary gland*
  - Cell-cell interaction
  - Stromal compartment
  - Extracellular matrix (ECM)
  - ECM-mammary epithelial cell interactions
  - Myoepithelial cells
- *Blood vascular system of the mammary gland*
  - Arterial Supply
  - Venous Drainage
  - Lymphatic system of the udder
- *Nerve Supply to the Udder*

Learning Objectives

- External anatomy of the mammary gland in cows, sheep, goats, pigs, and mares
- Functional histomorphology of the mammary gland
- Molecular mechanisms controlling cell–cell interactions
- Stromal factors controlling the growth and functions of mammary epithelial cells
- Mammary epithelial cells and extracellular matrix crosstalk

3.1 Introduction

Mammary gland is an exocrine gland modified from a sweat (sudoriferous) gland. During the course of evaluation, the number and anatomical features of the mammary glands gained their functional features from simple to complex type. Monotreme animals like platyplus hold a primitive type of mammary gland that does not have nipples but hairs and the young one laps the hairs to get milk. In marsupials, the teats are located within a pit and protected by a pouch-like skin fold and the young one attaches with the teat soon after birth. The bovines possess the most advanced type of mammary gland composed of different components like supportive components made of skin and fibroelastic tissue (ligaments), secretory components

Table 3.1 Comparative features of the mammary gland in different species

Species	Teat position			Total glands	Openings per teat
	Thoracic	Abdominal	Inguinal		
Cattle	–	–	4	2	1
Goat	–	–	2	2	1
Sheep	–	–	2	2	1
Pig	4	6	2	12	2
Horse	–	–	2	2	2
Red kangaroo	–	4	–	4	15
Opossum	–	13	–	13	8
Cat	2	6	–	8	3–7
Dog	2	6	2	10	8–14
Mouse	4	2	4	10	1
Rat	4	4	4	12	1
Rabbit	4	4	2	10	8–10
Whale	–	–	2	2	1
Elephant	2	–	–	2	10–11

Larson (1985) and Nickerson and Akers (2011) and Mukherjee et al (2023)

made up of mammary epithelial cells, and duct system, along with blood vascular, lymphatic, and nervous components. In general, the mammary glands are joined together and enclosed in a common envelope to form the udder from which the teats emerge. The udder conformation is reported to affect the milk production; hence, it is considered to be a good selection criterion for milch animals. In addition, the udder morphometric features are useful to predict the udder health and prognosis of udder infections. One of the primary reasons for culling the dairy animals is poor udder health. The number and functional morphology of the mammary gland vary considerably between different classes of mammals. Regarding the evolutionary strategy toward fewer offspring and better maternal care, a considerable variation is reported in the number of mammary glands form 2 (primates) to 25 in some opossums. The weight of the mammary gland is about body weight$^{0.8}$. There are striking differences among species in regard to gross morphology of the mammary gland, including the number of mammary glands and their anatomical location (Tables 3.1 and 3.2).

3.2 Cow

The bovine mammary gland consists of four separate glands grouped together as an udder with a teat in each gland. Two normal functional glands grouped as the quarters are situated on each side of the median line at the inguinal region. The right and left udder halves are separated by the longitudinal intermammary groove or sulcus intermammaricus. The front and rear quarters do not have gross anatomical barriers, but are rather separated by a thin connective tissue septum preventing direct

Table 3.2 Comparative gross morphology of the mammary gland in different species

Species	Udder width (cm)	Udder front depth (cm)	Udder rear depth (cm)	Udder height (cm)	Teat circumference (cm)	Fore teat length (cm)	Rear teat length (cm)	Teat diameter (cm)	References
Friesian cows	31.68	18.99	22.78	56.94	–	6.50	6.50	2.79	Saleh et al. (2023)
Sahiwal cows	56.84 ± 0.95	28.07 ± 0.79	–	53.92 ± 0.68	9.13 ± 0.17	6.27 ± 0.18	6.11 ± 0.18	1.81 ± 0.06	Sharma et al. (2024)
Gir cows	20.51 ± 0.99	20.29 ± 1.04	–	45.99 ± 2.07		7.07 ± 0.42	3.49 ± 0.21	–	Singhai et al. (2013)
Murrah Buffalo	50.6 ± 0.36	15.5 ± 0.10	–	54.2 ± 0.34	10.31 ± 0.38–11.90 ± 0.45	9.02 ± 0.45–10.42 ± 0.47	–	–	Thomas et al. (2004) and Prasad et al. (2010)
Sheep (Pelibuey ewes)	11.68 ± 1.55	–	–	13.91 ± 2.51		3.47	2.64 ± 1.41	1.58 ± 0.62	Arcos-Álvarez et al. (2020)
Goats (Tunisian local goats)	13.80	–	–	19.30	12.47	9.43	–	3.91	Ahlem et al. (2023)
Mares (Caspian)	8.25 ± 0.28	–	–	9.19 ± 0.21		1.125 ± 0.05	–	–	Abshenas et al. (2014)
Camel	40.0	28.0	32.0	46.0	4.5	5.0	6.0	5.0	Müller et al. (2024)

connections between the front and rear quarters. The rear quarter produces 60% of total milk. The mammary glands are connected to the abdominal cavity by inguinal canal. Apart from this, some paired narrow passages just above the udder allow nerve, blood, and lymph vessels into the udder quarters.

3.2.1 Characteristics of Good Udder

A good udder should have a large volume to produce more milk and be soft in touch to denote more epithelial tissue. It should be evenly balanced and symmetrical with moderate udder height.

Large-sized udder that has a greater number of glandular tissues should be one of the important selection criteria for dairy animals. Udder weight is positively correlated with milk production traits. The shape and depth of udder also affect the udder health in bovines. A pendulous type of udder is reported have more chances of udder infections compared to the non-pendulous types of udder (Sharma et al. 2017).

The udder depth is the distance between the udder floor to the point of the hock. It is generally desirable that the depth should never reach below the hock; otherwise, it may affect the gait and lead to udder injury. The distance between the base of the vulva and the top of the mammary gland is considered the rear udder depth, and less distance between these two points is desirable. Both the front and rear udder depth have high positive correlations with milk yield. Udder depth also has a significant impact on milking efficiency.

The udder should be firmly attached to the floor of the abdominal cavity. The median suspensory ligament is the main structure that attaches the medial surface of the udder to the body wall. A strong median suspensory ligament could be evaluated by a deep cleft between the left and right udder halves. A strong udder cleft is desirable.

Milk is extracted from each mammary gland through teats, which can be cylindrical or conical and lack sweat or sebaceous glands on their walls. Typically, one teat corresponds to each gland, although extra teats, known as supernumerary teats, can sometimes occur naturally, with a 50% incidence rate. It is one of the most common congenital anomalies in cattle. These additional teats are often removed for cosmetic purposes and prevent mastitis at the age of 4–6 months. Sometimes, a supernumerary teat may attach to the side of a primary teat. This is called web or conjoined teats. Teats lacking a streak canal are termed pseudo-teats. A desirable teat should possess moderate size, correct placement, and sufficient tension in the sphincter muscle around the teat opening to facilitate milking while preventing milk leakage between milkings. Teat diameter and distance between the front teats are moderately correlated with peak milk yield.

3.3 Mare

The equine udder is composed of two separate mammary gland complexes. Each gland has a separate duct system and teat openings. Each teat has two openings, and the milk produced from each gland remains separate till foal's mouth. Like bovines, the medial suspensory ligament is situated along the midline of the two udder quarters.

3.4 Sheep and Goats

Two separate mammary glands joined together to form an udder situated at the inguinal region at each side of the ventral midline. Udder halves are separated by the median intermammary groove. The shape of the udder is usually conical with a concave base. The convex lateral surfaces are covered with skin and hairs, whereas the medial surfaces are flattened. The medial and lateral suspensory ligaments attach the udder to the abdominal wall.

Knowledge Corner . . .
Among all mammals, the blue whale holds the record for the largest mammary glands—each can grow as long as 5 feet and weigh about 250 pounds, roughly the size of a grown human! Even more fascinating, these giant glands can pump out over 150 liters of super-rich, creamy milk every single day, giving the baby whale the energy it needs to grow at an incredible speed.

3.5 Supporting Structures of the Udder

Mammary gland is a skin gland situated externally. The base of the udder is attached partly to the abdominal wall (60%) and pelvic floor (40%). The supporting structures of the udder provide mechanical strength of the udder to hold it with the abdominal wall. The lactating mammary gland weight of a Holstein cow may exceed 50 kg, and the udder may become pendulous due to the weakening of the suspensory apparatus. So, strong suspensory structures are the desirable qualities in selecting good-quality udder. Other than good tensile strength, the supporting structure should also have a good stretchability that allows the udder to increase in length during the accumulation of milk.

Turner (1952) classified the mammary suspensory system into six different types of tissues, out of which skin and superficial fascia have poor suspension capabilities. The International Nomenclature of Veterinary Anatomy (Schaller 1992) classified the suspensory apparatus of the mammary gland into lateral and medial laminae (suspensory ligaments).

The supporting structures of udder are described as follows:

Skin The udder is covered by skin with thin hair that primarily protect the udder from external injury. However, very little mechanical support is provided by the skin when the udder is completely filled with milk.

Fine Areolar Subcutaneous Tissue or Superficial Fascia It is made up of fine areolar subcutaneous tissue beneath the skin. It is extended from the lateral surface of the udder in the hind quarter and joins with femoral fascia at the medial thigh region. Being loose connective tissue, superficial fascia allows the udder skin to move easily.

Coarse Areolar Subcutaneous Tissue It is a cord-like tissue beneath the skin that forms a loose band between the upper surface of the front quarters and abdominal wall. Though they do not provide major support to the udder but keep close attachment between the udder and abdominal wall.

Lateral Suspensory Ligaments They are one of the major suspensory apparatus of the udder. After originating from subpelvic tendon, it runs vertically to support the lateral surface of the udder. This ligament is nonstretchable. The lateral suspensory ligaments have two layers: superficial layer of the lateral suspensory ligaments is made of loose connective tissue and extends from the lateral surface of udder at the hind quarters to the femoral fascia at the medial surface of the thigh. The deep layer of the lateral suspensory ligament extends up to udder stroma and supports the lobes and lobules. This layer is divided into an abdominal (lamina lateralis pars abdominalis) and pelvic (lamina lateralis pars pelvinae) parts.

Median Suspensory Ligament This is the main supporting structure of the udder with the greatest tensile strength. It originates as two parallel connective tissue sheath and runs ventrally to the glandular tissue. Similar to lateral suspensory ligaments, it is also divided into abdominal (lamina medialis pars abdominalis) and pelvic (lamina medialis pars pelvinae) parts. Unlike the lateral suspensory ligaments, the medial one is elastic in nature and allows the mammary gland to stretch when filled with milk. This ligament becomes weaker in older cows and leads to pendulous udder and udder edema.

Sub-pelvic Tendon It is not a true supporting structure of the udder, but it gives rise to superficial and deep lateral suspensory ligaments.

3.6 Internal Structure of the Udder

Internally the udder is composed of secretory tissues, connective tissues, and ductular system. The secretory tissue produces the milk and drains through the ductular system. Connective tissue acts as a supporting system to the udder. The functional milk production of the mammary gland is alveoli composed of a layer of luminal alveolar cells on a basement membrane surrounded by contractile myoepithelial cells. The tubular acinar cells (34–168 in buffaloes) are embedded within adipose and connective tissues to form lobules (*Lobuli glandulae mammariae*). Several lobules are joined together to form lobes (*Lobi glandular mammariae*). The milk produced in the secretory tissue is drained by the ductal system that ends up in the teat cistern till milking or suckling.

3.6.1 Duct System

Duct systems deliver milk from alveoli to the teat. The duct system of the mammary gland is composed of alveolar duct, intralobular duct, interlobular duct, intralobar duct, and interlobar and lactiferous ducts. Individual ducts from each alveolus (alveolar ducts) merge to form interlobular ducts, which then combine to create interlobar ducts. Interlobular ducts merge to form larger ducts that drain into cisterns, the primary collecting spaces. Typically, 5–20 large ducts connect to the gland cistern of the udder. The branching points of the ducts feature a narrow opening that expands into a sinus-like enlargement before narrowing again. This constriction at the branching point prevents milk from flowing into the teat and gland cisterns due to gravity. The duct arrangement differs across species based on the number of openings per teat. Cattle, buffalo, sheep, and goats have a single opening per teat, resulting in one final duct per gland. Mares and sows have two main ducts with corresponding openings. In contrast, dogs and cats possess 10 or more openings per teat, each connected to a corresponding final duct.

Intralobar ducts are lined with simple cuboidal epithelium. Lobular ducts are lined by simple cuboidal epithelium near their origin, transitioning to two layers of cuboidal cells distally. Lactiferous ducts feature a bilayered cuboidal epithelium and drain into a lactiferous or gland sinus located at the teat's base. The gland sinus is lined with stratified cuboidal epithelium. Ductal myoepithelial cells are spindle-shaped and aligned parallel to the longitudinal axis, forming a continuous layer surrounding the luminal cells, particularly within the ducts.

Gland Cistern (sinus lactiferous or udder cistern) These are large cavities with variable size that act as a reservoir of milk between milking. The gland cistern of a cow can store 100–400 ml of milk. The gland cistern of a cow is circular in shape, but in buffaloes it appears as numerous pockets with ductal interceptions. The area of gland cistern varies considerably among species (Table 3.3).

3.6.2 Teat Cistern (Sinus Papillaris)

Teat cistern is the cavity inside the teat. It comes straight from the gland cistern and runs alongside it. The teat cistern has a storage capacity of 10–50 ml. The annular fold, a constriction made of thick connective tissue that ranges in thickness from 2 to 6 mm, is located at the junction of the gland and the teat cistern. Multiple overlapping longitudinal and circular folds in the mucosa give the teat cistern its

Table 3.3 Area of gland (cm^2) cistern in different species

Animal	Right front	Left front	Right rear	Left rear	References
Cow (Friesian)	13.20–32.21 (median 19.05)	3.03–51.00 (median 21.19)	2.61–25.23 (median 47.89)	11.24–26.77 (median 26.77)	Bonelli et al. (2020)
Sheep	16.92 ± 1.32	21.10 ± 1.86	–	–	Nudda et al. (2000)
Goat	12.28–79.01	4.48–62.86	–	–	Wójtowski et al. (2020)
Buffalo	11.85 ± 1.40		11. 84 ± 3. 09		Thomas et al. (2004)

honeycombed appearance. The double-layered epithelium that covers the teat cistern is made up of columnar (luminal) and cuboidal (basal) cells. In some cases, a horizontal septum develops at the annular fold and obstructs the milk flow from the gland cistern to the teat cistern and the condition is termed as "blind quarter."

3.6.3 Streak Canal (Ductus Papillaris)

It is the distal aperture of the teat cistern via which milk is extracted. The opening of the streak canal is guided by a sphincter made of circular smooth muscles. The sphincter retains the milk and keeps the orifice closed during periods between milking and prevents the entry of pathogens. The sphincter showed peristaltic contractions in response to teat stimulus that removes debris at the end of the canal and facilitates blood and lymph flow in the teats. Leaky teats are developed when these muscles become incompetent and lead to the occurrences of udder infections. The narrowing of streak canal interferes with milk flow, and the cows are called 'hard milkers." Buffaloes have longer teat canal length and narrower streak canal diameter. So, they require vacuum during machine milking compared to cattle. The diameter of the teat canal varied considerably among species. In cows, the teat canal diameters are 3.0 mm (1.6–5.1), 2.9 mm (1.1–4.5), and 2.4 mm (1.2–4.0) in the proximal, mid, and distal ends, respectively (Berteau et al. 2024). The length of teat canal in goat is about 4.01 ± 0.55 mm (Adam et al. 2017). In sheep, the length and width of teat canal are 5.7–10.3 mm and from 1.8–3.1 mm, respectively. The length and width of teat canal in buffaloes are 8.25–11.56 cm and 2.71 ± 0.10 cm (Mota-Rojas et al. 2024).

3.6.4 Fürstenberg Rosette

The mucosal folds at the proximal site of the streak canal form a petal-like structure called Fürstenberg rosette. It is also called squamocolumnar junction as the epithelial lining of teat canal becomes squamous to columnar epithelium at this point. In cows, Fürstenberg rosette is lined by double-layered columnar cells. The lining cells have

Table 3.4 Occurrence of plasma cells in Fürstenberg rosette and teat cistern in dry, calving, and lactating cows

Plasma cells types	Dry		Calving		Lactating	
	Fürstenberg rosette	Teat cistern	Fürstenberg rosette	Teat cistern	Fürstenberg rosette	Teat cistern
IgG1 (%)	90.2	79.5	85.4	82.5	89.1	65.0
IgM (%)	8.0	16.0	12.7	6.3	8.4	35
IgA (%)	1.8	4.5	1.9	11.3	2.5	0.0

Collins et al. (1986)

vacuolated cytoplasm indicative of lipid secretion. There are primary and secondary folds toward the lumen of the rosette, which vary 10–14 in crossbred cows and buffaloes, whereas in desi cows the projections are more. The more numbers of these connective tissue folds in Fürstenberg rosette of native cows protect them from microbial invasions. Subepithelial area of rosette comprises different leukocyte subpopulations, viz. lymphocytes, polymorphonuclear leukocytes, macrophages, and plasma cells. There is the presence of longitudinal and circular smooth muscle surrounding Fürstenberg rosette. The rosette acts as a mechanical seal and provides local defense against pathogens. The mucosal immune defense against pathogens in the streak canal is provided by Fürstenberg rosette-associated lymphoid tissue (FALT) in cows. FALT resembles a similar structure as gut-associated lymphoid tissue (GALT) and bronchus-associated lymphoid tissue (BALT). FALT contains centrum germinativum and follicle-associated epithelium. The subepithelial area of Fürstenberg rosette has B lymphocyte infiltrations that are subsequently differentiated into plasma cells. Among these plasma cells, IgG1-producing cells are predominantly followed by IgM and IgA-producing cells. The plasma cell population varies with the physiological state of the animals (Table 3.4). In sheep and goats, there are CD3-positive "T" lymphocytes in the intraepithelial region and lamina propria. The cells of Fürstenberg rosette are reported to produce biquitin, a cationic bactericidal protein.

The desquamation at this site forms keratin, which occludes the lumen of teat canal between milking and prevents bacterial entry.

3.7 Functional Histomorphology of the Mammary Gland

Alveoli The primary secretory unit of the mammary gland is the alveoli. Adult mammary gland is divided into two distinct compartments: epithelial compartment called parenchyma and stromal compartment. The epithelial compartment comprises of lobuloalveolar structure and the duct system that are embedded into the stroma made up of adipocytes, fibroblasts, vascular endothelium, immune cells, and extra-cellular matrix (ECM). Mammary acini/alveoli are lined by different types of cells such as stem and progenitor cells, basal and luminal epithelial cells, and myoepithelial cells. The proportion of these cells changes with the stage of lactation.

Leukocytes such as lymphocytes and plasma cells are often observed within the acini but neutrophils are rare in healthy glands. Out of these cells, mammary secretory epithelium and myoepithelial cells are of prime importance as mammary secretory epithelial cells produce the milk and contractile myoepithelial cells support the gland and help in milk secretion. The epithelial component of the mammary gland constitutes nearly 10–15% of its overall volume. These cells are cuboidal to columnar in shape, with a diameter of 50–250 mm depending upon the stage of lactation. The apical pole of mammary epithelial cells surrounds the lumen where the milk is accumulated and the basal poles are covered by cytoplasmic processes of mammary epithelial cells. These secretory tissue components are embedded within the stromal tissue comprising fibroblasts, adipocytes, extracellular matrix proteins, blood vessels, and lymphatics. The secretory epithelial cells are joined to each other by tight junctions. At the apical portion, desmosomes and adherens junction form the junctional complexes, whereas the joining of epithelial cells and myoepithelial cells is facilitated by hemidesmosomes. Tight junctions form the border between the apical and basolateral surface and prevent the paracellular transport of ions and other small molecules. It also contributes to maintaining the polarity of the cells by separating the plasma membrane into distinct protein and lipid domains.

The mammary epithelial cells consist of cytoplasm together and cell organelles surrounded by the plasma membrane. Important cellular organelles include nucleus, Golgi apparatus, rough endoplasmic reticulum, and mitochondria. The organelles are responsible for the synthesis, transport, and secretion of different milk constituents. The epithelial cells undergo remodeling of its ultrastructure in and around parturition under the influence of reproductive hormones and paracrine factors, whereas the secretory potential is lost during mastitis due to the shrinkage of the cytoplasm.

The endoplasmic reticulum (ER) attached to the ribosome is a dynamically regulated cell organelle that is responsible for the synthesis of lipids and proteins. The milk lipids are synthesized into the ER and packaged into lipid droplets in the cytoplasm. ER exists in two forms: both granular (rough) and agranular (smooth) endoplasmic reticulum. The ER undergoes marked structural and functional changes during lactation and involution.

Lactating mammary epithelial cells contained numerous mitochondria responsible for energy production and cellular metabolism. The shape of mitochondria varies from cup- or ring-shaped, some of which are extremely elongated. The mitochondria are localized either at the basal region or at the lateral margins associated with tonofilaments-desmosomal complex. The mitochondria contain cristae arranged as lattice pattern. Mitochondria contain enzymatic machinery responsible for ATP production by tricarboxylic acid (TCA) cycle and oxidative phosphorylation.

Lactating bovine mammary epithelial cells contain pleomorphic network of Golgi complex at supra and juxtanuclear regions of the cytoplasm. The shape of Golgi complex depends upon its localization. It appears as a hollow cone or cylinder when situated at juxta and supranuclear regions, but it is bowl-shaped when localized at the supranuclear region. The Golgi complex consists of a single dictyosome. Each dictyosome consists of 5–7 cisternae having a 1.5 μm width. The main function of Golgi complex is the packaging, sorting, distribution, and post-transcriptional modification of proteins and lipids.

Mammary lysosomes are membrane-bound intracellular organelle with highly acidic environment. Lysosomes are concerned with exocytosis, endocytosis, and apoptosis during mammogenesis, lactogenesis, and mammary gland involution. It contains several hydrolytic enzymes such as acid phosphatase (APase), aryl sulfatase (ASase), N-acetyl-pD-glucosaminidase (NAGase), P-glucuronidase (p-glu-ase), and cathepsin D. These enzymes are synthesized in rough ER and undergo post-translational modifications at Golgi apparatus before reaching the lysosomes. The lysosomes can be identified by the staining with marker enzyme ASase. Lysosomes that contain only ASase stain are considered primary lysosomes. The number of primary lysosomes is increased after parturition. Secondary lysosomes contain ASase stain along with vacuoles filled with products of ASase reaction and casein micelles. Their numbers are reported to increase after parturition, peak around lactation, and declined at the time of involution. Telolysosomes are the smaller subgroups of secondary lysosomes, also known as residual bodies. They have ASase reaction products along with other substrates of unknown origin. Their numbers are decreased at the end of gestation. Other groups of secondary lysosomes are the dense bodies identified with the granular ASase stain. Their numbers increased during involution.

The cytoskeleton of mammary epithelial cells is formed by actin microfilaments, keratin intermediate filaments, and α- and β-tubulin. The cytoskeletal network provides the integrity of the cell as well as facilitates the interactions between cells and extracellular matrix. This communication is mediated by the interaction of transmembrane proteins with intracellular proteins on neighboring cells or proteins in the extracellular space.

Corpora amylacea are hyaline glycoprotein-rich aggregates that appear as dense bodies in the alveoli and connective tissue. They appear as round and oval shaped to irregular shaped, resembling concentrically laminated cauliflower-like structures, with a few droplets at the center. They originate from desquamated epithelial cells undergoing lysis, accumulating as solid, clump-like materials within the alveolar lumen in cows. In cows, corpora amylacea are frequent during the later stages of lactation (95%), but their number reduces to 50% during involution. The location of corpora amylacea also varies during the stage of lactation. In lactating mammary glands, they are most abundant within the alveoli, but during periods 90% of corpora amylacea are present in the interstitial tissue. During gestation, they are situated outside the alveoli and within the interalveolar connective tissue. Corpora amylacea are seen in goats, ewes, and mares.

3.8 Cell–Cell Interaction

Proper functioning of the mammary epithelial cells depends upon cell–cell and cell–extracellular matrix interactions. The cell–cell interaction is facilitated by cell–cell interacting junctions, tight junctions, the adherens junctions, desmosomes, and gap junctions.

3.8.1 Tight Junctions

Tight junctions form a continuous seal at the apical pole of the mammary epithelial cells. It maintains different internal milieus between ducts and alveoli containing milk with high lactose, milk proteins, and low sodium and chloride, and the interstitial fluid with plasma proteins and high level of sodium and chloride by preventing interdiffusion through the paracellular pathway. There are several proteins associated with tight junctions (Table 3.5).

The shape of the tight junctions is dynamic in nature. It is leaky around pregnancy, but soon after parturition decreased progesterone level is associated with conformational changes in the tight junctions to form ridge-like structures that restrict the paracellular pathway so that the milk constituents accumulate inside the rumen. The permeability of tight junctions is affected by oxytocin and mastitis. Endotoxins such as lipopolysaccharide (LPS) produced from *E. coli* and lipoteichoic acid (LTA) from *Staphylococcus aureus* result in the opening of tight junctions and affect the barrier integrity.

Table 3.5 Major proteins associated with tight junctions in mammary alveoli

Name	Characteristics	Functions
Zonula occluden-1 (ZO-1)	A 210kD cytosolic peripheral membrane protein that acts as peripheral component of tight junctions	Restricts the permeability of solute at tight junctions
Zonula occluden-2 (ZO-2)	A 160 kD protein having structural similarity with ZO-1	Barrier function in tight junction
Occludin,	It is the only trans membrane protein with a MW of 65 kD	Nonbarrier functions such as epithelial cell survival and apoptosis
Cingulin	140 kD protein localized on the cytoplasmic side of tight junctions	Facilitates the interactions between tight junction and cytoskeleton

3.8.2 Adherens Junctions

They are involved in cell–cell adhesion, intracellular signaling, and regulation of the cytoskeleton. These junctions are composed of adhesion receptors and associated proteins in the cytoplasm. E-cadherin, a sticky transmembrane fiber, is a major adhesion receptor that forms calcium-dependent linkage with cytosolic proteins such as α-catenin, β-catenin, and p120 catenin. Adherens junction is formed when cadherin binds with β-catenin that in turn joins with cytoskeletal protein actin. The interaction of cadherin with β-catenin leads to the activation of NFκB, Wnt, and MAPK signaling pathways to regulate a variety of functions. Upregulation of E-cadherin was reported in goats after milk stasis.

3.8.3 Desmosomes

These are intercellular junctions between mammary epithelial cells and the basal myoepithelial cells. Desmosome is composed of two main proteins, namely desmoglein (Dsg) and desmocollin (Dsc) of the cadherin family. The desmosomes between two adjacent luminal pithelium contain Dsg2 and Dsc2, whereas the junction between luminal epithelium and myoepithelial cells is formed by Dsg3 and Dsc3.

3.8.4 Gap Junctions

Gap junctions allow the transfer of biomolecules up to 1500 Da between cells. These are hemichannels made of six connexin molecules. In the rodent mammary gland, there are four types of connexins such as Cx26, Cx30, Cx32, and Cx43 in luminal epithelial cells, whereas in myoepithelial cells, Cx43 has been identified. Studies have shown that Cx26 increased gradually from early pregnancy gland; in contrast, Cx32 is increased after parturition in mouse mammary gland. But both of them reached their maximum during the early lactation period.

3.9 Stromal Compartment

The stromal compartment of the mammary gland consists of different types of connective tissues such as adipocytes, fibroblasts, vascular endothelial cells, immune cells (macrophages and mast cells), and extracellular matrix (ECM).

3.9.1 Adipocytes

They are the most abundant cellular components of mammary stroma in rats and mice. However, in ruminants and humans, the stroma is fibro-adipose in nature comprising white adipose tissue and fibroblasts. The adipocytes mainly provide structural support and create a favorable microenvironment for mammary epithelial cells. They provide triglycerides to the developing mammary epithelial cells for energy generation. Adipocytes of the mammary stroma secrete a wide range of endocrine factors called adipokines that regulate the functions of mammary epithelial cells.

Adipokines are secreted locally and act via juxtacrine and paracrine fashion to modulate the growth and development of mammary epithelial cells. Important adiponectins secreted by stromal adipocytes are as follows:

3.9.1.1 Leptin

It is a nonglycosylated protein of 16 kDa encoded by the Ob gene. It is mainly concerned with the energy homeostasis and nutrient partitioning during pregnancy and lactation. The production of leptin by the adipocytes is under the control of several hormones such as prolactin, insulin, estradiol, and glucocorticoids. Prolactin is the main regulator of leptin secretion by controlling prolactin and prolactin receptor gene expression in mammary epithelial cells. Estradiol has been shown to regulate leptin levels in the human mammary gland. Leptin also increases the self-renewal capacity of mammary stem cells.

3.9.1.2 Adiponectin

Adiponectin is a 28–30 kDa protein with 240 amino acids secreted from stromal adipocytes. It interacts with adiponectin receptor (AdipoR) that has two isoforms, AdipoR1 and AdipoR2. Receptor activation leads to the activation of protein kinase through cyclic adenosine monophosphate. Adiponectin is primarily concerned with cellular energy metabolism, but unlike leptin, the concentration of adiponectin is inversely correlated with the body mass index.

3.9.1.3 Chemerin

It is a 16 kDa chemoattractant cytokine (chemokine) of white adipose tissue. It is also called retinoic acid receptor responder protein 2 (RARRES2). It acts through G-protein-coupled receptors such as chemokine receptor-like 1 (CMKLR1), G protein-coupled receptor 1 (GPR1), and C-C chemokine receptor-like 2 (CCRL2). The receptor activation leads to downstream signaling cascades by phospholipase C activation followed by the release of inositol triphosphate (IP3) and calcium mobilization. Chemerins are mainly involved in the regulation of lactogenesis in bovine mammary epithelium. Studies have shown that bovine mammary epithelial cells express CMKLR1 and CCRL2 during postpartum periods.

Retinoids (RARs) and pleiotrophin (PTN) are two paracrine factors secreted from adipocytes that regulate transcription and facilitate ductal branching in developing mammary glands.

3.9.2 Fibroblasts

Stromal fibroblasts play an important role in mammary development, regulation of mammary epithelial cell function, and production of ECM components. Mammary stromal fibroblasts can be identified by their surface markers such as fibroblast-specific protein 1 (FSP1), vimentin, and platelet-derived growth factor receptor α (PDGFRα). However, some common fibroblast markers are also expressed in mammary myoepithelial cells. Phenotypically, there are two different subpopulations of fibroblasts: lobular fibroblasts that showed higher expression of a CD105 and lower expression of CD26 or dipeptidyl peptidase-4. In contrast, interlobular fibroblasts are characterized by lower expression of CD105 and higher expression of CD26.

Mammary fibroblasts secreted paracrine growth factors during different stages of mammary gland development. At their quiescent state, mammary fibroblasts secrete ECM matrix proteins and matrix metalloproteinases (MMPs) to maintain the integrity of mammary ECM. During mammogenesis, the fibroblasts are activated and secrete fibroblast growth factors (FGFs) to facilitate mammary development. There are 18 different FGFs that interact with four different FGF receptors (FGFRs). Besides these, there are some intracellular FGFs (iFGFs) that play a significant role in the regulation of voltage-gated sodium channels. FGFs are involved in placode formation, branching morphogenesis, expansion of luminal epithelial cells, and myoepithelial cell differentiation. Pregnancy-associated lobuloalveolar development of the mammary gland is induced by FGFR2-IIIb.

Other than FGFs, mammary stromal fibroblasts secrete hepatocyte growth factors (HGF), transforming growth factor- β1 (TGF-β1), and stroma cell-derived factor-1 (SDF-1) involved in the development of mammary parenchyma. HGFs are involved in tubulogenesis and branching morphogenesis. It also helps in the proliferation of estrogen receptor-positive (ER+) mammary epithelial cells. Stromal fibroblast-derived TGF-β1 regulates glandular morphogenesis. The autocrine signaling of TGF-β on the fibrobasts induces the secretion of ECM proteins and angiogenic factors. SDF-1 is also an autocrine regulator of fibroblasts that facilitates the differentiation of fibroblasts into myofibroblasts.

Stromal fibroblasts synthesize the components of ECM such as collagens, elastin, integrins, fibronectin, and proteoglycans to maintain mammary tissue architecture. Matrix metalloproteinases (MMPs) such as MMP2, MMP3, and MMP14 are also released by the fibroblasts to regulate ECM remodeling.

Fibroblasts are also involved in the immune regulation of the mammary gland. It has been reported that inflammation-associated fibroblasts (INFs) during mastitis facilitate the up of tumor necrosis factor-α and interleukin-8 in epithelial cells.

3.9.3 Endothelial Cells

Vascular endothelial cells function as a semipermeable barrier to allow transport of oxygen and nutrients to the mammary tissue. The milk precursors such as glucose and amino acids are also transferred to epithelial cells via the endothelial barrier. The endothelial compartment comprises a single layer of squamous endothelium during pregnancy. During lactation, the endothelial cells become activated with an elevated number of mitochondria to support high energy demand at this stage. The growth and development of vascular endothelium during angiogenesis are mediated by matrix metalloproteinases (MMP-9) and vascular endothelial growth factor (VEGF) secreted from epithelial and stromal cells. During the onset of inflammation, vasoactive mediators such as nitric oxide (NO), endothelin-1, prostacyclin (PGI2), and histamine are produced by endothelial cells. The endothelial nitric oxide synthase (eNOS) produces NO that inhibits calcium influx and relaxation of the actin cytoskeleton to modulate endothelial surface area for efficient attachment, rolling, and migration of neutrophils during diapedesis to the site of infection. It has also been reported that endothelial cells secrete interleukins (IL-1, IL-6, IL-8) and granulocyte macrophage colony-stimulating factor (GM-CSF) during mastitis.

3.10 Extracellular Matrix (ECM)

ECM gives structural support to maintain mammary tissue architecture and provides a conducive microenvironment for the growth and biological activities of mammary epithelial cells. The ECM also separates mammary epithelial cells from supporting connective tissue. The components of ECM are synthesized from epithelial, fibroblasts, myoepithelial, adipocytes, endothelial, and immune cells of stroma.

The ECM is divided into interstitial and pericellular matrices. The matrix that surrounds the cells is called th interstitial matrix and the pericellular matrix is in close contact with the cells. The pericellular matrix comprises 20–100-nm-thick basement membrane or basal lamina. The basal lamina has three layers, namely lamina densa, lamina lucida externa, and lamina lucida interna. The lamina densa is an electron-dense layer situated in the middle between the lamina lucida externa and the lamina lucida interna. The term “lucida” denotes less dense “lucid” areas. The major components of basal lamina are glycoproteins (laminins, collagen IV, nidogens, and perlecan) and proteoglycans.

Laminin (LM) is heterotrimeric glycoprotein having a MW of 900 kDa. It exists as trimmers having 5 α, 3 β, and 3 γ subunits with 15 different combinations. There are four different LM isoforms in the mammary gland of humans: laminin-111 (LM-1; α1, β1, γ1), laminin-322 (LM-5; α3, β3, γ2), laminin-511 (LM-10), and laminin-521 (LM-11).

Collagen IV is also a trimeric glycoprotein that exists as six distinct chains. It acts as an anchor for mammary epithelial cell and regulates their viability.

Nidogen (entactin) is a 150 kDa sulfated glycoprotein secreted from stromal fibroblast and helps to form basal lamina.

Perlecan is a complex glycosaminoglycan comprising a core protein linked with heparin sulfate. It provides structural integrity of the basal lamina.

Fibronectin (FN) is a 500 kDa dimeric glycoprotein of ECM that acts as an adhesive for the attachment of the ECM to the basement membrane. It also plays a significant role in ductal morphogenesis and end but formation during mammogenesis.

Knowledge Corner...
Staphylococcus aureus contains fibronectin-binding proteins (FnBPs) that help to adhere the bacteria and facilitates their colonization of bovine mammary glands, thus leading to infectious mastitis.

Secreted protein acidic and rich in cysteine (SPARC/osteonectin) is a glycoprotein (32 kDa) that facilitates cell–matrix interactions by FN assembling and integrin-linked kinase activity.

Small leucine-rich proteoglycan (SLRP) such as decorin, lumican, biglycan, fibromodulin, and keratocan bind to collagen fiber. They are active components of the ECM and bind with growth factors, cytokines, and cell surface receptors to induce signal transduction pathways and regulate biomechanical properties of tissues.

Decorin is a small leucine-rich proteoglycan that binds to collagen I to regulate collagen fibrillogenesis. Studies in dogs showed that an increase in decorin protein leads to neoplastic mammary tumors.

Lumican is an 18 amino acid signal peptide under SLRP that interacts with $\alpha2\beta1$ integrin to stimulate cell adhesion. It also inhibits cell migration and prevents metastasis.

Biglycan is composed of a core protein (38 kDa) that attaches with chondroitin sulfate/dermatan sulfate side chains to give an overall MW of 150–240 kDa. It controls the elasticity of the tissue by inducing fibrillin-1, an elastic fiber-associated protein.

Fibromodulin binds with collagen type I fibrils and regulates collagen fibrillogenesis.

Keratocan is a keratan sulfate proteoglycan that helps to maintain mammary gland integrity.

Tenascins (TN) is an extracellular matrix glycoprotein that regulates cellular differentiation and morphology. Studies have shown that TN inhibits β-casein expression in the mammary epithelium. Higher expression of TN is seen in breast carcinoma in humans.

3.11 ECM–Mammary Epithelial Cell Interactions

The interaction between mammary epithelial cells and ECM is crucial for the development and survival of mammary epithelial cells. These interactions are facilitated by transmembrane receptors in the mammary epithelial cells and their ligands in the ECM components.

Integrins are the major transmembrane receptors in the mammary epithelial cells that facilitate cell–ECM interaction in the mammary gland. These are heterodimers composed of α and β subunits. There are 18 α and 8 β subunits identified that form 24 different integrins. α2, α3, α6, β1, and β4 subunits are localized in both luminal and myoepithelial cells, but α1, α5, and αv subunits are only prevalent in myoepithelium. Integrin receptor has cytoplasmic, transmembrane, and extracellular domains. Other than integrins, α-dystroglycan, discoidin domain receptor 1 tyrosine kinase, and syndecans also interact with a variety of ECM components.

Different types of integrin receptors and their ligands are detailed in Table 3.6.

Integrins, being mechanosensors, are activated in response to biophysical and biochemical cues from the matrix and actin cytoskeleton. Activated integrin binds with ECM ligands and activates protein complexes at their cytosolic domains. These protein complexes comprise focal adhesion kinase (FAK), Src family kinases, and integrin-linked kinases.

Integrin-linked kinases facilitate prolactin-induced transcription of β-casein gene during lactogenic differentiation of the mammary gland.

Focal adhesion kinase (FAK) regulates adhesion, migration, proliferation, and survival of cells. FAC also phosphorylates adapter protein paxillin (PAX). PAX-induced activation of guanine nucleotide exchange factors (GEFs) regulates Rho GTPases activity and promotes phagocytosis.

Cytoskeletal actin-binding proteins such as talin (TLN) and vinculin (VCL) also activate integrins to form FAK that regulates actin polymerization and cytoskeletal tension.

Table 3.6 Types of integrin receptors and their ligands

Integrin receptors	Ligands
α1β1	Collagen
α2β1	Collagen and laminin
α6β1	Laminin
α6β4	Laminin
α3β1	Laminin 5, uPAR
α5β1	Fibronectin
αvβ3	Vitronectin
αvβ5	Vitronectin
α-Dystroglycan	Laminin-1
Discoidin domain receptor 1 tyrosine kinase	Collagen
Syndecans	Fibronectin, laminin, collagen, and growth factors

3.12 Myoepithelial Cells

These are hybrid cells having smooth muscle and epithelial cell characteristics. They are prevalent in both acini and ducts. The acinar myoepithelial cells have long cytoplasmic projections that form a basket-like network surrounding the luminal epithelial cells, whereas in ducts the cells are spindle-shaped and arranged parallel to the long axis. They contain actin and myosin like smooth muscle and contract in response to oxytocin that causes milk letdown.

3.12.1 Structure of Myoepithelial Cells

The myoepithelial cells are adhered to the basement membrane by hemidesmosomes and to the adjacent epithelial cells by desmosomes. Adhesion proteins such as desmoglein (Dsg)2 and desmocollin (Dsc)2 are present in the desmosomes between epithelial cells and myoepithelial cells, whereas desmosomes between two myoepithelial cells contain Dsg3 and Dsc3.

The plasma membrane of myoepithelial cells has a serrated appearance due to small projections toward the stroma. Caveolae are pinocytic vesicles present in the plasma membrane of myoepithelial cells. The nucleus has an irregular outline due to the presence of small invaginations. The nuclear chromatin appears as patches or thread-like structures. The cytoplasmic organelles are mostly prevalent around the para- or perinuclear areas. The mitochondria are smaller (diameter, 240 mμ) compared to normal epithelial cells (770 mμ) located in the granular portion of the cytoplasm.

The cytoplasm contains contractile proteins like α-smooth muscle actin (α-sm actin) and heavy chain-myosin (hc-myosin), responsible for oxytocin-induced contraction of myoepithelial cells. Besides these two, myoepithelial cells also express other contractile proteins such as calponin 1 (CNN1) and tropomyosin 2 (TPM2) specific for smooth muscles.

Myoepithelial cells contain cytokeratins (CK) that contribute to the cytoarchitecture. CK 5, CK 14, and CK 17 are important cytokeratins present in the myoepithelial cells and are the characteristic markers of these cells.

3.12.2 Functions of Myoepithelial Cells

The contraction of myoepithelial cells in response to oxytocin facilitates milk ejection. Besides this, they help communicate between the luminal and stromal compartment to regulate tissue functions.

3.12.2.1 Milk Ejection

Oxytocin-induced contraction of smooth muscle alpha-actin (ACTA2) present in the myoepithelial cells generates the contractile force for ejection of milk. The contraction is facilitated by the activation of phospholipase C (PLC)/Ca^{2+} signaling pathways where phospholipase C (PLC) generates inositol 1,4,5-trisphosphate (IP3) that in turn increases intracellular calcium.

3.12.2.2 Regulation of Tissue Polarity

The key mediators of luminal cell polarity and tissue morphogenesis are laminin-1 and desmosomal proteins. Desmosomal proteins specific to myoepithelial cells are desmocollin 3 (Dsc 3) and desmoglein 3 (Dsg 3) that help in the formation of acinar-like structures by joining adjacent myoepithelial and luminal epithelial cells.

3.12.2.3 Synthesis of Basement Membrane Components

Myoepithelial cells produce basement membrane components such as collagen IV, laminin (laminin-1, laminin-5), and fibronectin to organize new basement membrane. Matrix metalloproteinases (MMPs) such as MMP2 and MMP3 synthesized by myoepithelial cells help in the molding of a new basement membrane.

3.12.2.4 Regulation of Ductal Morphogenesis

Various growth and morphogenic factors are produced by myoepithelial cells that act in a paracrine manner to regulate mammary gland morphogenesis (Table 3.7).

3.12.2.5 Tumor Suppression

Myoepithelial cells act as a physical barrier between the tumor cells and the stroma to prevent tumor cell progression. They also inhibit the growth of tumor cells and angiogenesis by expressing various tumor suppressor genes (Table 3.8).

3.13 Blood Vascular System of the Mammary Gland

The precursors of milk are obtained from blood by the mammary gland. With an average blood flow rate of 280 milliliters per second, a high-yielding cow needs 400–500 units of blood to produce one unit of milk (Pandey et al. 2018). Eight percent of the total blood volume is received by the lactating udder. The mammary gland needs a highly developed blood circulatory system in order to supply this enormous demand.

Table 3.7 Paracrine factors secreted by myoepithelial cells and their function in morphogenesis of the mammary gland

Paracrine factors	Functions
Neogenin	Helps in cell clustering during the formation of the terminal end buds
Ephrin	Adhesion and migration of mammary epithelial cells
Pleiotrophin (PTN)/ heparin affin regulatory peptide (HARP)	Delays the maturation of epithelial cells by inhibiting their differentiation
Epimorphin	Helps in branching and tubular morphogenesis

Table 3.8 Tumor suppressor genes expressed in myoepithelial cells and their functions

Tumor suppressor genes	Functions
Maspin	Anti-angiogenic, protease inhibitor
Tissue inhibitor of metalloproteinases (T1MP-1)	Presents invasion of tumor cells by inhibiting MMP
Caveolin-1	Inhibition of tumor growth and metastasis by suppressing growth factor signaling pathways
Cytokeratin-5/6	Decreases survival potential of tumor cells by controlling cytoskeletal structure
Alpha-smooth muscle actin (αSMA)	Presents cell growth and survival by modulating cytoskeletal structure
Relaxin	Suppression of tumor by producing nitric oxide (NO)
Activin	Presents cell proliferation and induces apoptosis
Connexin-43	Inhibits tumor cell proliferation
Thrombospondin-1 (TSP-1)	Suppressions of angiogenesis
Myoepithelium-derived serine proteinase inhibitor (MEPI)	Inhibition of growth and invasion of tumor cells
Neogenin	Proliferation and migration of cancer cells

Pandey et al. (2010)

Arterial Supply Blood from the heart flows through the posterior dorsal aorta, which transitions into the abdominal posterior dorsal aorta upon entering the abdominal cavity. This aorta runs parallel to the vertebral column and, at the level of the sixth lumbar vertebra, bifurcates into the right and left iliac arteries, further branching into the internal and external iliac arteries. The external iliac artery gives rise to the external pudendal artery, also known as the mammary artery, which reaches the dorsal surface of the udder via the inguinal canal. Upon emerging from the inguinal canal, the mammary artery and the associated milk vein follow an S-shaped path, accommodating the stretching of blood vessels caused by the distension of the udder as the median suspensory ligament stretches. The mammary artery continues as the subcutaneous abdominal artery, which branches into anterior and posterior mammary arteries. The subcutaneous abdominal artery supplies the anterior dorsal portion of each side of the udder. The anterior and posterior mammary arteries penetrate vertically into the parenchyma of the fore and rear quarters on each side, terminating in a capillary network surrounding the alveoli. The teats receive blood supply from papillary arteries, which originate from the mammary arteries. At the teat, the papillary artery and venous plexus form the corpus cavernosum.

Venous Drainage Veins draining the mammary gland run parallel but opposite in direction to the corresponding arteries. There are three main veins responsible for carrying blood away from the mammary gland:

1. *External pudic vein (middle mammary vein):* This vein runs alongside the external pudic artery, ascending through the inguinal canal to join the external

iliac vein. While its route mirrors that of the artery, the blood flow is in the opposite direction.
2. *Subcutaneous abdominal vein (milk vein/anterior mammary vein)*: This vein exits the mammary gland at the anterior end of the front quarters and runs along the abdominal wall. It is visible under the skin on the cow's abdomen and enters the body cavity through a depression at the xiphoid process, known as the "milk wells," before emptying into the internal thoracic vein.
3. *Perineal vein (posterior mammary vein)*: This vein drains the rear halves of the gland, running parallel to the perineal artery in an upward and backward direction. After curving around the ischial arch, it connects to the internal pudic vein.

An anterior–posterior venous circle is formed by the anterior and posterior mammary veins at the base of the udder. This venous circle helps maintain blood drainage even when the cow is lying down. Additionally, papillary veins, which drain the teat, connect to the mammary veins at the venous circle at the udder's base.

Compared to cows, buffaloes have more noticeable anterior connecting veins. The venous system of the buffaloes had many big branches that connected the circulation in the left and right portions of the udder. Native cattle and Friesians displayed smaller branches from the major veins that improve blood flow to the udder.

3.14 Lymphatic System of the Udder

The lymphatic system is primarily responsible for circulating interstitial fluids that come from the mammary parenchyma's capillaries and removing the waste materials from the udder. The majority of the afferent lymphatic ducts go toward the dorsal parts of the udder after merging to produce bigger lymphatics. The lymphatic vessels terminate at the supramammary lymph nodes, located on both the right and left sides of the udder. There are typically 1–7 supramammary lymph nodes positioned above the caudal border of the mammary gland, with sizes ranging from 4 to 10 cm. The branches of the lymphatic vessels then pass through the inguinal, iliac and pre-femoral lymph nodes, eventually joining the lumbar lymph trunk. From there, the lymph continues to the thoracic duct, where it drains into the anterior vena cava.

The shape and lobulation of the supramammary lymph glands varied significantly between species. Buffaloes have nonlobulated glands that are disc- and kidney-shaped. In contrast, cows have lobulated glands consisting of separate lobules, although one lobule is typically large enough to constitute the majority of the gland. Within each breed, there are noticeable individual variations in both the size and lobulation of the glands. Additionally, differences are also observed between the two halves of the udder in terms of the number and location of the lobules.

High-yielding cows often develop udder edema, which is the accumulation of fluid between the skin and glandular tissue during the periparturient period. The cause of udder edema is an imbalance between hydrostatic and osmotic pressures, leading to fluid leakage from the capillaries into the interstitial spaces. Increased capillary permeability, due to damage to the capillary walls, and obstruction of the lymphatic system are also contributing factors. To address udder edema, massaging the udder in the direction of the supramammary lymph nodes helps facilitate lymph movement toward these nodes (since lymph always moves dorsally toward the supramammary lymph nodes), preventing the buildup of lymphatic fluids.

3.15 Nerve Supply to the Udder

The sensory (afferent) nerves of the udder transmit information from the udder to the brain, playing a key role in initiating the milk ejection reflex. The motor supply is entirely autonomic or sympathetic, consisting of motor fibers that control the smooth muscles of the arterial walls and the teat sphincter. These nerves regulate blood flow to the udder by adjusting the diameter of blood vessels and are involved in inhibiting the milk ejection reflex.

The primary spinal nerves that supply the udder are the first, second, third, and fourth lumbar nerves, along with the external spermatic nerves. The first lumbar nerve innervates the anterior part of the udder, excluding the parenchyma. The second, third, and fourth lumbar nerves merge to form the inguinal nerve. The caudal part of the udder is supplied by the perineal nerve, which consists of fibers from the second, third, and fourth sacral spinal nerves. The highest density of innervation is found in the dermis of the teats, with terminal endings sensitive to physical stimuli such as pressure, touch, and stretching.

Sympathetic nerve fibers originate in the lateral horns of the spinal cord. The circular smooth muscles of the udder contract rhythmically between milkings, relaxing during milking to allow the dilation of the teat canal and the flow of milk, all regulated by sympathetic nervous control.

Exercises

Objective Questions

1. The rear quarter produces ________________% of total milk produced by a cow.
2. The desirable age to remove supernumerary teats is ________________.
3. The main supporting structure of the udder is ___________________.
4. The constriction made of thick connective tissue at the junction of the gland and the teat cistern is called _______________.
5. The mucosal folds at the proximal site of the streak canal form a petal like structure called________________________.
6. ___________________________ are hyaline glycoprotein-rich aggregates appear dense bodies in the alveoli and connective tissue.

7. Occludin is a protein associated with ________________________ junction.
8. Chemoattractant cytokine (chemokine) produced by the stromal adipose tissue is ________________.
9. ____________________ enzyme produces NO in the endothelial cells.
10. ________________________are the major transmembrane receptors in the mammary epithelial cells that facilitate cell-ECM interaction in the mammary gland.
11. __________________________ are pinocytic vesicles present in the plasma membrane of myoepithelial cells.

Subjective Questions

1. Describe the role of stromal tissue in the development and survival of mammary epithelial cells.
2. Name the vasoactive compounds produced by endothelial cells.
3. How cell–ECM interactions are operating the mammary gland?
4. Describe in brief the cell–cell interacting junctions in the mammary alveoli.
5. What are the functions of mammary epithelial cells?

Answers to Objective Questions

1. 60%
2. 4 to 6 months
3. Median suspensory ligament
4. The annular fold
5. Fürstenberg rosette
6. Corpora amylacea
7. Tight junctions
8. Chemerin
9. Endothelial nitric oxide synthase (eNOS)
10. Integrins
11. Caveolae

References

Books

Larson BL (1985) Biosynthesis and cellular secretion of milk. In: Larson BL (ed) Lactation. Iowa State University Press, Ames

Mukherjee J, Das PK, Banerjee D (2023) Lactation physiology. In: Das PK, Sejian V, Mukherjee J, Banerjee D (eds) Textbook of veterinary physiology. Springer, Singapore. https://doi.org/10.1007/978-981-19-9410-4_25

Schaller O (1992) Illustrated veterinary anatomical nomenclature [Stuttgart] Ferdinand Enke! Verlag[

Research Article

Abshenas J, Sajjadian SM, Taghavi M (2014) Ultrasonographic examination of mammary glands in Caspian mares during the lactation and dry period. Iran J Vet Surg 9(1):Serial No:20

Adam ZEAS, Ragab GAN, Awaad AS, Tawfiek MG, Maksoud MKMA (2017) Gross anatomy and ultrasonography of the udder in goat. J Morphol Sci 34(3):137–142

Ahlem A, Carabaño MJ, Aicha L, Mouldi A, Farah BS, Sghaier N (2023) Major udder morphology traits and their relationship with milk production in Tunisian local goats. Iran J Appl Anim Sci 13(2):297–306

Arcos-Álvarez D, Canul-Solís J, García-Herrera R, Sarmiento-Franco L, Piñeiro-Vazquez Á, Casanova-Lugo F, Tedeschi LO, Gonzalez-Ronquillo M, Chay-Canul A (2020) Udder measurements and their relationship with milk yield in Pelibuey ewes. Animals (Basel) 10(3):518. https://doi.org/10.3390/ani10030518

Berteau M, Pepler PT, Broadhurst A, Hammond G, Zadoks RN, Viora L (2024) Assessing teat canal morphology in the dry period and during lactation by high-resolution ultrasound. J Dairy Res 91(1):57–64. https://doi.org/10.1017/S0022029924000098

Bonelli F, Orsetti C, Turini L, Meucci V, Pierattini A, Sgorbini M, Citi S (2020) Mammary Cistern size during the dry period in healthy dairy cows: a preliminary study for an ultrasonographic evaluation. Animals 10(11):2082. https://doi.org/10.3390/ani10112082

Collins RA, Parsons KR, Bland AP (1986) Antibody-containing cells and specialized epithelial cells in the bovine teat. Res Vet Sci 41:50–55

Mota-Rojas D, Napolitano F, Chay-Canul A, Ghezzi M, Braghieri A, Domínguez-Oliva A, Bragaglio A, Álvarez-Macías A, Olmos-Hernández A, De Rosa G et al (2024) Anatomy and physiology of water Buffalo mammary glands: an Anatomofunctional comparison with dairy cattle. Animals 14:1066. https://doi.org/10.3390/ani14071066

Müller A, Wernery U, Kinne J, Nagy P, Juhász J, Appelt A, Wittek T (2024) Study on anatomical structures of the dromedary udder. Animals 14(11):1674. https://doi.org/10.3390/ani14111674

Nickerson SC, Akers RM (2011) Mammary gland. Anatomy In book: Encyclopedia of Dairy Sciences, pp.328–337. https://doi.org/10.1016/B978-0-12-374407-4.00290-9

Nudda A, Pulina G, Vallebella R, Bencini R, Enne G (2000) Ultrasound technique for measuring mammary cistern size of dairy ewes. J Dairy Res 67:101–106

Pandey PR, Saidou J, Watabe K (2010) Role of myoepithelial cells in breast tumor progression. Front Biosci (Landmark Ed) 15(1):226–236. https://doi.org/10.2741/3617

Pandey Y, Taluja JS, Vaish R, Pandey A, Gupta N, Kumar D (2018) Gross anatomical structure of the mammary gland in cow. J Entomol Zool Stud 6(4):728–733

Prasad RM, Sudhakar K, Raghava Rao E, Ramesh G, Mahender M (2010) Studies on the udder and teat morphology and their relationship with milk yield in Murrah buffaloes. Livest Res Rural Dev 22:Article #20

Saleh AA, Easa AA, El-Hedainy DK, Rashad AMA (2023) Prediction of some milk production traits using udder and teat measurements with a spotlight on their genetic background in Friesian cows. Sci Rep 13:16193. https://doi.org/10.1038/s41598-023-43398-y

Sharma T, Das PK, Ghosh PR, Banerjee D, Mukherjee J (2017) Association between udder morphology and in vitro activity of milk leukocytes in high yielding crossbred cows. Vet World 10(3):342–347. https://doi.org/10.14202/vetworld.2017.342-347

Sharma N, Revanasiddu D, Kumar S, Gowane GR, Gupta ID, Verma A (2024) Factor analysis for udder and teat type traits in Sahiwal and Karan Fries cows. Indian J Anim Sci 94(2):173–178

Singhai SK, Ravikala K, Murthy KS, Gajbhiye PU, Vataliya PH, Savsani HH (2013) Udder teat morphology and body measurements and their relationship with milk yield and milking traits in Gir cows. Indian J Anim Prod Mgmt 29(1–2):5–11

Thomas CS, Svennersten-Sjaunja K, R Bhosrekar M, Bruckmaier RM (2004) Mammary cisternal size, cisternal milk and milk ejection in Murrah buffaloes. J Dairy Res 71:162–168

Thomas C S, Svennersten-Sjaunja K, Bhosrekar M R, Bruckmaier R M (2004) Mammary cisternal size, cisternal milk and milk ejection in Murrah buffaloes. J Dairy Res 71: 162–168

Turner CW (1952) The mammary gland: 1. The anatomy of the udder of cattle and domestic animals. Lucas Brothers, Columbia, MO

Wójtowski J, Ślósarz P, Junkuszew A, Milerski M, Szymanowska A, Szymanowski M (2020) Application of ultrasound technique for cistern size measurement in dairy goats (short communication aluation). Animals (Basel) 10(11):2082. https://doi.org/10.3390/ani10112082

Immune Responses of the Mammary Gland 4

Contents

J. Mukherjee et al., *Veterinary Lactation Physiology*,
https://doi.org/10.1007/978-3-032-21123-1_4

Abstract

The mammary gland has various defense mechanisms that protect it from infections, ensuring the production of safe and clean milk. These defense mechanisms can be categorized into anatomical, cellular, and humoral factors. Anatomical defenses include the streak canal, keratin plug, teat orifice, teat sphincter, and Fürstenberg rosette, which all help prevent pathogen entry. Cellular defense is provided by leukocytes (polymorphonuclear neutrophils, macrophages, lymphocytes) and mammary epithelial cells. Leukocytes can be either resident (macrophages) or recruited from the bloodstream (PMNs, lymphocytes) through chemoattractant factors released by pathogens. Several humoral factors, including immunoglobulins, complement proteins, lactoferrin, transferrin, lysozymes, cytokines, and chemokines, are produced locally or transported from the blood, providing immune surveillance. These defense factors work together to maintain optimum udder health. There are various tools available to modulate the immune response in the mammary gland as preventive measures, such as genetic selection, micronutrient supplementation, cytokine immunotherapy, genetic engineering, herbal therapy, intramammary probiotics, and vaccination. These methods can help reduce the need for unnecessary antibiotic use.

Graphical Abstract

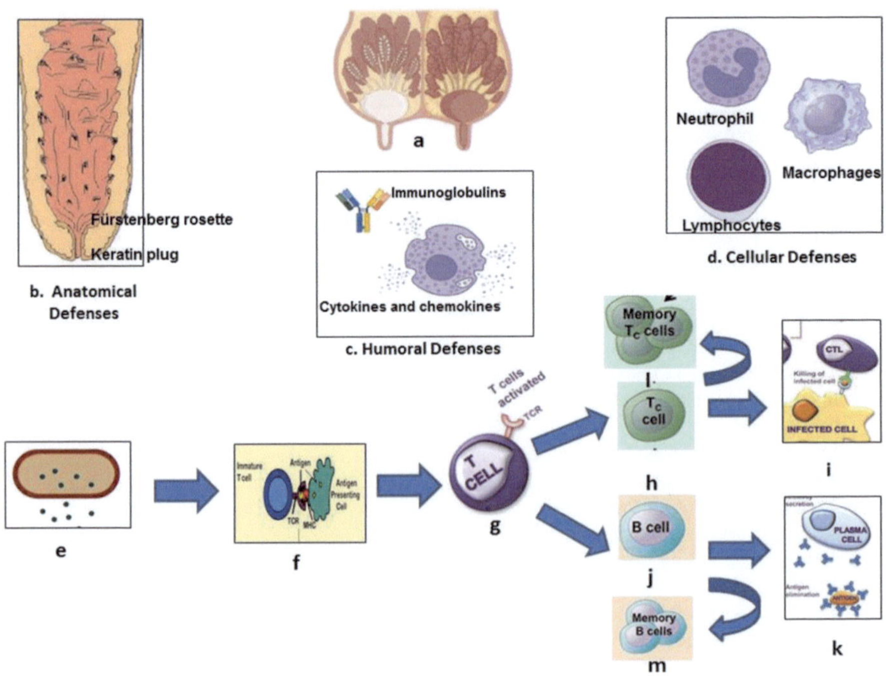

Description of the graphic: The mammary gland (**a**) is equipped with anatomical (**b**), humoral (**c**), and cellular (**d**) defense factors. Anatomical defenses (keratin plug, teat orifice, teat sphincter, and Fürstenberg rosette) prevent the entry of pathogens into the mammary gland. The antigens produced by invading pathogens (**e**) are processed within macrophages and B-lymphocytes in association with MHC class I or II (**f**). Antigen presented with MHC-II activates T-lymphocytes, macrophages and other immune cells (**g**) to induce cell-mediated or humoral responses. In cell-mediated immune response, cytotoxic T lymphocytes (**h**) cause lysis of infected cells (**i**). In humoral response, B-lymphocytes are differentiated into plasma (**j**) that facilitates opsonization of antigens (**k**). Memory T (**l**) and B (**m**) cells persist in the body for a long time to provide lifelong protection against reinfection by the same pathogen

Keywords

Mammary gland · Immunity · Neutrophils · Macrophages · Lymphocytes · Cytokines · Chemokines · Antimicrobial peptide · Immunoglobulins

Inside the Chapter

- *Components of mammary gland immunity*
- *Anatomical defenses*
  - Streak canal
  - Keratin plug
  - Teat sphincter
  - Fürstenberg's rosette
- *Cellular defenses*
  - Polymorphonuclear neutrophils (PMN)
  - Macrophages
  - Lymphocytes
  - Mammary epithelial cells
- *Humoral defenses*
  - Immunoglobulins (Ig)
  - Complement System (CS)
  - Transferrin [TF]
  - Lactoferrin
  - Lysozyme
  - Lactoperoxidase (LPO)
  - Myeloperoxidase (MPO)
  - Cytokines
  - Chemokines
  - Xanthine oxidase
- *Integration of Innate and Adaptive Immune response of mammary gland during infections*
- *Modulation of mammary gland immunity*
  - Genetic selection
  - Micronutrient supplementation

- Cytokine immunotherapy
- Genetic engineering
- Herbal therapy
- Live bio-therapeutics (Intramammary probiotics)
- Vaccination

Learning Objectives

- Different components of mammary gland immunity
- Integration of innate and adaptive immune response of the mammary gland during infections
- Molecular mechanisms leading to host–pathogen interaction
- Immune functions of mammary epithelial cells
- Modulation of mammary gland immunity

4.1 Components of Mammary Gland Immunity

The MG has evolved to provide nutrition to the offspring. But this organ plays a pivotal role in the transfer of passive antibodies to the newborn, particularly ruminants, pigs, and horses, where placental transfer of immunoglobulins is not possible due to syndesmochorial or epitheliochorial placentation. Milk, being a nutritious liquid, attracts the microorganisms for colonization in the cisterns, ducts, and alveoli. It was estimated that milk favors higher growth of bacteria (10^9 cfu/mL) with a doubling time of less than 30 min (Kornalijnslijper et al. 2004). Therefore, the mammary gland has to protect itself from possible intramammary infection or mastitis. Mastitis is the costliest disease in dairy animals, and the protection against mastitis is one of the prime concerns in the dairy industry. It has also been documented that cows selected for higher milk production are vulnerable to mastitis that lowers producers. Hence, improvement of mammary gland immunity should be taken into consideration while selecting cows for higher milk production.

The immunity of the mammary gland is mediated by the interplay between nonspecific and specific immune components, which includes anatomical, cellular, and humoral defense mechanisms (Table 4.1). The immune function of the mammary gland varies considerably during different stages of lactation, and endocrine milieu of the animals plays a significant role in controlling the immune function of the mammary gland.

Table 4.1 Components of mammary gland immunity

Classification	Components	Probable mechanisms
Anatomical defenses	Streak canal	Physical barrier restricts the entry of bacteria
	Keratin plug	Immobilization and lysis of bacteria
	Teat sphincter	Closure of the teat canal between milkings
	Fürstenberg rosette	Mechanical seal at teat canal Local immune cell defense
Cellular defenses	Polymorphonuclear neutrophils (PMNs)	Diapedesis, chemotaxis, and phagocytosis
		Antigen (Ag) processing and presentation
	Macrophages	Phagocytosis
	Lymphocytes	Recognition of Ag and production of corresponding Ab (B-lymphocytes)
		Cell-mediated cytotoxicity (T-lymphocytes)
	Mammary epithelial cells	Leukocyte migration by the production of chemokines (IL-8)
Humoral defenses	Complement system (alternative pathway)	Opsonization (C3b and C3bi)
		Neutrophil migration (C5a)
	Lactoferrin	Bacteriostatic (reduces iron availability to microorganisms)
	Transferrin	Alters the membrane permeability of Gm (−) ve bacteria with the release of lipopolysaccharides (LPS)
	Lysozymes	Causes cell wall damage in Gm (+)ve bacteria by cleaving β 1,4-glycosidic bond in cell wall proteoglycans.
	Lactoperoxidase and myeloperoxidase	Bactericidal to both Gm-positive and -negative bacteria by the production of reactive oxygen species
	Cytokines	Mediators of inflammation
	Chemokines	Recruitment of leukocytes during inflammation
	Antimicrobial peptides (AMP), host defense peptides (HDPs)	Antimicrobial and immune-regulation

Mukherjee and Das (2019) and Mukherjee et al. (2023)

4.2 Anatomical Defenses

As the pathogens enter the mammary gland via teat orifice, teat is considered to be the first line of defense against the pathogens into the mammary gland.

4.2.1 Streak Canal

Streak canal is the initial site for infection or mastitis as it is the primary site for the entry of pathogens. The streak canal infection serves as a source of pathogens entering the mammary gland. Hence, it is considered the most natural barrier against intramammary infections. Apart from providing a physical barrier, the secretions from the epithelial lining of the streak canal also inhibit bacterial growth. The patency and size of the streak canal are important factors controlling the bacterial invasion into the teat. It has been shown that udders with more patent streak canal had greater changes of intramammary infection. There was a significant positive correlation between the occurrence of mastitis and external diameter of teat orifice. It has also been documented that milk collected from short and wide streak canals had higher somatic cell counts. The specialized stratified squamous epithelium of streak canal secretes keratin that also has antibacterial properties.

4.2.2 Keratin Plug

Keratin is a fibrous protein secreted from the keratinocytes of the basal layer of the epidermis. In cows, the keratin layer is 30 and 300 μm thick. This layer provides a physical barrier against the pathogens by entrapping them before reaching the teat sinus. During the lactation period, this lining is desquamated and the entrapped bacteria also flushed out during the milking. It has been reported that 24–45% of keratin was removed during the milking process, which are replaced by a new keratin with a regeneration time of 2–4 week. The cessation of milking during the dry period allows the keratin plug to persist and seals the teat orifice till parturition. It may take 16–50 days to complete the sealing after the cessation of milk. The important proteins of keratin lining are cationic proteins, S100 groups of proteins, and xanthine oxidase that have bactericidal and bacteriostatic properties. The cationic protein present in the keratin plug alters the cell wall composition of the bacteria and kills them by osmotic lysis. The lipid composition of teat keratin also differs between the stages of lactation. In lactating cows, keratin contains a higher proportion of lipids than nonlactating cows. In lactating cows, cholesterol and triglycerides were 23% and 50%, respectively, whereas, during dry periods, they changed to 39% and 31%, respectively. Studies have shown that the removal of keratin increased the risk of mastitis in dairy cows.

4.2.3 Teat Sphincter

It is the smooth muscle sphincter at the teat ends that controls the opening and closing of the teat duct. Hence, this sphincter retains the milk and also acts as a barrier against pathogens as well. This sphincter is made of circular and longitudinal smooth muscles. The sphincter goes to the flaccid state at the time of milking and returns to its normal tone after 2 h. This time is very crucial for the entry of pathogens. The peristaltic contraction of teat sphincter from proximal to distal end also flushes the bacteria between milking. The muscle tone of the teat sphincter decreases with the age and makes the older cows more susceptible to intramammary infections. Parturition-induced hypocalcemia also reduces the tone of teat sphincter and makes the cows prone to mastitis during this time.

4.2.4 Fürstenberg Rosette

The Fürstenberg rosette contains a series of mucosal folds and cellular structures just above the streak canal primarily present in ruminants. It is one of the important natural defense systems of the mammary gland against pathogens.

Physical Barrier to Pathogens Fürstenberg rosette consists of a series of folds that form a physical "seal" or "valve" that prevents the entry of pathogens from external sources.

Immune Surveillance The Fürstenberg rosette-associated lymphoid tissue (FALT) present in the mammary gland of the cow plays a pivotal role in mucosal immune defense. The Fürstenberg rosette is populated with antigen-presenting cells (MHC class II), lymphocytes, plasma cells, polymorph nuclear neutrophils, and mononuclear phagocytes (macrophages) in the stroma and migrates to the teat lumen upon infection. The plasma cells are mostly IgA positive. There is also the presence of epithelial M cells. CD3-positive 'T' lymphocytes were identified in the Fürstenberg rosette of sheep and goats. The antigen-presenting cells of FALT help to detect the antigens and initiate an immune response by producing antibodies.

> **Knowledge Corner...**
> The recent detection of highly pathogenic avian influenza (H5N1) clade 2.3.4.4b in dairy cattle has revealed the virus's ability to replicate within the mammary gland, induce mastitis, and generate substantial viral concentrations in milk.

Enhancing Local Inflammatory Response In case of an infection, Fürstenberg rosette contributes to a localized inflammatory response by releasing cytokines and other immune factors. This helps to mobilize additional immune cells to the site of infection, which can help to contain and fight off the invading pathogens. Studies have shown that IL-2 plays a greater role in increasing the plasma cell populations in the infected quarters.

4.3 Cellular Defenses

The resident leukocytes of the mammary gland, along with mammary epithelial cells, provide cellular defense of the mammary gland against pathogens. The mammary gland leukocytes comprise polymorphonuclear neutrophils (PMNs), macrophages, and lymphocytes (Table 4.2). The leukocytes are either resident (macrophages) or recruited from peripheral circulation (PMN, lymphocytes) under the influence of chemoattractant factors released by pathogens. The activity of freshly recruited leukocytes into the mammary gland determines the pathogenesis

Table 4.2 Cellular components in milk and colostrum in different species

Total cells/mL	Species		
	Cow	Pig	Human
Colostrum	5×10^5	10^6–10^7	10^6–10^7
Mature milk	<4.5×10^5	1–5×10^6	10^4–10^5
Monocyte/macrophage (%)			
Colostrum	21–46	1–11	47–66
Mature milk	25–45	2–22	44
Neutrophils (%)			
Colostrum	37–40	45–92	21–60
Mature milk	5–40	14–33	16
Lymphocytes (%)			
Colostrum	17–23	10–26	5–11
Mature milk	<20	0.5–13	2
Lymphocyte subsets (% of total lymphocytes)			
B-cells (total)	3.5	10–30	7–35
T-cells (total)	88	70–90	50–88
CD4(+)	21	25–33	43
CD8(+)	51	45–57	48
NK	15	No report	9
Epithelial cells (%)			
Colostrum	<1	0.4–20	<1
Mature milk	<25	30–99	10–90

and establishment of intramammary infection. During the migration of leukocytes from the blood to the mammary gland, epithelial cells are desquamated and secreted into the milk. The leukocytes, along with the mammary epithelium, are called milk somatic cell count (SCC) and are considered an important indicator of udder and milk quality. In normal healthy mammary gland, the total somatic cell populations are below 100×10^3 cells/ml of milk, which may increase up to several million per ml of milk during intramammary infections. Leukocytes perform a wide array of functions for immune surveillance. They secrete some immune components such as chemokines, cytokines, antimicrobial peptides, and reactive oxygen species (ROS). Leukocytes also help to repair the damaged epithelial cells. At the time of involution, resident phagocytes of the mammary gland engulf the cellular debris. Mammary epithelial cells produce dimeric IgA in monogastric animals and help in leukocytes' migration at the time of inflammation.

4.3.1 Polymorphonuclear Neutrophils (PMN)

These are the predominant cell type constituting more than 90% of total leukocytes during the early stage of inflammation. They usually migrate from peripheral

Table 4.3 Neutrophil granules and their contents

	Name of granule			
	Primary/ azurophilic (peroxidase positive)	Secondary/specific (peroxidase negative)	Tertiary/gelatinase (peroxidase negative)	Secretory vesicles (peroxidase negative)
Granular contents	Myeloperoxidase, defensins, elastase, lysozyme, proteinase 3, α-mannosidase, β-Glucuronidase, azurocidin	Lysozyme, lactoferrin, collagenase, gelatinase, cathelicidins, alkaline phosphatase, cytochrome b558, histaminase CD11b/CD18	Gelatinase, lysozyme, acid phosphatase, acetyltransferase, cytochrome b558, CD11b/CD18	Alkaline phosphatase, CD11b/ CD18, cytochrome b558, plasma proteins
Functions	Phagocytic killing	Migration and killing	Migration	Adhesion

Gullberg et al. (1999)

circulations under the influence of different inflammatory mediators like cytokines, chemokines, complements, and prostaglandins. Bovine PMN is characterized by multilobulated nucleus within the plasma membrane. The multilobed nucleus of PMN allows rapid migration through endothelial cells. The plasma membrane of PMN has receptors like L-selectin and β2-integrin that allow binding of PMN with endothelial cells and facilitate diapedesis. Neutrophils also have the receptors for Fc component of the immunoglobulins (IgG2 and IgM) and complement (C3b) that favor phagocytosis. The granular cytoplasm of PMN contains glycogen (20% of the cell on a dry weight basis) and numerous granules. The granules of neutrophils are called primary, secondary, and tertiary granules and secretory vesicles. These granules contain several proteins involved in the phagocytic killing of microorganisms (Table 4.3).

4.3.1.1 Comparison Between Blood and Milk Neutrophils

As the blood PMNs are migrated into the mammary gland, mammary PMNs are in more advanced stage of development compared to blood PMNs. Immature neutrophils or band cells are common in blood, whereas they seldom appear in milk. Neutrophils constitute 5–20% of the total SCC in normal bovine milk, whereas in goat milk neutrophils constitute up to 50–70% of the total SCC. The size of blood and milk neutrophils is similar (10–15 μm in diameter), but blood PMN has 2–3 lobed nuclei, whereas the majority of milk PMNs have segmented multilobed nuclei. The phagocytic potential of milk neutrophils is comparatively less (one-third of that in blood neutrophils) than blood neutrophils because

1. Milk PMNs have lower energy reserve than blood neutrophils. It was reported that milk PMN contains 38% less glycogen than blood PMN.

2. The viability of milk neutrophils (70.34%) was less compared to blood neutrophils (91.8%) studied in goats (Tian et al. 2005).
3. In milk, the majority of PMNs are at their terminal apoptotic stages (28.47%) compared to blood (7.60%) documented in goats (Tian et al. 2005).
4. Milk PMN has less surface area of plasma membrane required for the formation of pseudopodia for engulfment of the bacteria. Milk PMN has an additional role to phagocytose milk fat and casein molecules. So, the plasma membrane is already preoccupied with engulfing these particles.
5. Inhibition of phagocytic killing by milk components as the lysosomes are already fused with phagosomes containing milk fat and casein molecules instead of bacteria.
6. Reduced number of primary and secondary granules in milk PMN compared to blood. The release of gelatinase in milk neutrophils is significantly lower than the blood neutrophils of goats (Tian et al. 2005).

4.3.1.2 Functions of PMN

The primary function of PMN is the phagocytic killing of bacteria. The bovine PMN requires 10–14 days to mature in the bone marrow and then enter the circulation. The half-life of PMN in the blood is short (about 8.9 h) because they enter the tissue and reside 1–2 days as phagocytes. The influx of PMN from the blood to milk is low under normal conditions, but rapid migration of neutrophils occurs in response to bacterial infection. The killing of bacteria by neutrophils is a multistep process that involves adherence of neutrophil with the endothelium, binding of chemokines to neutrophil receptors (chemotaxis), ingestion of bacteria (phagocytosis), and organism killing.

Neutrophil Adherence

The first step of PMN recruitment is the adherence of PMN with the endothelium. The migration of neutrophils occurs through two different routes: paracellular (between endothelial cells) or transcellular (through endothelial cells). In post-capillary and collecting venules, PMNs adhere to the endothelial surface after stimulated by suitable chemoattractants. The chemoattractants for bovine PMN are complements (C5a), lipopolysaccharides (LPS), and interleukins (IL-1, IL-2, and IL-8). These chemoattractants bind with their receptors on the plasma membrane of PMN and activate adhesion receptors on the neutrophils for binding with the endothelium.

The capturing of neutrophils to the endothelium is mediated through some inducible cell adhesion molecules like selectins and integrins.

Selections are involved in the initial interaction between neutrophils and endothelium. There are three classes of selectins: L-selectin (leukocytes), E-selectin (endothelium), and P-selectin (platelets and endothelial cells). P-selectin glycoprotein ligand-1 (PSGL-1) is the primary ligand in the endothelium that binds with L-selectin.

Chemotaxis

Chemotaxis is the guided movement of neutrophils in response to certain chemoattractants released from a distant source. The chemoattractants are the chemical substances that guide the neutrophil for its migration toward the site of infection by modulating cytoskeleton, change in cell shape, and polarization. Chemoattractants are present either within the vasculature or extravascularly. Within the vascular wall, chemoattractants are immobilized by glycosaminoglycans (GAGs) or heparin sulfate on the endothelial membrane. Extravascularly, they can be attached to the extracellular matrix. The chemoattractants for neutrophil chemotaxis are of four types: lipids, N-formylated peptides, complement anaphylotoxins, and chemokines.

Lipid Chemoattractants They are derived from arachidonic acid (AA) through multiple enzymatic pathways. Leukotriene B4 (LTB4) is one of the strongest lipid chemoattractant synthesized from AA by the action of 5-lipoxygenase (5-LO). LTB4 interacts with two G protein-coupled receptors (GPCRs), namely BLT1 and BLT2.

N-formylated Peptides N-formyl-l-methionyl-l-leucyl-l-phenylalanine (FMLP) is an N-formylated peptide generated by bacteria that acts as a chemoattractant. Formyl peptide receptors, FPR1/2/3, are also GPCRs in neutrophils that recognize formylated peptides. FMLP is called "end target" chemoattractant as neutrophils will prefer to migrate toward FMLP compared to other chemoattractants in a complex chemoattractant gradient.

Complement Anaphylotoxins C5a is an important chemoattractant derived from the C5 complement protein. C5a interacts with the neutrophils by two complement GPCRs, viz. C5aR1 and C5aR2. C5a is also considered "end target" chemoattractant for neutrophils.

Chemokines These are low-molecular-weight (8- to 12-kDa) chemotactic cytokines. They are classified into four subfamilies on the basis of the presence of a cysteine residue at the amino terminal end (Table 4.4). Chemokines facilitate neutrophil trafficking by generating a gradient-guided signal. There are two functional classifications of chemokines: end target and intermediary chemoattractants. End target chemoattractants (N-formylated peptides and C5a) are dominant over intermediary chemoattractants (lipid chemoattractants).

Firm Adhesion and Spreading

Integrins facilitate firm attachment of neutrophils with the endothelium and favor their migration by interacting with the extracellular matrix. The integrins are heterodimers consisting of α and β subunits. The α (CD11) and β (CD18) subunits are expressed independently from independent precursors. There are four α subunits, namely CD11a, b, c, and d. CD11b/CD18 (αMβ2 or Mac-1) is the main integrin expressed on the neutrophils that interacts with intercellular adhesion molecules (ICAM-1) expressed on the endothelium.

Table 4.4 Chemokine subfamily with examples

Chemokine subfamily	Structure	Examples	Receptors
α subfamily (CXC subfamily)	Two cysteine residues are separated by a single amino acid	CXCL1 (growth-related gene product-α or GRO-α) CXCL2 (GRO-β) CXCL3 (GRO-γ) CXCL5 (epithelial cell–derived and neutrophil activating 78-amino-acid peptide or ENA-78) CXCL6 (granulocyte chemotactic protein-2 or GCP-2) CXCL7 (neutrophil activating peptide.2 or NAP-2) CXCL8 (interleukin 8 or IL8)	CXCR1 and CXCR2
β subfamily (CC subfamily)	They have two cysteine residues	CCL3 (macrophage inflammatory protein-α or MIP-1α) CCL4 or MIP-1β	CCR2
γ subfamily (C subfamily)	They have only one cysteine residue	XCL1 (lymphotactin) and XCL2 (single C motif 1β; SCM-1β)	CR1
δ subfamily (CX3C superfamily)	They have two cysteine residues separated by three amino acid	CX3CL1 (fractalkine)	CX3CR1

The migration of neutrophils toward a chemotactic gradient is achieved by alterations in the cell polarity, nature of adhesion, and retraction. The chemotactic gradient provides two types of information to the neutrophils, the position that depends on the concentration of the chemotactic agent and the direction that is governed by the ability of neutrophils to perceive the direction of the gradient toward the source. The polarized neutrophils are characterized by the formation of pseudopods by actin polymerization in the leading edge and uropod, a highly contractile portion at the rear edge where protrusions are suppressed along the lateral sides.

Extravasation and Diapedesis

The extravasation of neutrophils is operated via two different routes:

Transendothelial migration: It occurs prominently at the borders of endothelial cells rich in P-selectin. Transendothelial migration of PMN is achieved through two cell adhesion molecules such as platelet endothelial cell adhesion molecule-1 (PECAM-1 or CD31) expressed on both neutrophils and epithelial junctions and junctional adhesion molecule (JAM) present at tight junctions between the endothelial cells but absent on neutrophils.

Migration within interstitial tissues: The process of interstitial migration of PMN is called haptotaxis. Here, the movement is governed by the gradient of immobilized chemoattractants unlike soluble chemoattractants in chemotaxis.

In haptotaxis, the chemoattractants generated by bacteria or inflamed tissue are attached to extracellular matrix components. Upon stimulation by the chemoattractants, neutrophil granules express some receptors for laminin-, fibronectin-, and vitronectin (*$\alpha6\beta1$, $\alpha5\beta1$, and $\alpha v\beta3$*) of the extracellular matrix.

Diapedesis of neutrophils is mediated by the continuous formation of new adhesive contacts at the front and detachment in the rear. At the leading edge, vitronectin receptor ($\alpha v\beta3$) is expressed, then it undergoes endocytosis at the rear edge and again recycled at the front that facilitates attachment at the front and detachment at the rear. Antiadhesive molecules such as leukosialin (CD43) are also expressed at the rear edge that also favors detachment.

4.3.1.3 Molecular Mechanism of Neutrophil Migration

The migration of neutrophils is regulated by the Rho GTPase family of proteins. They exist in two forms: a guanosine diphosphate (GDP)-bound inactive form and guanosine triphosphate (GTP)-bound active form. Guanine nucleotide exchange factors (GEF) remove GDP from Rac and favor binding with GTP to activate. In contrast, GTPase-activating proteins (GAPs) convert GTP to GDP and switch off the activity. There are three Rho GTPases involved in neutrophil migration, namely Rho, Rac, and Cdc42. Rac is involved in actin cytoskeleton organization. RhoA operates from the rear end of the cell and favors retraction of the trailing edge. Cdc42, on the other hand, stabilizes the migration at the leading edge by actin–myosin contraction.

Two inositol lipids, viz. phosphatidylinositol 4,5-bisphosphate [PI(4,5)P2] and phosphatidylinositol 3,4,5-trisphosphate [PI(3,4,5)P3], are reported to regulate the cytoskeleton and motility of cells.

When chemoattractants bind with G protein-coupled receptor (GPCR) at the surface of neutrophils, GPCR activation stimulates Rac GEF for the activation of Rac. Rac stimulates phosphoinositide 3-kinase (PI3K) that converts PI(4,5)P2 into PI(3,4,5)P3 at the leading edge. PI(3,4,5)P3 favors actin polymerization to push the cell forward. At the rear end, phosphatase and tensin homolog (PTEN) negatively regulates PI3K; hence, PI(3,4,5)P3 formation decreases and inhibits actinomyosin contractility.

4.3.1.4 Neutrophil Migration into the Mammary Gland

In response to the acute inflammatory reaction, neutrophils rapidly migrate into the mammary gland and subsequently into the milk. At first, neutrophils are adhered to capillary endothelial cells and subsequently penetrate the endothelial layer to reach subepithelial stromal tissues. Then they migrate between the basal cells of the epithelium by penetrating the basal lamina. The motility of neutrophils across the luminal epithelial lining may be facilitated either by the lysis of individual surface epithelial cells or breaking the tight junctions between the luminal cells or by separating the luminal cell layer from basal epithelia to cause sloughing of the cells, allowing the neutrophils to enter the lumen.

The chemoattractants recruit neutrophils into the mammary gland during mastitis and are components (C5a and C3a), lipopolysaccharide (LPS), and interleukins (IL-1, IL-2, and IL-8). IL-8 plays a major role in neutrophil migration into the mammary gland during mastitis and also facilitates the release of alkaline phosphatase from the secondary granules for phagocytosis.

4.3.1.5 Opsonization

Before the process of phagocytosis, the contact and immune recognition of the bacterium by the neutrophils must occur. The process of immunological recognition of the bacteria is called opsonization. Opsonization is mediated by specific antibodies. Predominant opsonizing antibodies for bovine PMN are IgM and IgG2; however, IgM is the most important for phagocytosis. Other than the antibodies, complement C3b also opsonizes bacteria and binds with CR1 receptor on the PMN plasma membrane. The antibody has two sites: one for recognizing the bacterium (Fab regions) and the other to bind with PMN via Fc-receptors (FcR) on the plasma membrane.

At the neutrophils, two classes of receptors are present: one for antibodies and the other for complement. Predominant FcR on the neutrophils are FcγRIIA (CD32) and FcγRIIIB (CD16) and complement receptors, viz. CR1 (CD35) and CR3 (or CD11b/CD18 integrin). In contrast to the human PMN, bovine PMN lacks FcγRI and FcγRII but has a distinct receptor for IgG2. The expression of CR1 receptor on the PMN is induced upon their migration to the mammary gland and their expression is more in mammary PMN compared to blood PMN.

However, nonopsonic phagocytosis also occurs in the case of Gram-negative bacteria where carbohydrate-rich pili of Gram-negative bacteria interact with the carbohydrate receptors on the PMN plasma membrane through lectin–carbohydrate interaction.

4.3.1.6 Phagocytosis

After opsonization, the complement components and immunoglobulins-coated bacteria interact with the receptors on neutrophils. Subsequently, these opsonized particles are engulfed by the neutrophils to form phagosomes. The phagosomes are a distinctive organelle developed when the opsonized particles are encircled by an invagination of the PMN plasma membrane. Then the phagosomes are fused with intracellular granules to form a phagolysosome where the bacterial killing occurs with the help of reactive oxygen species (ROS) and antimicrobial peptides.

Phagosomes Formation

The engulfment of IgG-coated pathogenic particles is mediated after their encounter with FcR and complement receptors (CR1).

FcR generates immunoreceptor signaling pathways that promote the phosphorylation of their cytoplasmic domain immunoreceptor tyrosine-based activation motifs (ITAMS) by Src-tyrosine kinases. Phosphorylated ITAMS induces several downstream signaling pathways that facilitate activation of PI3-kinase and Rho proteins (RhoA). The activation of RhoA facilitates F-actin polymerization that ultimately leads to phagocytic cup formation that encircles pathogens. PI3-kinase, on the other hand, promotes closure of phagocytic cup by myosin-induced "purse-string-like" contraction of pseudopods.

But the engulfment of C3bi-opsonized particles involves a separate pathway through the activation of Rho only without the involvement of Rac or Cdc42. Here, the ingestion occurs independently in response to increased Ca^{++} with the rise of inositol phosphate.

Phagosomes Maturation

Phagosomes undergo sequential steps of migration: early phagosomes, intermediate phagosomes, and late phagosomes, and finally the phagolysosome through the interactions with early endosomes, late endosomes, and lysosomes. The maturation process begins with the separation of new phagosomes from the plasma membrane. During the process of maturation, the phagosomes acquire an acidic environment for the lysis of foreign particles. A number of proteins are associated with this maturation process such as Ras-associated binding GTPase (Rab GTPase), vacuolar ATPase (V-ATPase), major histocompatibility complex (MHC) class II molecules, and acid hydrolases.

The early phagosome formation begins with the activation of Rab22a, a GTP-bound protein that recruits an endosomal fusion protein Rab5 guanine nucleotide exchange factor (GEF) Rabex-5 at the phagosomal membrane. Rabex-5 in turn activates Rab5 by conversion of GDP to GTP. Activated Rab5 stimulates Rabaptin-5 that converts phosphatidylinositol (PI) into phosphatidylinositol 3-phosphate (PI(3) P), which in combination with Rab5 recruits early endosome antigen 1 (EEA1) that facilitates the interactions between endosomes and phagosomes. Activated Rab5 also promotes tethering complexes CORVET (Class C Core Vacuole/Endosome Tethering) to strengthen the fusion.

Bactericidal and Respiratory Burst Activity

Bactericidal activity of PNM depends upon two different mechanisms. The generation of reactive oxygen species (ROS) is called respiratory burst (oxygen dependent), and the release of enzymatic or antimicrobial protein content in the granules is called degranulation (oxygen independent).

Respiratory Burst Activity

This mechanism includes a series of enzymatic events that increase oxidative metabolism and results in the conversion of molecular oxygen to its univalent reduction product superoxide anion ($O^{-\cdot}{}_2$), along with other toxic species such as hydrogen peroxide (H_2O_2), singlet oxygen ($^1O_2$), hypochlorous acid (HOCl), and hydroxyl radical ($OH^{\cdot}$).

NADP Oxidase-Dependent Mechanism

The oxidative response is initiated with the activation of NADPH-oxidase complex. The NADPH oxidase complex consists of cytosolic (p40phox, p47phox, and p67phox, phox stands for phagocyte oxidase) and membrane (p22phox and gp91phox) proteins. Two membrane proteins, namely p22phox and gp91phox, together form a heterodimeric flavohemoprotein known as cytochrome b558. There are three small GTPase proteins, namely Rac2, Cdc42, and Rap1A, that are also associated with the activation of the NADPH oxidase complex. Upon activation, cytosolic p47phox, p67phox, and p40phox are phosphorylated and translocate into the membrane to interact with cytochrome $b_{558.}$ p29 peroxiredoxin, a newly identified protein, is also reported to be associated with p67phox of NADPH-oxidase. Activated enzyme complex then converts O_2 to H_2O_2 with three intermediates like superoxide anion ($O^{-\cdot}{}_2$), H_2O_2, and the hydroxyl radical (OH°).

Myeloperoxidase (MPO)–Halide–Hydrogen Peroxide Antibacterial System

Myeloperoxidase is a hemoprotein present in the azurophil granules. MPO is synthesized in promyelocytes and promonocytes stages of myelopoiesis. The synthesis of MPO includes the formation of pre-MPO after primary translation in the endoplasmic reticulum (ER). Pre-MPO turns into apo-pro-MPO after co-translational cleavage and addition of high-mannose oligosaccharide side chains. Apo-pro-MPO is then associated with molecular chaperones (calreticulin and calnexin) at ER and acquires a heme group to form pro-MPO. This pro-MPO undergoes protein hydrolysis after leaving the ER to form MPO dimers.

MPO utilizes H_2O_2 produced during respiratory burst and produces hypochlorous acid (HOCl) with chloride ion. HOCl also produces chloramines, a long-lived oxidant generated after chlorination of taurine. HOCL causes oxidation of DNA, RNA, proteins, and lipids. The MPO-generated HOCl in the ECF causes severe tissue damage and inflammation.

Nitric Oxide-Synthase-Derived Reactive Nitrogen Intermediates

Reactive nitrogen species such as nitric oxide (NO) is produced from L-arginine by NO-synthases (NOS). The oxidant activity of NO is moderate, but it forms stronger oxidants such as nitrogen dioxide (NO_2) and peroxynitrite (ONOO-) after reacting with oxygen and superoxide, respectively. But very little NO is generated in the human PMN; hence, its antimicrobial role is controversial.

4.3.1.7 Secretion of Antimicrobial Proteins

Neutrophils release several antimicrobial peptides to destroy the microorganisms. These proteins are stored in the granules of neutrophils. Different antimicrobial peptides secreted from neutrophils are listed in Table 4.5.

4.3.1.8 Modification of Extracellular Matrix

Neutrophils secrete a wide array of proteases from their granules that alters the ECM by degrading major ECM components. Serine proteinases and metalloproteinases are two main classes of proteases involved in the degradation of ECM at natural pH. These are different serine proteinases and metalloproteinases secreted by neutrophils (Table 4.6).

Table 4.5 Antimicrobial peptides secreted from neutrophils and their function

Antimicrobial peptide	Source	Functions
Bactericidal/ permeability increasing protein (BPI)	Azurophilic granules	Destroys gram-negative bacteria after binding with LPS
Defensins	Azurophilic granules	Causes membrane permeabilization of both gram-positive and gram-negative bacteria Regulation of the inflammation by interacting with protease inhibitors such as alpha-1-antitrypsin and alpha-1-antichymotrypsin Helps in wound healing by inducing fibroblasts proliferation
Cathelicidin (hCAP-18)	Specific granules	Interferes with bacterial cell membrane and destabilizes it
Lactoferrin	Specific granules	Interferes with the iron transport in bacteria
Phospholipase A2	Specific granules	Membrane hydrolysis of gram-positive bacteria
Lysozyme	Specific granules	Hydrolysis of,4-beta-linkages between N-acetylmuramic acid and N-acetylglucosamine in the cell wall of gram-positive bacteria
Secretory leukoproteinase inhibitor (SLPI)	Specific granules	Inhibition of serine proteinases Antimicrobial activity
Protegrins	Specific granules of pig neutrophils	Toxic activity against bacteria, fungi, and enveloped viruses

Table 4.6 Proteages released from neutrophils that modify ECM

Class	Name	Source	Functions
Serine proteinases	Cathepsin G	Azurophil granules	Cleavage of ECM proteins like type IV collagen, laminin, tenascin C, and cell-adhesion proteins Modulation of inflammation by stimulating the production of cytokines and chemokines
	Elastase	Azurophil granules	Cleavage of elastin, fibronectin, laminin, vitronectin, and collagen type I
	Proteinase 3	Azurophil granules	Degradation of fibronectin, type IV collagen, and laminin
	Azurocidin or CAP-37	Azurophil granules	Chemotactic activity for monocytes Stimulates PKC in endothelial cells
Metalloproteinases	MMP-8	Specific granules	Cleavage of type I collagen
	MMP-9	Secretory	Degrades native type V collagen

Knowledge Corner...

The reduced susceptibility of herbivores to mammary cancer, compared to omnivores and carnivores, is due to a range of morphological and metabolic adaptations that have evolved since the Jurassic period, driving phylogenetic divergence among these species. One such adaptation is the dense stromal structure in the bovine mammary gland, which may provide a protective, anticancer barrier for developing mammary cells.

4.3.1.9 Production of Cytokines

Neutrophils produce different classes of cytokines, chemokines, and growth factors that are actively involved in the regulation of inflammation and immunity (Table 4.7).

Table 4.7 Cytokines, chemokines, and growth factors released from neutrophils

Class	Name	Functions
Proinflammatory cytokines	TNF-α	Triggers the release of leukocyte adhesion molecules that favor immune cell infiltration
	L-1-a, IL-1-b	Stimulation and differentiation of $CD4^+$ cells
	IL-12	Proliferation and differentiation of Th1 cells
Anti-inflammatory cytokines	IL-1 receptor antagonist (IL-1Ra)	Decreases inflammatory reaction by blocking IL-1
Chemokines	IL-8	Chemoattractant cytokine
	Macrophage infiltrating protein-1α (MIP-1α)	Recruitment of inflammatory cells
	Cytokine-induced chemoattractants (CINC)	Chemoattractant effects on neutrophils
	Growth-related gene product-α (GRO-α),	Chemoattractant effects on neutrophils
Other cytokines and growth factors	Interferon-α (IFN-α)	Immune-regulatory protein involved in antiangiogenic, antiproliferative, and proapoptotic activities
	Granulocyte colony-stimulating factor (G-CSF)	Stimulates the proliferation, differentiation, and survival of neutrophil precursors
	Fas ligand (FasL)	Induces apoptosis of activated T-cells
	CD30 ligand (CD30L)	Induces IL-8 production
	Vascular endothelial growth factor (VEGF)	Angiogenesis
	Hepatocyte growth factor (HGF)	Stimulates the growth and differentiation of hepatocytes, endothelial and epithelial cells, melanocytes, and keratinocytes

Cassatella (1995)

4.3.1.10 Neutrophil Extracellular Traps (NETs)

These are large web-like structures made up of cytosolic and granular proteins of neutrophils assembled on decondensed chromatin materials. It is a novel mechanism to eliminate microorganisms without phagocytosis. The trap is formed soon after the activation of neutrophils through a series of events such as nuclear delobulation, chromatin decondensation, and loss of nuclear membrane degranulation, which ultimately leads to the mixing of nuclear and cytosolic contents. Now the cellular content is ejected out of the cells that form a NET-like structure that is 10–15 times larger than the volume of neutrophils. NET causes immobilization of microorganisms and their elimination. NETosis is therefore a kind of programmed cell death associated with the release of chromatin bound to cytosolic contents. However, the NETosis is different from apoptosis in many ways; unlike apoptosis NETosis, it does not require activation of caspases and results in the destruction of the plasma membrane.

Other than neutrophils, NETosis can be seen in other immune effector cells like eosinophils and mast cells, basophils, monocytes, and macrophages. The mechanism of NETosis can be induced by pathogens (bacteria, fungi, protozoa, viruses), cell wall components (lipopolysaccharides), antibodies, immune complexes, cytokines and chemokines (IL-8, TNF), microcrystals, and other physiological stimuli.

Types of NETosis

Based on the morphological features of PMN, NETs can be classified into three types.

Classical of suicidal NETosis: In this mechanism, the cell's death occurs. This mechanism is triggered by the formation of NADPH-dependent ROS that ultimately leads to the dissociation of granules and mixing of granular content with condensed chromatin.

The early step of classical NETosis is the respiratory burst. The production of ROS through respiratory burst activity causes the release of serine proteases and MPO from azurophilic granules. The serine proteases, particularly neutrophil elastase (NE), cause dissociation of cytoskeletal elements and gradually reach the nucleus to damage the lamin and histones to induce chromatin condensation, followed by the destruction of the nuclear lamina to release nuclear chromatin into the cytoplasm. At the final step of NETosis, the granular proteins are bound to the decondensed chromatin by electrostatic interaction. These complexes are released from the cells through large pores formed by gasdermin D protein (GSDMD).

Vital NETs: In vital NETosis, the cells remain viable along with their vital functions. It is an oxidant-independent process and mediated by a TLR2-dependent mechanism. Vital NETosis starts earlier than classical NETosis. In this mechanism, the chromatin condensation is brought about by a process called citrullination of histones by peptidyl arginine deaminase 4 (PAD4). In this mechanism, the NET is released without damaging the cytoplasmic membrane by some unknown mechanism. As the cytoplasmic membrane remains intact, the cells are able to preserve their integrity; hence, it is called vital NETosis.

Mitochondrial NETs: In this mechanism, PMN releases mitochondrial DNA to form NET. The release of mitochondrial DNA is ROS dependent. The exact mechanism of mitochondrial NET formation is yet to be explored.

Blood neutrophils retain their ability to form NET after migration to the mammary gland. It has been studied in dairy cows that the formation of NET can affect the quality and quantity of milk production in two ways: firstly, the NET attracts more neutrophils to the mammary glands and milk SCC is increased. Secondly, the formation of NETs results in the disruption of the blood–milk barrier and alters the permeability to affect the milk composition. Further, it increases the chances of mastitis as well. Hence, it is recommended by some authors that the formation of NET could be used as a diagnostic tool for the early detection of mastitis in dairy cows.

4.3.2 Macrophages

Macrophages are the predominant leukocytes in the milk comprising 10–80% of total cell populations in healthy animals. They are derived from the blood and differentiate within the mammary gland. Based on their preferential locations, mammary macrophages can be classified into ductal macrophages (between mammary epithelial cells) and bovine mammary macrophages (in the lumen within milk). Macrophages perform a dual role both in innate and adaptive immunity. Phagocytosis of the invading pathogens and secretions of pro-inflammatory cytokines are the innate functions of macrophages, while they can also act as antigen-presenting cells to facilitate adaptive immune responses. The macrophages also play a pivotal role in mammary involution by digesting cellular debris and milk components.

Macrophages are derived from erythromyeloid progenitor in embryonic yolk sac during organogenesis. They are located in different tissues as long-lived resident macrophages. The resident macrophage populations are maintained from blood monocytes derived from bone marrow during adulthood in response to infection, tissue injury, and inflammation.

4.3.2.1 Structure

Macrophages are large mononuclear cells having a diameter of 10–30 μm. They have a large horseshoe-shaped nucleus with coarse chromatin. The large size of the nucleus hinders their migration between endothelial cells. The structure of macrophages varies considerably during different phages of inflammatory reaction. At the initial stage of inflammation (24 h), the majority (90%) of macrophages resemble circulating monocytes and are called monocyte-like macrophages. In bovines, they are 12–15 μm in size with spherical nucleus and fine granular cytoplasm. The cytoplasm occupies most of the cell as indicated by the nucleoplasmic index. These macrophages are myeloperoxidase-negative (MPO-negative). There are numerous short and thin pseudopodia along the cell surface. During the time of resolution of inflammation (48–168 h), the mammary gland showed larger proportion of MPO-positive macrophages with large numbers of vacuoles. These macrophages contain phagosomes and phagolysosomes with apoptotic neutrophils (in some cases, more than 10 phagocytosed apoptotic neutrophils can be seen in the cytoplasm). The size is considerably increased to 20 μm or more. The nucleoplasmic index is toward the cytoplasmic side. The number of lysosomes is decreased. These macrophages contain a large pseudopodia.

The macrophages isolated from nonlactating ewe mammary glands were 13–30 μm in diameter, with an eccentric oval- or kidney-shaped nucleus and basophilic cytoplasm. The cytoplasm contains short and rough endoplasmic reticulum, large number of spherical mitochondria, and membrane-bound vacuoles. The Golgi bodies are also present along with lysosomal granules of 0.1–0.5 μm in diameter. There is the presence of phagosomes throughout the cytoplasm of the macrophages. The macrophages of involuting mammary glands have lipid droplets compared to nonlactating glands.

Macrophages Receptors

Both monocytes and macrophages express different types of receptors on their membrane, vacuoles, and cytoplasm that help them for pathogen recognition, uptake, and phagocytosis of foreign bodies and clearance by endocytosis (Table 4.8).

Table 4.8 Macrophage receptors and their functions

Receptor family	Name	Function
Scavenger (collagenous)	SR-A	Phagocytosis (bacteria and apoptotic cells) endocytosis of polyanionic ligands (LDL) Adhesion
	Macrophage receptor with collagenous structure (MARCO)	Phagocytic clearance of pathogens
Scavenger (noncollagenous)	CD36	Phagocytosis (apoptotic cells) Recognition of bacterial diacyl lipid M2-induced macrophage fusion and giant cell formation
Integrin	CR3 (CD18/11b)	Complement-mediated phagocytosis Endothelial adhesion
GPI-anchored	CD14	Interaction with LPS Recognition of apoptotic cell Pro-inflammatory signaling
Ig superfamily	FcR (ITAM/ITIM)	Phagocytosis (antibody-mediated)
	TREM-1 (ITAM)	Regulation of inflammation
Seven transmembrane	CCR2	Receptor for MCP-1
	C5aR	Chemotaxis, degranulation
	EMR2 (EGF-TM7)	Myeloid cell adhesion chondroitin sulphate binding

(continued)

Table 4.8 (continued)

Receptor family	Name	Function
NK-like C-type lectin-like	Dectin-1	Fungal recognition through β-glucan in their wall
C-type lectin (single CTLD)	DC-SIGN	Mostly expressed in dendritic cells Pathogen recognition
	CD206 (macrophage mannose receptor)	Clearance of glycoproteins with mannosyl terminal
Multiple CTLD	MR	Phagocytosis
Toll-like receptors (leucine-rich repeats)	TLR2	Recognition of peptidoglycans Peptidoglycan
	TLR4	Recognition of LPS
Carbohydrate-binding lectins and scavenger receptors	F4/80	Induction of regulatory T-cells Interaction between macrophage and NK cells
	CD68 (pan-macrophage marker)	Phagocytosis
	CSF1 receptor	Proliferation and differentiation of macrophages
	Mer-TK	Regulation of cytokine secretion Survival of macrophages
	CD64	Antibody-dependent cell-mediated cytotoxicity Immune complex clearance
Sialoadhesin	Siglec-1 (CD169)	Recognition of sialic acid

Gordon and Plüddemann (2017) and Taylor et al. (2005)

4.3.2.2 Functions of Macrophages

Activation

The activation of macrophages is facilitated by cytokines secreted by lymphocytes. There are two pathways of activation depending on the immune environment. The macrophages activated through classical activation pathway are called M1 or “classically activated” macrophages and the alternative pathway-derived macrophages are designated as M2 or “alternatively activated” macrophages. M2 macrophages are further subdivided into M2a, M2b, and M2c types. These macrophages differ in their cell surface markers, secreted cytokines, and biological functions (Table 4.9).

The process of activation of macrophage into M1 or M2 is called polarization. M1 macrophages are characterized by pro-inflammatory, antimicrobial, and antigen-presenting properties, whereas M2 macrophages have anti-inflammatory and anti-microbial properties. Activation of M1 macrophages is induced by interferon-gamma produced from TH1 lymphocytes, and M2 phenotype is induced by TH2 lymphocytes secreting IL-4 and IL-13. Activation stimuli and the changes that occur during M1/M2 polarization are summarized in Table 4.10.

Table 4.9 Types of macrophage and their characteristic features

Types of macrophages		Surface marker	Cellular marker	Cytokine production
M1 (classically activated)		CD68, CD80, CD86, IL-1R, TLR2, TLR4, iNOS, IFNγR, MHC II^{high}, Fc-RI/II/II	NF-κB, STAT1, STAT5, interferon regulatory factor (IRF3), IRF5	IL-1α, IL-1β, IL-6, IL-12, IL-18, TNFα, M-CSF
M2 (alternatively activated)	M2a	CD200, IL-1RII, Dectin-1, MHC II^{low}	(IRF) 4, PPARγ, STAT6	IL-10, IL-1Ra, TGFβ
	M2b	CD86, MHC II^{low}	IRF4, suppressor of cytokine signaling (SOCS3)	IL-1β, IL-6, IL-10, TNFα
	M2c	CD163, CD206, TLR1	IRF4, SOCS3	IL-10, TGFβ

Gordon and Plüddemann (2017) and Taylor et al. (2005)

Table 4.10 Functional attributes of classical and alternative activation of macrophages

Attributes	Macrophage activation	
	Classical activation	Alternative activation
Stimuli	LPS, IFNγ, TNFα, GM-CSF	IL-4/13
Effects on surface antigens	Increase MHC class II, CD86, decrease mannose receptor	Increase mannose receptor, Dectin-1, CD23 decrease CD14, CD163
Metabolic changes	Increase inducible nitric oxide synthase (iNOS) and respiratory burst activity	Increase arginase activity
Secretory responses	TNFα, IL-12, IL-1, IL-6, IP-10, MIP-1α, MCP-1, and low MW mediators	IL-1RA, IL-10, chemokines (AMAC-1), chitinase-like proteins (Ym1/2)
Functional effects of activation	Increase antigen processing presentation and phagocytic killing of pathogen	Cell growth, collagen formation, and tissue repair Allergic response and parasite killing

Gordon and Plüddemann (2017) and Taylor et al. (2005)

Antibody-Dependent Cellular Phagocytosis (ADCP)

Like neutrophils, macrophages are also able to internalize particles followed by the killing of pathogens by ROS or enzymes. This process is called antibody-dependent cellular phagocytosis (ADCP). Like neutrophils, the recognition and internalization of the pathogen depend upon opsonization by complement factors or antibodies. Thus, macrophages have two distinct classes of surface receptors for antibody and complement proteins (Table 4.11). The Fcγ receptors bind with the Fc component of the immunoglobulin G (IgG) molecule located opposite to the antigen-binding site. Complement receptors are specific for complement proteins.

ADCP is classified into two categories based on recognition by Fc or complement receptors.

Table 4.11 Macrophage receptors for antibodies and complements

Receptor family	Ligand	Affinity
Fcγ receptor		
FcγRI (CD64)	IgG1, IgG3 (IgG4, IgG2)	High
FcγRII (CD32)	IgG1, IgG3 (IgG4, IgG2)	Low
FcγRIII (CD16)	IgG1, IgG3	Low
Complement receptor		
CR1 (CD35)	C3b, C4b, iC3b	C3b > C4b > iC3b
CR2 (CD21)	C3d/C3g, iC3b	C3d/C3g > iC3b
CR3 (CD11b/CD18)	iC3b; ICAM-1	iC3b = ICAM-1
CR4 (CD11c/CD18)	iC3b	iC3b

Lendeckel et al. (2022)

Fc Receptor-Mediated Phagocytosis In this process, the internalization of particles is mediated by the activation of Fcγ receptor. These receptors have three domains: extracellular domain for binding with the Fc component of IgG, transmembrane domain, and cytoplasmic domain having immunoglobulin gene family tyrosine activation motif (ITAM). Binding of receptors with ligands leads to the phosphorylation of tyrosine (Y) residues in the ITAM domain through the src family kinases. Activated ITAM leads to the activation of PI3-kinase and phospholipase C, which results in actin polymerization. As a result of actin polymerization, a small piece of cell membrane protrudes over the surface and forms pseudopodia to internalize the particle.

Complement Receptor-Mediated Phagocytosis Unlike Fc receptor-mediated phagocytosis, this is relatively passive with little involvement of pseudopodia. Here, the complement-coated particles directly sink into the cell. Further, complement-mediated phagocytosis does not induce the release of inflammatory mediators as Fc receptor-mediated phagocytosis.

Generation of reactive oxygen and nitrogen species (ROS/RNS): The macrophages destroy the foreign particle by the generation of ROS and RNS similar to neutrophils. This is called oxidative burst activity and facilitated by NADPH oxidase. Receptor-mediated activation of NADPH oxidase occurs when the cytosolic subunits of NADPH oxidase (p40, p47, and p67) are fused with membrane subunits (p22 and gp91) in the phagosome. Superoxide anion ($O^{\cdot -}{}_2$) in the phagolysosome is converted to H_2O_2 by superoxide dismutase (SOD). H_2O_2 further generates other toxic ROS such as $OH^{\cdot}$ and OCl^-. The RNS includes nitrogen oxides, particularly $NO^{\cdot}$ from L-arginine by the action of inducible NO synthase (iNOS). $NO^{\cdot}$ further reacts with $O^{\cdot -}{}_2$ to form peroxynitrite ($ONOO^-$). The acidic form of peroxynitrite called peroxynitrous acid (ONOOH) is highly reactive and facilitates antimicrobial action.

Antigen Processing and Presentation

Macrophages play a pivotal role in the processing and presentation of antigen. The antigen presentation is mediated by major histocompatibility complex (MHC) class II molecules (MHCII) expressed on the surface of the macrophages, and the processed antigen is presented to helper T-cells. There are two distinct classes of MHC, namely MHCI and MHCII. Functionally they are almost identical in delivering a peptide to be recognized by cytotoxic (CD8+) and helper (CD4+) T-cells, respectively. But the origin of these peptides differs in their source. MHC class I molecules deliver endogenous or intracellular peptides; in contrast, MHC class II delivers exogenous or extracellular peptides. However, cross-presentation may also occur.

Antigen presentation by macrophages is mediated to MHCII molecules. The antigen is taken up by the macrophages and stored temporarily into the endosomes. When these endosomes are fused with lysosomes, the protein antigen is depleted into smaller fragments. Simultaneously the MHCII is synthesized in the endoplasmic reticulum and subsequently transported into vesicles. The nascent MHCII contains a peptide that occupies its antigen-binding site. This is called class II invariant chain peptide (CLIP). When the two vesicles containing MHCII and antigen fragments are fused together, CLIP is removed from the antigen-binding site of MHCII in exchange for antigen fragments. Now the MHC-II/peptide complexes are channelized into the plasma membrane to interact with CD4+ cells.

Pathogen Recognition

Macrophages have a pattern recognition receptor (PRR) for the recognition of pathogens. These PRRs act at the initial state of innate immune response and further stimulate adaptive immune responses. Macrophages express several pattern recognition receptors detailed in Table 4.12.

Cytokine Secretion

Macrophages help in immune cell recruitment and their subsequent activation by releasing some pro-inflammatory cytokines, anti-inflammatory cytokines, and chemokines. The secretion of these cytokines is mediated by interorganellar exchanges through vesicular trafficking and cytoskeletal remodeling. Proteins such as N-ethylmaleimide-sensitive factor attachment protein receptor (SNARE) family and synaptotagmins (Syt) regulate cytokine secretion by macrophages. Different cytokines secreted by the macrophages are summarized in Table 4.13.

4.3.3 Lymphocytes

Lymphocytes mediate specific responses by recognizing antigens of invading pathogens through membrane receptors. Lymphocytes are generally small round cells containing a large nucleus. The primary roles of lymphocytes are the

Table 4.12 Pattern recognition receptors (PRRs) of macrophages and their ligands

Class	Name	Ligands
Class A scavenger receptor family	Scavenger receptor AII II (SR-A)	Lipopolysaccharides (LPS) and lipoteichoic acid (LTA)
	Macrophage receptor with collagenous structure (MARCO)	LPS
	Scavenger receptor with C-type lectin-I/II (SRCL)	Gram (+) and gram (−) bacteria, yeast
C-type lectin receptor (CLR)		
C-type lectins containing a single carbohydrate recognition domain (CRD)		
DC-SIGN		Glycoprotein envelope of viruses, coronavirus S 70 protein, glycan antigen, mannose-capped surface lipophosphoglycan, Iipoarabinomannan, *Candida albicans, Aspergillus fumigatus*
Deetin-2		Capsular polysaccharide, HIV-1 gp120, *Candida albicans*
C-type lectins containing multiple CRDs		
Mannose receptor (MR)		Glycoprotein A, *Klebsiella pneumoniae* lipopolysaccharide, capsular polysaccharide, Influenza A virus
NK-like C-type lectin-like receptors (NKCL)		
Dectin-1		β-glucan, *Pneumocystis carinii*
LOX-1		*Staphylococcus aureus, Escherichia coli*
Toll-like receptors (TLRs)		
TLR-2		Peptidoglycans of Gram (−) bacteria, Lipoproteins, ipoarabinomannane, Zymosan
TLR-3		dsRNA
TLR-4		LPS
TLR-5		Flagellin
TLR-9		Bacterial DNA

Mukhopadhyay et al. (2009) and Lendeckel et al. (2022)

production of antibodies against invading pathogens (B-cells), whereas T-cells are involved in cell-mediated immunity. In healthy mammary gland, the total lymphocyte count was <50,000/mL and the proportion was higher in foremilk than other milk fractions.

Table 4.13 Cytokines secreted by the macrophages

Class	Name	Functions
Pro-inflammatory cytokines	Tumor necrosis factor (TNF-α)	Stimulates the acute phase of the immune response Induces vasodilation and decreases vascular permeability that facilitates the infiltration of neutrophils, lymphocytes, and monocytes at the site of inflammation Stimulates chemokines such as CXCL1, CXCL2, and CXCL5 to mediate neutrophil attraction Stimulates diapedesis by augmenting cell adhesion molecules
	IL-1	Stimulates the production of acute-phase proteins Stimulates histamine release to promote vasodilation and inflammation Favors chemoattraction of neutrophils and stimulates the expression of cell adhesion molecules
	IL-6 (both pro- and anti-inflammatory cytokine)	Stimulates differentiation of B-cells into plasma cells Activates cytotoxic T-cells Regulates bone homeostasis
	IL-12	Stimulates Th1 cells Produces IFN-γ Inhibits angiogenesis
	IL-18	Produces IFN-γ Activates T-cells and NK cells
	IL-23	Produces IFN-γ Activates T-cells
	IL-27	Favors the differentiation of T-cells to Th1 cells
Anti-inflammatory cytokines	IL-10	Suppresses macrophage activation Inhibits antigen processing and presentation by suppressing MHC-II expression Inhibits the production of IFN-γ
	TGF-β	Suppresses the effects of TNF-α, IL-1b, IL-2, and IL-12 Inhibits the functions of both Th1 and Th2 cells
Chemokines	CXCL1 and CXCL2 (macrophage inflammatory protein 2-a, MIP-2a)	Angiogenesis and development of melanoma
	CCL5 (RANTES)	Attracts T-cells, basophils, eosinophils, and dendritic cells to the site of inflammation
	CXCL8 (IL-8)	Chemoattraction of neutrophils
	CXCL9 (MIG)	Chemoattraction of T-cells
	CXCL10 (IP-10)	Attracts T-cells, N K cells, dendritic cells Anticancer activity
	CXCL11 (IP-9)	Chemoattraction of T-cells

4.3.3.1 Lymphocyte Subsets in the Mammary Gland

The lymphocyte subsets in the mammary gland are divided into two distinct categories, T- and B-lymphocytes. The T-lymphocytes can further be classified into $\alpha\beta$ T-cells and $\gamma\delta$ T-cells. The $\alpha\beta$ T-cells are of two types, namely CD4+ (T-helper) and CD8+ cells. Helper T-cells can be subdivided into Th1 and Th2 cells. CD8+ lymphocytes comprise T-cytotoxic and T-suppressor cells. B-lymphocytes are classified into plasma cells and memory cells. Ruminant $\gamma\delta$ T-cells also express a specific surface glycoprotein called WC1. Based on this surface glycoprotein, mammary $\gamma\delta$ T-cells can further be classified into two distinct subpopulations: one is $WC1^+$ and $CD2^-$ and the other is $WC1^-$, but $CD2^+$. In the mammary gland, the ratio of γ/δ to α/β T-cells is twice that in blood.

The distribution of T-lymphocytes in mammary tissue varies considerably. CD4+, and CD8+ cells are mainly localized in the parenchyma with close apposition to the alveolar epithelium. CD4+ T-lymphocytes were equally distributed in the epithelial and connective tissue areas. However, clusters of CD4+ and CD8+ T-lymphocytes can be seen in interalveolar connective tissue. In the epithelial area of the mammary gland, it showed lower CD4+ T-lymphocytes compared to CD8+ T-lymphocytes. In the gland cistern, CD4+ and CD8+ T-lymphocytes are almost equally distributed.

In healthy mammary glands, lymphocytes comprise about 10–28% of total somatic cells, out of which T-lymphocytes are higher (40–50% total lymphocytes) compared to B-lymphocytes (20–25% of total lymphocytes). Among the T-lymphocytes, CD8+ subsets are predominant, accounting for 50–60% of total T-lymphocyte population. During intramammary infections, the lymphocyte percentage is reduced to 14–24%, with higher proportion of CD4+ T-cells to recognize Ag-MHC class II complexes. However, under chronic infections, CD8+ are predominant.

The proportion of different lymphocyte subsets varies between different stages of lactation. During the dry period, CD4 predominates over CD8 in the blood, but their ratio alters during lactation in cows and ewes. The proportion of CD4+ in the milk increases with the advancement in parity. The proportion of B-cells is relatively lower in milk throughout lactation. The $CD21^+$ MHC II^+ B comprises less than 5% of milk lymphocytes in cows.

4.3.3.2 Lymphocytes Recruitment in the Mammary Gland

Lymphocytes that are recruited in the mammary gland are CD4+, CD8+, αβ T-lymphocytes, $\gamma\delta$ T-cells, and few B-lymphocytes. The recruitment of these lymphocytes is facilitated by some cytokines and chemokines produced mainly by the inflammed mammary epithelial cells. The chemokines responsible for the lymphocytes migration are CCL28, CXCL8, CCL2, CCL5, CXCL10, and CCL20. These chemokines induce the upregulation of vascular adhesion molecules, which interacts with the lymphocytes. CCL28 and CCL2 are the two main chemokines involved in lymphocyte migration in the mammary gland. In the lymph nodes, two adhesion molecules, namely glycosylation-dependent cell adhesion molecule-1 (GlyCAM-1) and mucosal addressin cell adhesion molecule-1 (MAdCAM-1), facilitate lymphocyte migration. GlyCAM-1 interacts with the L-selectin of lymphocyte, whereas MAdCAM-1 interacts with lymphocyte integrin α4ß7. In the mammary gland, both GlyCAM-1 and MAdCAM-1 are expressed, but mammary GlyCAM-1 produced by mammary does not have the ability to bind with L-selectin because of the differences in the glycosylation. Hence, MAdCAM-1 interacts with lymphocytes. The endothelial cells of small mammary vessels in the mammary lobules express MAdCAM-1, which interacts with integrin α4ß7 on lymphocytes to facilitate lymphocyte migration to the mammary gland.

Prolactin has a significant role in lymphocyte migration into the mammary gland. It stimulates the production of chemoattractants that facilitate the migration of IgA-secreting B-lymphocytes in the mammary gland.

In a healthy mammary gland, the ratio of CD4/CD8 is nearly 0.68, which is increased to 1.39 in staphylococcal mastitis, but it is decreased to 0.65 in streptococcal mastitis. The ration of $\gamma\delta$ T-cells / $\alpha\beta$ T-cells is also increased in mastitis.

4.3.3.3 Antigen Recognition by T- and B-Lymphocytes

Both T- and B-lymphocytes are the only cells that have the ability to recognize specific antigen. Thus, both of these cells are involved in antigen-mediated immune responses, which plays a pivotal role in adaptive immunity. The antigens are recognized by the membrane receptors present in both B- and T-lymphocytes called B-cell receptors (BCR) and T-cell receptors (TCR). The BCR are specific for exogenous antigen to form antibody, whereas TCR recognizes antigen binding with MHCI to cause cytotoxicity. The properties of antigens recognized by BCR and TCR are summarized in Table 4.14.

Antigen Recognition by BCR

The BCR is a macromolecular complex with two different structural and functional components, namely membrane-bound immunoglobulins (mIgs) and heterodimer of α (alpha) and β (beta) peptide chains. The mIg facilitates antigen recognition and αβ heterodimer helps in signal transduction. The mIg is extracellular and composed of four polypeptide chains and an anchoring unit to form a "Y"-shaped structure. The anchoring unit helps to fix the mIg in lipid bilayer of plasma membrane. Generally, IgM and IgD act as a membrane receptor of mIg and hydrophobic CH4 domain of

Table 4.14 The properties of antigens recognized by BCR and TCR

Properties	Antigens recognized by BCR	Antigens recognized by TCR
Interaction	The interaction of antigen with BCR forms a binary complex of Ag-Ab	The interaction of antigen with BCR forms a ternary complex of Ag-MHC-Ab
Types of Ag	BCR binds with soluble antigens	TCR does not bind the soluble antigen
Involvement of MHC	No	Yes
Chemical nature of Ag	Proteins, polysaccharide, and lipids in nature	Mostly protein in nature

IgM is anchored into the B-cell membrane. Fab component of IgM is situated outside the cell, and Fc component is involved in signal transduction.

The αβ heterodimer is composed of two polypeptide chains, namely alpha and beta, with a long cytoplasmic tail. The cytoplasmic tail of α and β chains is composed of 61 and 48 amino acids, respectively. In the cytoplasmic component, there is an immunoreceptor tyrosine-based activation motif (ITAM). Upon binding with specific antigens, the tyrosine residue of ITAM is phosphorylated by tyrosine kinases to induce signal transduction.

Signal Transduction by BCR

The binding of BCR with specific ligands (Ag) activates SRC family kinase (SFK) or nonreceptor tyrosine kinases, which phosphorylates tyrosine residue of ITAM. Activation of ITAM leads to the formation of a molecular complex called "signalosome" composed of BCR, tyrosine kinases, together with some adaptor proteins such as CD19, B-cell linker protein (BLNK) and signaling enzymes such as phospholipase C gamma-2 (PLC γ2) and phosphatidylinositol 3-kinase (PI3K). The signalosome activates multiple signaling cascades through GTPases and several transcription factors such as nuclear factor-kappa B (NF-kB), Bcl6, nuclear factor of activated T-cellsn (NFAT), and forkhead box O transcription factor (FoxO). All the mechanisms affect cell metabolism, gene expression, and the organization of the cell cytoskeleton.

Antigen Recognition by TCR

TCR is a complex of multiprotein molecules composed of two variable antigen-binding sites (αβ or γδ) and accessory proteins such as CD3γε, CD3δε, and CD247 ζζ chains. The polymorphic α and β chains of TCR recognize a wide range of peptides. Each chain is composed of a variable (V) and a constant domain (C) connected by a joining segment (J). Additionally, β chain has diversity segment (D). Each (V) domain has three complementarity-determining regions (CDRs), namely CDR-1, -2, and -3. These hypervariable CDRs can generate several combinations of TCR to identify a wide range of diversified antigens. CDR1α and β bind to an Ag through amino and carboxy-terminal motifs, whereas CDR3α and β regions bind to the central region of the peptide. The transmembrane domain of TCR is also associated with a CD3 component composed of three different chains, namely gamma (γ), delta (δ), and epsilon (ε). These chains form both homodimer (δδ) and heterodimers (γε and δε). The cytoplasmic portion of CD3 is associated with ITAM, which is responsible for downstream signaling cascade. There are 10 ITAMs associated with CD3, each CD3δ, γ, and ε chains have one ITAM, whereas each CD3ζ contains three ITAMs. Unlike BCR, the αβ-TCR does not recognize Ag in its natural form; rather, they identify processed Ag presented with MHC-I or MHC-II. The MHC-I is specific for intracellular small peptides (8–10 amino acids), whereas MHC-II is specific for longer peptides (13–25 amino acids) of extracellular origin. CDR-1 and CDR-2 interact with MHC molecules.

Signal Transduction by TCR

TCR recognizes processed Ag; hence, T-cells are associated with an antigen-presenting cell (APC). The molecular interaction between T-cells and APC is called immunological synapse or kinapse. The immunological synapse is divided into three zones, namely central, peripheral, and distal supramolecular activation clusters. In the central zone, TCR complex, co-stimulatory and co-inhibitory molecules, and co-receptors are present. The peripheral zone consists of adhesion molecules LFA-1-ICAM-1 and CD2-LFA3. In the distal zone, F-actin and phosphatase CD45 are present.

Binding of Ag with TCR leads to the activation of tyrosine kinases such as Fyn and lymphocyte-specific protein tyrosine kinase (Lck) associated with the CD3ε and the co-receptors CD4/CD8. These kinases phosphorylate ITAM moieties of the δε chains and CD3. Activated ITAMs attract ZAP-70, which in turn bind with phospholipase C γ1 (PLC γ1) or linker for the activation of T-cells (LAT) and induces two different signaling pathways.

In the first pathway, PLC-γ1 facilitates the conversion of the phosphatidylinositol biphosphate (PIP2) into inositol triphosphate (IP3) and diacylglycerol (DAG). IP3 induces the release of calcium from sarcoplasmic reticulum. Intracellular calcium binds with calmodulin, a serine/threonine-kinase that activates calcineurin. Calcineurin is a phosphatase that dephosphorylates transcription factor called nuclear factor of activated T-cell (NF-AT) to induce gene expression. DAG, on the other hand, activates protein kinase C (PKC), which activates transcription factor NF-κB for transcription of target genes.

In the second pathway, ZAP-70 phosphorylates LAT that activates a family of GTP-binding proteins called Ras. The Ras protein facilitates several phosphorylation pathways to activate mitogen-activated protein kinases (MAPK), which in turn activates a transcription factor called activator protein 1 transcription factor (AP1).

The activation of transcription factors such as NF-AT, AP-1, and NF-κB leads to their translocation into the nucleus to induce the transcription of IL-2 genes to promote cytotoxic activity of T-cells, integrins to facilitate cellular adhesion and expression of costimulatory molecules (CD40L), and antiapoptotic proteins.

4.3.3.4 Differentiation of B-Cells into Plasma Cells

Most of the B-cells are localized in the follicles of lymphoid organs. They are called follicular B-cells. Another specialized B-cell subset is present in the junction between the red and white pulp in the spleen called marginal zone B-cells. Follicular B-cells are surrounded by T-cell zones in the interfollicular region. In this region, B-cells encounter antigens, and proliferate and migrate to the interfollicular region to interact with antigen-specific CD4+ T-cells for full activation. A group of activated B-lymphocytes migrates to extrafollicular foci to form short-lived plasmablasts, which secrete low-affinity antibodies. Another group returns to follicle and proliferate to form germinal centers (GCs) where the antigen affinity of these B-cells increases to produce long-lived plasma cells and memory B-cells.

Different subsets of B-cells express different transcription factors during their course of development. Mature follicular B-cells express paired box protein

5 (PAX5), PU.1 interferon-regulatory factor 8 (IRF8), and BTB and CNC homologue 2 (BACH2). The antigen-induced activated B-cells that differentiated into short-lived plasma blast express high levels of IRF4 and X-box-binding protein 1 (XBP1), and intermediate (mid) levels of B-lymphocyte-induced maturation protein 1 (BLIMP1). The long-lived plasma cells express long-lived plasma cells, which express high levels of BLIMP1, IRF4, and XBP1.

4.3.3.5 Plasma Cells in the Mammary Gland

The immunoglobulins in the mammary secretions are mainly derived from blood. In general, 40% of colostral IgA and 85% of IgM directly derived from serum. However, mammary gland is capable of producing local antibodies by the plasma cells documented in cows, sheep, goats, pigs, and laboratory animals. The plasma cells are localized mainly in the interalveolar stroma below the secretory epithelial cells, intraepithelial region of teat end, adjacent to tight junctions between the epithelial cells, squamocolumnar junction at the Fürstenberg rosette. Before the pathogens gain access to the mammary gland through teat meatus and enter the streak canal, they have to encounter the interior mucosal surfaces of the udder. This mucosal immune system and associated lymphoid cells are in close apposition with the epithelia of the distal teat end where initial antigen priming occurs. These cells are mostly IgA lymphoblasts that differentiate into plasma cells to synthesize local secretory antibodies.

There are discrepancies regarding the sources of plasma cells in the mammary gland. The widely accepted hypothesis is that the lymphoblasts migrated from gut-associated lymphoid tissues (GALT) via the mesenteric lymph node (MLN) and thoracic duct to the mammary gland during pregnancy and lactation. The dendritic cells of Peyer's patch of GALT and MLN act as antigen-presenting cells and processed orally administered antigens and present it to B-cells. These B-cells are now differentiated into antigen-secreting lymphoblasts with the expression of gut-homing receptors $\alpha 4\beta 7$ and CCR9. These lymphoblasts then leave the lymphoid tissue and reach the mammary gland through the postcapillary venules. The endothelial cells of postcapillary venules express addressin cell adhesion molecule called MadCAM-1 that interact with the $\alpha 4\beta 7$ integrin (homing receptor) of gut-derived lymphocytes. The maximum expression of MadCAM- 1 on endothelial cells of the mammary gland is seen at the end of pregnancy.

Apart from these cell adhesion molecules, some chemokines are also reported to be involved in the lymphocyte recruitment into the mammary gland. Epithelial chemokine CCL28 helps in the homing of IgA-secreting cells into the mammary gland to interact with their receptor CCR10.

The plasmocytes of the mammary gland synthesize mainly IgA and IgM, but IgG-secreting cells are also present.

4.3.3.6 Functions of T-Lymphocytes in the Mammary Gland

After the recognition of antigen and MHC complex, helper T-cells produce some cytokines to activate B-lymphocytes, macrophages, and other immune effector cells to induce immune response.

The helper T-cells are activated by antigen-presenting cells (APC) through two signals. In signal 1, APC with MHC molecule and a foreign peptide interacts with TCR. In signal 2, stimulatory proteins, namely B7 proteins (CD80 and CD86) of APC, interact with CD28 on the surface of the T-cells. The expression of co-stimulatory proteins is induced by pathogens. Signal 2 is required to activate downstream intracellular signaling pathways for effector functions. If a T-cell receives signal 1 without signal 2, it will undergo apoptosis. This is one of the methods to achieve tolerance to self-antigens. If a T-cell receives both signal 1 and signal 2, it will activate (see "Signal transduction by TCR"). Activated T-cells express high-affinity IL-2 receptors and release IL-2 as well. This IL-2 acts in an autocrine manner to the T-cells itself to induce proliferation and differentiation of helper T-cells to form effector helper T-cells. There are two different subsets of effector helper T-cells (T_H1 cell and T_H2 cells) based on the cytokine they produce. If the helper T-cells differentiate into TH1 cells, they secrete interferon-γ (IFN-γ) and tumor necrosis factor-α (TNF-α) cytokines to activate macrophages (see "Activation of macrophages") and cytotoxic T-cells to kill pathogens. They can also stimulate B-cells to secrete specific IgG antibodies. The differentiation of helper T-cells into T_H2 cells: they secrete interleukins 4, 5, 10, and 13 (IL-4, IL-5, IL-10, and IL-13) that stimulate B-cells to produce antibodies.

Cytotoxic T-cells destroy virus-infected cells by inducing apoptosis and subsequently killing the viruses. Cytotoxic T-cells recognize the antigen on the surface of the infected cells and cause the release of lytic granules through a calcium-dependent mechanism. These granules are derived as modified lysosomes that contain several lytic proteins (Table 4.15). Two main lytic proteins are perforin and granzyme. Perforin polymerizes to form transmembrane pores in target cell membranes. Another group of granules contains granzymes, a group of enzymes under the serine proteases (SP) family that cleave the cell's internal proteins.

Table 4.15 Proteins of lytic granules of cytotoxic T-cells and their functions

Class	Granular proteins	Functions
Lysins	Perforin	Pore formation in infected cells
Granzymes	SP A	DNA fragmentation, tryptase protease
	SP B	DNA fragmentation, caspase protease
	SP C	Tryptase proteases
	SP D, E, F	Tryptase proteases
	SP G	Tryptase protease
	Met-ase	Metase protease
	Leukophysin	Lntracellular processing of cytotoxic granules
Other molecules	Leukolexin	DNA fragmentation
	Calreticulin	Chelates-free calcium
	TIA-1	RNA-binding protein/endonuclease activator
	TIAR	RNA-binding protein/endonuclease activator
	Proteoglycans	Bind activated granule constituents

Trapani (1995)

4.3.4 Mammary Epithelial Cells

Epithelial cells in the mammary gland are the primary active secretory cells. While these cells are mainly involved in milk production, they also play important roles in the mammary gland's immune functions. The viability of milk epithelial cells, measured by trypan blue exclusion, is high in humans (over 90%) but only about 40% in goats. A significant number of epithelial cells are damaged during mammary gland infections due to the effects of lysosomal enzymes, oxidative by-products from phagocytosis, and cytokines released during the immune response.

4.3.4.1 Synthesis and Processing of Dimeric Immunoglobulins

Mammary epithelial cells are crucial in the synthesis and processing of dimeric IgA in monogastric animals and 90% of the mammary gland IgA is synthesized locally. Epithelial cells of the mammary gland express poly-Ig receptor at their basolateral surface, which capture IgA followed by transcytosis of poly-Ig receptor-IgA complex to the apical surface of the cell. Intracellular enzymes cleave IgA from poly Ig receptors and the receptors are recycled. The IgA accumulates in the mammary parenchyma and passively transferred via the colostrum. Additionally, mammary epithelial cells contribute to leukocyte migration during inflammation by producing cytokines (IL-6, M-CSF, TGFs, and EGF) and chemokines (IL-8).

4.3.4.2 Pathogen Detection

The mammary epithelium can detect microbe-associated molecular patterns (MAMP) through the expression of pathogen recognition receptors (PRR) (Table 4.16) to detect bacteria such as *streptococci, staphylococci*, and *E. coli*.

The recognition of pathogens and subsequent signal transduction by mammary epithelium differ between pathogens.

Table 4.16 PRR of mammary epithelial cells and associated MAMP

PRR	MAMP
TLR2/TLR1 heterodimer	Triacylated lipopeptides and lipoproteins
TLR2/TLR6 heterodimer	Diacylated lipopeptides and lipoproteins
TLR3	Double-stranded RNA, polyinosinic –polycytidylic acid (polyI:C)
TLR4	Lipid A part of Lipopolysaccharide
TLR5	Flagellin
TLR9	Single-stranded DNA
NOD1 (CARD4)	γ -D-glutamyl-meso-diaminopimelic acid (iE-DAP)
NOD2 (CARD15)	Muramyl dipeptide (MDP)
C-type lectin receptors	β-glucan
Inflammasome NLRP3	Uric acid, extracellular ATP, invasive bacteria

Rainard et al. (2022)

Gram-negative bacteria such as *E. coli* are detected through the lipid A moiety of LPS (endotoxin), which activate the transcription factors NF-kB, AP-1, and TRF3. The activation of these transcription factors helps in the expression of a large number of chemokines and antimicrobial peptides (AMPs) genes by MECs and pro-inflammatory cytokines (TNF-α and IL-1β) genes in macrophages (brown cells).

In case of Gram-positive bacteria, which lack endotoxin, they are perceived through lipopeptides, lipoteichoic acid, protein A and α-toxin to produce IL-1β, and TNF-α through the transcription factor NF-kB. However, they elicit lesser reactions.

4.3.4.3 Phagocytosis

Mammary epithelial cells are considered nonprofessional phagocytes that exhibit pathogen-induced phagocytosis and xenophagy (foreign-eating). Unlike preferential phagocytes such as neutrophils and macrophages, they use different mechanisms. Mammary epithelial cells do not express Fcγ receptors (FcγR) and the complement receptors (CRs); so, they are unable to recognize opsonic particles; rather, the pathogen itself triggers its entry into the cells with the active participation of host cells.

The internalization of pathogens occurs through the "trigger" or "zipper" mechanisms. In the "trigger" mechanism, pathogens secrete effector proteins that modulate the actin cytoskeleton of the host cells to facilitate internalization of pathogens. Intracellular killing is mediated by the production of reactive nitrogen species and reactive oxygen species. Nitric oxide (NO^{+}) is produced by inducible nitric oxide synthases (iNOS).

4.3.4.4 Production of Antimicrobial Peptides (AMPs)

Mammary epithelial cells produce a large number of antimicrobial peptides against pathogens. These AMPs act by permeabilization of membrane of pathogens along with some secondary actions. These AMPs are of two groups, namely β-defensins and cathelicidins (Table 4.17).

4.3.4.5 Production of Chemokines

Mammary epithelial cells secrete CXC chemokines such as CXCL1, CXCL2, CXCL3, CXCL5, and CXCL8 that help in the attraction of neutrophils and CCL chemokines such as CCL2, CCL5, and CCL20 to attract mononuclear leucocytes.

4.3.4.6 Modulation of Inflammation

Mammary epithelial cells play significant roles in inflammation by secreting some pro-inflammatory cytokins (IL-6, IL-1a, IL-1b, TNF-a), production of lipid mediators of inflammation (oxylipids), and modulation of leukocyte response (TGF-β).

Table 4.17 Antimicrobial peptides synthesized from mammary epithelial cells

Group	Name of AMP	Functions
β-defensins	Tracheal antimicrobial peptide (TAP)	They are cationic proteins interact with bacterial membranes to form pores
	Lingual antimicrobial peptide (LAP)	Antimicrobial (gram-positive and gram-negative) and antifungal activities
	Bovine neutrophil β-defensins (BNBD)	Bactericidal activity against two major mastitis pathogens, *Escherichia coli* and *Staphylococcus aureus* by membrane disruption
Cathelicidins		Kill microorganisms by membrane disruption
Lactoferrin		Binds to iron and make it unavailable to bacteria
Acute-phase protein	Haptoglobin	Antioxidant and antibacterial activity
	Serum amyloid A3 (SAA3)	Antibacterial, modulation of inflammation by activating TLR4 and acting as chemoattractant for monocytes
	Pentraxin-3 (PTX3)	Acts as a sensor to recognize microbial patterns and antimicrobial activity
S100 calcium-binding proteins	S100A8, S100A9, S100A12	Antimicrobial role, acts as alarmins (damage-associated molecular pattern, DAMPs), pro-inflammatory stimulation, chemoattractants, and metal scavengers

4.4 Humoral Defenses

Several humoral factors are associated with cellular defense factors in mammary immunity.

4.4.1 Immunoglobulins (Igs)

Immunoglobulins (Igs) are the most important humoral defense factors of the mammary gland that link the cellular and humoral immune responses. They are a part of adaptive defense mechanism and specific. The major functions of immunoglobulins include opsonization of bacteria prior to phagocytosis, inhibition of metabolism of bacteria, activation of complement-mediated bacteriolytic mechanisms, and neutralization of toxins and viruses. The total immunoglobulins account for 70–80% of the total protein content in colostrum (20–150 g/L) and 1–2% of total protein (0.5–1 g/L) in milk. The concentration varies between species (Table 4.18), during lactation cycle, and inflammatory conditions. The concentration of Ig in the milk increases at the end of lactation and during inflammatory condition. Major portions of immunoglobulins are transported from the blood via a selective receptor-mediated intracellular route. A small portion is produced from localized plasma cells. There are four important immunoglobulins concerned with mammary

Table 4.18 Immunoglobulin concentration in colostrum, milk, and serum in different species

Species	Immunoglobulin	Concentration (mg/mL)		
		Colostrum	Mature Milk	Serum
Rat	IgG	2.6	1.06	24.6
	IgG2a	0.67	0.8	6.91
	IgG2b	0.05	0.26	0.89
	IgA	1.15	1.02	0.18
	IgM	0	>0.002	0.95
Mouse	IgG (total)	N.D.	0.12	2.8–4.8
	IgG2a	–	–	0.4–1.5
	IgG2b	–	–	0.2–0.6
	IgA	0.05	0.3	0.6
	IgM	0.2	0.59	0.2
Rabbit	IgG	1.5	0.1	5–10
	IgA	~30.0	~5.0	0.01
	IgM	0.01	Trace	0.01
Dog	IgG (total)	12.1	0.15	15.6
	IgA	3.6	1.75	0.94
	IgM	0.6	0.13	1.6
Swine	IgG (total)	61.8	1.6	24.0
	IgA	11.3	4.1	2.0
	IgM	3.8	1.5	2.5
Cattle	IgG1	46.4	0.58	11.2
	IgG2	2.87	0.05	9.2
	IgA	5.36	0.10	0.37
	IgM	6.77	0.09	3.1
Sheep	IgG1	94–162	1.0	18.1
	IgG2	2.0	0.1	7.9
	IgA	3.5	0.2	0.2
	IgM	1.3–21.2	0.2	3.6
Horse	IgGa	82	0.2	3.4
	IgGb	183	0.3	19.6
	IgGc	0.3	N.D.	0.2
	IgG3	44	0.1	4.0
	IgA	9	0.7	0.4
	IgM	2.3	0.07	1.6
Cat	IgG	26.5	N.D.	14.7
	IgA	0.64	N.D.	2.2
	IgM	0.48	N.D.	5.3

Butler et al. (2015)

gland defense such as IgG1, IgG2, IgM, and IgA, out of which IgG1, IgG2, and IgM are involved in opsonization and IgA is concerned with toxin neutralization and agglutination of bacteria.

The main function of immunoglobulins is the opsonization to facilitate phagocytosis by macrophages and polymorphonuclear leukocytes. The predominant immunoglobulin that is involved in the opsonization is IgG.

Each immunoglobulin has antigen-binding sites at the light and heavy chains that facilitate the binding with antigen like "a lock and key." After binding with antigens, the stem region of the immunoglobulin binds with the receptor on the surface of phagocytes and is subsequently engulfed by lysosomes.

4.4.2 Complement system (CS)

Complement system involves a group of proteins synthesized from liver, tissue macrophages, monocytes, and locally by mammary tissue. This system plays pivotal roles in innate immunity by inducing inflammation and pathogen destruction by opsonization, chemotaxic, and intracellular killing. The complement system contains around 29 plasma and membrane proteins. Activation of the complement system leads to a cascade of reactions that sequentially activate other components to exert effector functions. There are three pathways of complement activation: the classical pathway (CP), the alternative pathway (AP), and the lectin pathway. In the mammary gland, CP is absent due to the lack or lower concentrations of C1q; hence, AP is the main pathway of complement activation. The concentration of different complement components also varies considerably between mastitic and healthy glands (Table 4.19). In a healthy mammary gland, the concentration is relatively low, but, during mastitis, a significant increase in complement proteins is noted due to the transudation from plasma.

Different components of the complement system have distinct roles (Table 4.20). The C3 and C4 components of the complement system are mainly involved in

Table 4.19 Concentrations of different complement components in the serum and milk of healthy and mastitic dairy cows

Component	Serum concentration	Mature normal milk	Mastitic milk		References
			Subclinical	Clinical	
C1q (μg/mL)	200	0.2	ND	ND	Rainard and Poutrel (1995)
C3 (% of serum)	100	ND	5	5–18	Mueller et al. (1983)
C5 (μg/mL)	ND	ND	ND	ND	Rainard and Poutrel (2000)
C5a (ng/mL)	15.4	0–0.12	0.18	5.5–50	Rainard et al. (1998) and Shuster et al. (1997)

Table 4.20 Functions of the complement system

Functions	Complement components
Bactericidal and hemolytic activities in normal milk	Membrane attack complex (MAC) made of C5b, C6, C7, C8 and several copies of C9
Bactericidal and hemolytic activities in mastitic milk	C3
Opsonization	C3 and C4
Recruitment of phagocytes	C4a, C3a, and C5a
Activation of phagocytes	C5a
Histamine release and vasodilation	C3a, C5a

opsonization and aid phagocytosis, whereas the C3a and C5a components promote the release of histamine to induce vasodilation and increase vascular permeability.

4.4.3 Transferrin [TF]

It is an iron-binding protein synthesized locally in the mammary gland (pigs, rodents, and rabbits) or transported from the blood (ruminants). The localization of transferrin was reported in the basal membrane of the secretory cells near the capillary vessels in sheep. The concentration of TF is 1.07 mg/mL, 0.02–0.04 mg/mL, and 4-5 mg/mL, respectively, in colostrum, normal milk, and serum. Higher values of lactoferrin in milk were reported in quarters having SCC more than 10^6 cells/mL. The concentration of TF is highest in the first milking (1.07 mg/mL), which decreased sharply on the first day of lactation and reached a steady state during the third week post partum (0.02 mg/ml). A significantly higher level of TF is reported in the serum of cows suffering from acute mastitis. TF is a glycoprotein having two lobes, each capable of binding one Fe^{+3}. TF disrupts the microbial membrane potentials by iron sequestration to exert bacteriostatic and bactericidal effects on a variety of pathogens such as *Pseudomonas aeruginosa*, *Klebsiella pneumonia*, *Yersinia pseudotuberculosis*, *Acinetobacter baumannii*, *Bacillus anthracis*, and fungal pathogens like *Candida species* and *Histoplasma capsulatum.* TF also interferes with bacterial adhesion and inhibits biofilm formation.

4.4.4 Lactoferrin

It is an iron-binding protein produced in epithelial cells and leukocytes. It interferes with the iron availability of some bacteria such as staphylococci and coliforms and requires iron for growth. Lack of iron also prevents the production of dismutase of bacteria that inactivate ROS, thus making them more prone to phagocytic killing. Lactoferrin acts synergistically with IgG1 to limit the growth of *Escherichia coli* and *Klebsiella pneumonia.* The activity of lactoferrin is increased by bicarbonate, whereas citrate acts as a lactoferrin inhibitor. Lactoferrin also causes the disruption of the outer membrane of Gram (−) bacteria by interacting with the lipid A portion of LPS. Lactoferrin affects the protein transport system of *E. coli* and exerts bactericidal effects. Bacterial proteases required for cell survival and replication are inhibited by lactoferrin. Mastitis-causing bacteria sensitive to lactoferrrin are *Streptococcus uberis, Klebsiella pneumonia, Staphylococcus aureus,* and *Prototheca zophii.*

The concentration of lactoferrin in the colostrum of cows is 5 mg/mL, but mature milk contains much less (200–485 μg/mL) lactoferrin. The concentration of lactoferrin is increased (20–30 mg/mL) after 3–4 weeks of involution that inhibits bacterial growth to prevent mammary infections during the dry period.

In mastitis milk, the concentration of lactoferrin is increased. Higher expression of lactoferrin mRNA is also reported in mammary tissues in experimentally induced mastitis. The concentration of lactoferrin is more in acute mastitis than pre-acute form. Application of lactoferrin as intramammary infusion also showed promising results. Infusion of 100 mg lactoferrin/10 ml/quarter achieved 91.7% cure rate in mastitis-infected Holstein-Friesian cows compared to control (48.3%). Lactoferrin hydrolysate solution (@ 0.5 g/quarter) reduced bacterial load by the 14th day with decreased SCC. In chronic mastitis, 200 mg lactoferrin/10 ml/quarter induces infiltration of granulocyte, T-cell, and B-cell in the mammary gland.

4.4.5 Lysozymes

It is a bactericidal protein in milk that cleaves β 1,4-glycosidic link between N-acetylmuramic acid and N-acetyl-D-glucosamine residues in peptidoglycans present in the cell wall of Gram (+) bacteria and outer membrane of Gram (−) bacteria. The binding of cationic lactoferrin to lipoteichoic acid of staphylococci makes them more susceptible to lysozyme. It also augments the activity of complement and secretory IgA in porcine and human milk. However, this mechanism is absent in ruminants as they contain less amount of IgA and lysozyme as well. The lysozyme is transported from the blood or synthesized locally. However, during infections, leukocytes are the predominant source of lysozyme in milk. The concentrations of lysozyme in the milk of humans, cows, and buffaloes are 10 mg/dL, 0.0004 g/L, and 0.000152 g/L, respectively. The concentration of lysozyme varies with the stage of lactation. The concentration of lysozyme is highest (0.72 mg/L) at the seventh day and decreased around the second week post partum. A significant increase in lysozyme concentration was reported during mastitis in cows (10–50 fold) and buffaloes (1000-fold). The activity of lysozyme in buffalo milk also varies with season. The lysozyme activity was highest during summer and winter compared to spring. The lysozyme activity was higher in primiparous cows compared to multiparous cows. The lysozyme activity was reported to increase with the advancement of lactation in cows but no such changes were seen in buffaloes.

4.4.6 Lactoperoxidase (LPO)

It is the second most abundant enzyme in milk after xanthine oxidase. The concentration of lactoperoxidase in milk is 30 mg/L, constituting 0.5% of the total whey proteins. LPO promotes phagocytic killing of pathogens by the production of hypothiocyanite and hypothiocyanous acid from the oxidation of thiocyanate in the presence of hydrogen peroxide. It also helps to produce hypoiodite and hypoiodous acid from the oxidation of I^-. These compounds interact with sulfhydryl groups of microbes to affect cellular functions. The activity of LPO increased from 1.44 U/mL to 3.28 U/mL from 14th before drying off to seventh day after drying off and decreased to 0.87 U/mL at 18th day after calving. Decreased LPO activity was seen from 0 to 4 months post partum in primiparous cows. Higher activity of LPO activity was associated with increased SCC in both cows and goats. The LPO activity in goats is measured from 0.49 to 1.07 units/mL.

4.4.7 Myeloperoxidase (MPO)

It is a lysosomal enzyme (heme protein) present in the primary granules of neutrophils and facilitates oxygen-dependent killing of pathogens. The reaction catalyzed by myeloperoxidase is similar to LPO, but, additionally, it catalyzes chloride oxidation to kill pathogens. However, the bactericidal effect of MPO is restricted during the dry period as proteins in milk inhibit MPO activity. The concentration of MPO in milk neutrophil lysate isolated from bovine milk is 0.45 ng/ml in healthy animals that reached 1.56–3.52 ng/mL in subclinical and 5.92 ng/mL in clinical mastitis (Alhussien and Dang 2020).

4.4.8 Cytokines

These are immunoregulatory peptides synthesized from mammary epithelial cells and leukocytes involved in the onset, progression, and resolution of inflammation. Cytokines act via specific receptors with high affinity; so, they are highly potent even at very low concentrations. There are several cytokines isolated from udders (Table 4.21), but their functions during intramammary infection are complex and depend upon several other factors. Cytokines act as a link between innate and adaptive immune responses.

4.4.9 Chemokines

They are the chemotactic cytokines that facilitate leukocytes trafficking in the mammary gland. Mammary tissue and epithelium express chemokines such as CXCL1, CXCL2, CXCL3, and CXCL8 in response to lipoteichoic acids from Gram (+) bacteria. Chemokines such as RANTES, CXCL5, CXLX8, MCP-1,

Table 4.21 Cytokines of the mammary gland

Name	Source	Functions	Concentration
IL-1	Macrophages, lymphocytes, monocytes, endothelial cells, and fibroblasts	Proinflammatory cytokine Increases neutrophil recruitment to udder Stimulates secretion IL-6, IL-8, IL-12, TNF-α, and IL-1	Normal milk: 55.36 pg/mL Mastitic milk: 263.03 pg/mL Serum of mastitic cow: 55.25 pg/mL
IL-2	CD4+ cells (Th1)	Proliferation of B-lymphocytes Increases cytotoxic activities of T-lymphocytes	
IL-4	CD4+ cells (Th1), CD8+/T-suppressors, B-lymphocytes	Differentiation of T-lymphocytes Inhibitory effect on IFN-γ production	
IL-6	Macrophages, lymphocytes, monocytes, neutrophils, mammary epithelium, and endothelial cells	Both pro- and anti-inflammatory roles Regulates the production of acute-phase proteins Favors the influx of monocytes into udder Induces B-cell differentiation Exerts anti-inflammatory action by inhibiting the expression of IL-1β and TNF-α	
IL-8	Monocytes, T-lymphocytes, macrophages, neutrophils, mammary epithelium, and endothelial cells	Induces inflammatory response Favors neutrophil migration into MG Induces neutrophil degranulation	Normal milk: 131.82 pg/mL Mastitic milk: 298.34 pg/mL Serum of mastitic cow: 164.22 pg/mL
IL-10	Th2 cells, B-lymphocytes, monocytes, eosinophils, mast cells	Principal anti-inflammatory cytokine helps resolution of inflammation Prevents production of proinflammatory cytokines and chemokines, Impairs antigen presentation by downregulating MHC class II	
IL-12	Macrophages, B-lymphocytes, monocytes, neutrophils	Differentiation of T-lymphocyte Acts as growth factor for activated NK cells Causes polarization of of CD4+ and CD8+ T-cells into Th1 and cytotoxic IFN-γ	Normal milk: 139.17 pg/mL Mastitic milk: 604.10 pg/mL Serum of mastitic cow: 70.34 pg/mL

(continued)

Table 4.21 (continued)

Name	Source	Functions	Concentration
		producers Stimulates the production of IFN-γ to activate macrophages Upregulates other cytokines as TNF-α, IL-8, and IL-10	
TNF-α	Macrophages, neutrophils, and mammary epithelium	Stimulates the generation of febrile and acute-phase responses Promotes neutrophil phagocytosis and bactericidal activity Induces expression of adhesion molecules on endothelial cells Stimulates secretion of IL-8 by different cells	Normal milk: 78.82 pg/mL Mastitic milk: 460.86 pg/mL Serum of mastitic cow: 104.78 pg/mL
G-CSF, M-CSF, GM-CSF	Fibroblasts, endothelial cells, macrophages, and T-lymphocytes	Increases numbers of both blood and milk neutrophils Induces phagocytosis and bactericidal activity of leukocytes Chemoattraction of macrophage and neutrophils to udder	
IFN-γ	T-lymphocytes, NK cells, monocytes	Links the innate and adaptive immune response Stimulates microbicidal activity of neutrophils and macrophages Induces production of IL-12 Upregulates cell-surface MHC-I and MHC-II molecules	

MCP-2, and MCP-3 are induced in response to lipopolysaccharides of Gram (−) bacteria. CXCL3 is the main chemotaxin of normal milk.

4.4.10 Xanthine Oxidase

Xanthine oxidase originated from the apical membrane of mammary epithelium and is primarily found in milk fat globule membrane. The bactericidal activity of xanthine oxidase is mediated by the production of nitric oxide from inorganic nitrite, which is further converted into peroxynitrite. The bacteriostatic action of xanthine oxidase is mediated through the production of hydrogen peroxide in the presence of a reducing substrate.

4.5 Integration of Innate and Adaptive Immune Response of the Mammary Gland during Infections

The entry of pathogens into the mammary gland and their toxic products causes irritation and tissue damage to release inflammatory mediators. The inflammatory mediators released from the damaged tissue stimulate local leukocytes to release pro-inflammatory cytokines such as IL-1β, IL- 6, and IL-17. These cytokines, together with IL-8 and TNF-α, are the main effector proteins to initiate inflammatory responses. Arachidonic acid (AA) metabolites such as prostaglandins (PGs) and leukotrienes (LTs) promote increased circulation to the mammary gland. The migration of neutrophils into the mammary gland results from the combined effects of chemoattractants, selectins, and integrins. IL-17 enhances the migration of leukocytes by regulating the expression of IL-8 and other chemokines for neutrophils (CXCL3 and CXCL8) and mononuclear leukocytes (CCL2, CCL20). Complement fragments (C3a andC5a) trigger neutrophil migration. Inflammatory mediators induce several physiological responses such as generation of febrile condition (TNF-α, IL-1β, and IL-6), initiation of acute-phase responses to produce acute-phase protein from the liver (interleukin-1, IL-6, IL-8, and TNF-α), and alterations in the vascular permeability (TNF-α). Simultaneously, B-lymphocyte differentiation is induced by IL-2 and IL-6. The antigens produced by invading pathogens are processed within macrophages and B-lymphocytes in association with MHC class I or II. The upregulation of MHC-I and II is stimulated by IFN-γ. Antigen presented with MHC-II on B-lymphocytes or macrophages facilitates the recognition of foreign peptides by T-cells and CD4+ cells are activated to induce polarization of B- and T-lymphocytes, macrophages, and other immune cells. T-cell-mediated response can be of cell-mediated (Th1 type) or humoral (Th2 type) based on the cytokines produced by T-helper cells. Cytokines such as IL-2 and IFN-γ secreted by Th1 cells to promote cell-mediated immune responses against intracellular pathogens, whereas IL-4, IL-5, and IL-10 produced by Th2 lymphocytes induce humoral responses and macrophage functions. Induction of humoral response causes differentiation of the B-lymphocytes into plasma or mammary cells. Activated macrophages release chemotactic signals, which favors further neutrophil migration to amplify the inflammatory response. The resolution of the infection is facilitated by the upregulation of anti-inflammatory cytokines such as IL-10 IL-6, IL-4. IL-10, and TGF-β. The generation of T-helper cells is inhibited by IL-6 and IL-4. Il-10 inhibits the production of IFN- γ, IL-1, and TNF-α by the Th1 cells. TGF-β inhibits the production of IFN- γ and other inflammatory mediators like chemokines, proinflammatory cytokines, nitric oxide, and ROS. TGF-β also increases IL-1 receptor antagonist. Other than the resolution of inflammation, TGF-β also promotes extracellular matrix deposition, fibrosis, and scarring. TGF-α, on the other hand, favors tissue repair by inducing epithelial proliferation and tissue remodeling to restore normal function.

4.6 Modulation of Mammary Gland Immunity

Modulation of innate and adaptive immune responses of the mammary gland is one of the prime concerns in the dairy industry. Indiscriminate uses of antibiotics to treat mastitis increase antimicrobial resistance, which is now a global concern. The antibiotic residues in the food chains through dairy products are also alarming. Thus, improving host defense is a goal in mastitis management. There are several tools to improve host defense that could be an alternative to conventional antimicrobial therapy of mastitis.

4.6.1 Genetic Selection

The milk production potential of an animal and resistance to mastitis is negatively correlated. Therefore, genetic selection to augment milk production decreases mammary gland immunity. The mastitis resistance is polygenic in nature; so, single genes with a high potentiality need to be discovered. One such gene is the CD18 subunit of the Mac-1 glycoprotein that plays an important role in leucocyte adhesion and migration, and point mutations in an allele of this gene result in bovine leucocyte adhesion deficiency (BLAD) syndrome. Studies in Holstein cows showed that single-nucleotide polymorphism (SNP) in CXCR2 gene was associated with impaired neutrophil function and mastitis susceptibility. Therefore, genes involved in neutrophil migration and different aspects of phagocytosis need to be explored. However, heritability of these factors was reported to be low. Direct selection of animals against mastitis incidence may be a promising approach to generating more resistant animals. An interesting study was conducted in Norway where two selection groups, viz. high protein yield (HPY) and low clinical mastitis (LCM), resulted in a 8.6% less incidence of clinical mastitis in LCM after three generations.

There are about 22 candidate genes for mastitis resistance in dairy cattle (Table 4.22) that could be used for selection.

4.6.2 Micronutrient Supplementation

Supplementation of vitamins and microminerals showed promising effects to augment udder immunity in cows. Important microminerals concerned with the udder immunity are copper, zinc, and selenium, along with vitamin E and vitamin A. The optimum effect of the micronutrient is dependent on the time of supplementation. In most of the trials, supplementation during the prepartum periods had a significant positive impact on the postpartum udder health. The effects of different micronutrients on the udder immunity are summarized in Table 4.23.

Table 4.22 List of candidate genes for mastitis resistance

Gene name	Gene	Chromosome
Major histocompatibility complex, class II, DRB3	*BoLA-DRB3*	23
Complement C6	*C6*	20
Complement C9	*C9*	20
Calcium voltage-gated channel auxiliary subunit alpha2delta 1	*CACNA2D1*	4
Caspase recruitment domain family member 6	*CARD6*	20
CD14 molecule	*CD14*	7
C-X-C motif chemokine ligand 8 (interleukin 8)	*CXCL8*	6
Chemokine (C-X-C motif) receptor 1	*CXCR1*	2
C-X-C motif chemokine receptor 2	*CXCR2*	2
Deoxycytidine kinase	*DCK*	6
Diacylglycerol O-acyltransferase 1	*DGAT1*	14
GC vitamin D binding protein	*GC*	6
Lactotransferrin	*LTF*	22
Lysophosphatidic acid receptor 3	*LPAR3*	3
Mannose binding lectin, liver (A)	*MBL1*	28
Mannose binding lectin 2	*MBL2*	26
Milk fat globule EGF and factor V/VIII domain containing	*MFGE8*	21
Neuropeptide FF receptor 2	*NPFFR2*	6
Suppressor of cytokine signaling 2	*SOCS2*	5
Signal transducer and activator of transcription 5 A	*STAT5A*	19
Toll-like receptor 2	*TLR2*	17
Toll-like receptor 4	*TLR4*	8

Table 4.23 The effects of different micronutrients on the udder immunity

Name of micronutrient	Mechanism of action	Effects on the udder immunity
Copper	It is a component of the antioxidant enzyme superoxide dismutase that protects the cells from reactive oxygen produced due to respiratory burst activity during phagocytosis	Improves phagocytic potential of neutrophils Decreases severity of mastitis
Zinc	It helps to establish keratin in the teat canal Regulates the integrity and toughness of mammary epithelial barrier to infection	Improves leukocyte function Decreases mastitis incidence
Vitamin E	Antioxidant, prevents lipid peroxidation to protect cell membranes	Increased neutrophil bactericidal activity Decreases mastitis incidence along or in combination with selenium
Selenium	Component of the antioxidant enzyme glutathione peroxidase that prevents lipid peroxidation	Improves bactericidal capabilities of neutrophils Decreases severity and duration of mastitis
Vitamin A and β-carotene	Induces proliferation of mammary epithelial cells	Decreases somatic cell counts in milk
Chromium	Influences the metabolism of glucose under stress	Improves immunity in cows under stress conditions

Table 4.24 Cytokine therapy in different mastitis models

Name	Mastitis model	Effects	References
G-CSF	*S. aureus*	No effect	Kehrli Jr et al. (1991)
	S. aureus	Reduced incidence (47%) of new IMI	Nickerson et al. (1989)
GM-CSF	*S. aureus*	Prevents new infections	Daley et al. (1993)
IFN-γ	*E. coli*	Reduction in rate, duration, and severity of mastitis	Sordillo and Babiuk (1991)
IL-2	*S. aureus*	Improves efficacy of antibiotic	Daley et al. (1992)
IL-1 and IL-2	*S. aureus*	Prevents new infections	Nickerson et al. (1989)

4.6.3 Cytokine Immunotherapy

Cytokine immunotherapy could be a promising therapeutic intervention to reduce the use of antibiotics in mastitis. The immunomodulatory effects of some recombinant cytokines were studied, and their effects on udder defense were explored in different mastitis model (Table 4.24). But the complex interactions between host and pathogen and variable responses of this therapy need to be explored under field conditions. The cost-effectiveness and side effects of cytokine therapy are also required to be considered before their application under field conditions.

4.6.4 Genetic Engineering

In recent years, manipulation of genome in cattle has emerged as a new era in mastitis therapeutics. Different components of innate immune system are the potential targets for biological manipulation. It is much easier to target proteins and peptides as their expression is under the control of milk protein gene promoters, whereas glycoconjugates and lipids require several enzyme cascades that are difficult to manipulate. Host defense peptides are the potential targets as they are a natural component of host defense and majorities are secreted in milk. Transgenic mice was produced that expresses TAP, a β-defensin-related peptide in their mammary gland. Transgenic cows were developed to secrete human lactoferrin in their milk, and thus, the cows are used as bioreactors for the large-scale production of lactoferrin. Lysostaphin, a glycylglycine enzyme of the cell wall of *staphylococci*, specifically cleaves the peptidoglycan pentaglycine bridges in the cell wall of *staphylococci*. The expression of lysostaphin is regulated by a -lactoglobulin promoter. Transgenic lysostaphin-secreting cows were developed that have less susceptibility against staphylococcal mastitis (14% in transgenic vs. 71% in the control animals). Mastitis-resistant transgenic cows were produced by targeting human lysozyme (hLYZ) gene to bovine β-casein locus, resulting in hLYZ knock-in cows. The milk secreted by transgenic hLYZ knock-in cows had the ability to kill

Staphylococcus aureus. Gene-edited dairy (GED) anti-mastitic goat was created that had increased lysozyme expression. This goat had reduced severity of mastitis by preventing the destruction of mammary epithelial cell (PANoptosis) and blood–milk barrier.

4.6.5 Herbal Therapy

The active principles of some medicinal plants showed anti-inflammatory effects against mastitis (Table 4.25). But their application in the clinical practice is limited due to limited in vivo trials.

4.6.6 Live Bio-therapeutics (Intramammary Probiotics)

Probiotic bacteria (lactic acid bacteria) have PAMP similar to some mastitis-causing pathogens. Hence, these probiotic bacteria interact with PRRs of the mammary epithelium and induce inflammatory reactions and leukocyte migration into the

Table 4.25 Active principles of some medicinal plants with anti-inflammatory effects

Name of the active principle/medicinal plant	Effects
Curcumin	Alleviates LPS-induced inflammation in a mouse mastitis model
Lipid-rich extract from Mexican avocado seed (*Persea americana var. drymifolia*)	Reduces *Staphylococcus aureus* internalization Induces immune response in bovine mammary epithelial cells
Nuciferine (in lotus leaf)	Reduces the severity of LPS-induced mastitis in mice via suppressing the TLR4-NF-B signaling pathway
Thymus vulgaris	Inhibits *Staphylococcus aureus* internalization by inhibiting NF-kappa B activation.
Tea tree oil extracts	Reduces the pro-inflammatory response caused by *S. Aureus* and promote the migration of neutrophils
Dandelion extract	Alleviates LPS-induced oxidative stress through the Nrf2 pathway
Stevioside	Anti-inflammatory effect mediated by regulating the NF-kappa B and MAPK pathways in *S. aureus* induced mastitis in mouse mammary glands
Citral and linalool (orange oil)	Inhibits the growth and biofilm formation of *S. aureus*
Vanillin	Protects blood–milk barrier Inhibits the inflammatory response in LPS-induced mastitis in mice model
Panax ginseng	Reduces *Staphylococcus aureus* internalization into bovine mammary epithelial cells

mammary gland. Intramammary administration of *Lactococcus lactis* showed 47% cure rate in clinical mastitis compared to 50% cure rate in antibiotic control. Intramammary infusion of live lactococcal culture enhanced recruitment of PMN to the udder.

4.6.7 Vaccination

Immunization protocols that are capable of potentiating antimicrobial defense could be an appropriate and convenient prophylactic measure to control mastitis. Effective immunization against mastitis may eliminate chronic infection, protect the gland from new pathogens, and reduce the severity of infection. Major mastitis-causing pathogens are *Staphylococcus aureus*, *Streptococcus uberis*, *Streptococcus agalactiae*, *Streptococcus dysgalactiae*, *Escherichia coli*, and *Klebsiella pneumonia.* Considerable research has been made to develop an effective mastitis vaccine against mastitis caused by coliform and streptococci (Table 4.26) that are able to reduce the incidence and severity of mastitis but major drawbacks are variability in response and insufficient antibody titer.

Table 4.26 *Coliform and Streptococcal*mastitis vaccines

Major pathogens	Vaccine antigen	Efficacy	References
Coliform	*Escherichia coli* J5 bacterins	Decreased severity in coliform mastitis in field trial	Cullor 1991
	Salmonella Re-17 bacterin toxoid	Decreased coliform mastitis severity in field experiment	McClure et al. (1994)
	E. coli J5 bacterin with killed *Staphylococcus aureus* (StartVac, Hipra)	Decreased mastitis severity in field study	Bradley et al. (2015)
	Enterobactin FepA	Reduction in bacterial growth in dry mammary secretion	Lin et al. (1999)
	Siderophore receptor FecA	Insufficient antibody titer	Takemura et al. (2002)
	Whole *E. coli* (P4), intramammary booster with bacterial extract	Augmentation in Th17 response	Herry et al. (2017)
	Klebsiella siderophore receptors and porin proteins (KlebVax)	Ineffective in a large-scale study	Tomazi et al. (2021)
	Klebsiella recombinant YidR	Reduced incidence of *Klebsiella* clinical mastitis	Tomazi et al. (2021)

(continued)

Table 4.26 (continued)

Major pathogens	Vaccine antigen	Efficacy	References
Staphylococcus aureus	Killed vaccine	Reduced severity	Watson (1992)
	Live vaccine	Better response than killed vaccine, promote recruitment of neutrophils	Colditz and Watson 1982
	Capsular polysaccharides (CP5, CP8, teichoic acid)	No protection study	Lee et al. (2005)
	Slime on killed bacteria, StartVac (Hipra)	Reduction in bacterial counts in milk	Schukken et al. (2014)
	Live VraG mutant small-colony variant	Humoral and cell-mediated response (Th1/Th17 type)	Côté-Gravel et al. (2016)
	Protein A (SpA)	Facilitated spontaneous cure of *Staph. aureus* infection	Pankey et al. (1985)
	Recombinant IsdB and IsdH	IgG2 antibodies and antigen-specific lymphoproliferation	Ster et al. 2010

Exercises

Objective Questions

1. A series of mucosal folds and cellular structures just above the streak canal primarily present in ruminants is called ________________.
2. In normal healthy mammary gland, the total somatic cell populations are ________________.
3. Predominant opsonizing antibody for bovine PMN are ____________ and ____________________.
4. ____________________ is a hemoprotein present in the azurophil granules of neutrophils.
5. Nitric oxide (NO) is produced from L-arginine by the enzyme ______________.
6. ________________ is a classical chemoattractant cytokine.
7. The novel mechanism to eliminate microorganisms without phagocytosis is __________________.
8. The process of activation of macrophage into M1 or M2 is called ____________________.
9. The nature of antigen binds with B-cell receptors (BCR) is ____________________.
10. Iron-binding protein synthesized locally in the mammary gland and secreted into milk is ________________________.

Subjective Questions

1. Briefly describe the molecular mechanism of neutrophil migration.
2. Write a short note on NETosis.
3. Describe some alternate therapeutic approach to reduce the use of antibiotics in mastits.
4. Describe in brief the interactions between innate and adaptive immune responses during intramammary infection.
5. Write a short note on milk somatic cells as an indicator of udder health and milk quality.

Answers to Objective Questions

1. Fürstenberg rosette
2. Below 100×10^3 cells/ml of milk
3. IgM and IgG2
4. Myeloperoxidase
5. NO-synthases (NOS)
6. IL-8
7. Neutrophil extracellular traps (NETs)
8. Polarization
9. Soluble antigen
10. Transferrin

References

Books

Butler JE, Rainard P, Lippolis J, Salmon H, Kacskovics I (2015) The mammary gland in mucosal and regional immunity. In: Mestecky J, Strober W, Russell MW, Kelsall BL, Cheroutre H, Lambrecht BN (eds) Mucosal Immunology, 4th edn. Academic, pp 2269–2306, ISBN 9780124158474, https://doi.org/10.1016/B978-0-12-415847-4.00116-6

Mukherjee J, Das PK (2019) Immune responses of mammary gland. In: Sar TK (ed) Mastitis: symptoms, triggers and treatment, 1st edn. Nova Science Publishers, New York, p 89

Mukherjee J, Das PK, Banerjee D (2023) Lactation physiology. In: Das PK, Sejian V, Mukherjee J, Banerjee D (eds) Textbook of veterinary physiology. Springer, Singapore. https://doi.org/10.1007/978-981-19-9410-4_25

Research Articles

Alhussien MN, Dang AK (2020) Sensitive and rapid lateral-flow assay for early detection of subclinical mammary infection in dairy cows. Sci Rep. Article no: 10:11161. https://doi.org/10.1038/s41598-020-68174-0

Bradley AJ, Breen JE, Payne B, White V, Green MJ (2015) An investigation of the efficacy of a polyvalent mastitis vac cine using different vaccination regimens under field conditions in the United Kingdom. J Dairy Sci 98:1706–1720

Cassatella MA (1995) The production of cytokines by polymorphonuclear neutrophils. Immunol Today 16:21–26

Colditz IG, Watson DL (1982) Effect of immunisation on the early influx of neutrophils during staphylococcal mastitis in ewes. Res Vet Sci 33:146–151

Côté-Gravel J, Brouillette E, Obradovic N, Ster C, Talbot BG, Malouin F (2016) Characterization of a vraG mutant in a genetically stable Staphylococcus aureus small-colony variant and preliminary assessment for use as a live-attenuated vaccine against intrammamary infections. PLoS One 11:e0166621

Cullor JS (1991) The Escherichia coli J5 vaccine: investigating a new tool to combat coliform mastitis. Vet Med 86:836–844

Daley MJ, Furda G, Dougherty R, Coyle P, Williams T, Johnston P (1992) Potentiation of antibiotic therapy of *Staphylococcus aureus* mastitis by recombinant bovine interleukin-2. J Dairy Sci 75: 3330

Daley MJ, Williams T, Dougherty R, Furda G, Hayes P, Coyle P (1993) Prevention and therapy of *Staphylococcus aureus* infections with recombinant cytokines. Cytokine 5:276

Gordon S, Plüddemann A (2017) Tissue macrophages: heterogeneity and functions. BMC Biol 15: 53. https://doi.org/10.1186/s12915-017-0392-4

Gullberg U, Bengtsson N, Bülow E, Garwicz D, Lindmark A, Olsson I (1999) Processing and targeting of granule proteins in human neutrophils. J Immunol Methods 1999(232):201–210

Herry V, Gitton C, Tabouret G, Reperant M, Forge L, Tasca C, Gilbert FB, Guitton E, Barc C, Staub C, Smith DGE, Germon P, Foucras G, Rainard P (2017) Local immunization impacts the response of dairy cows to Escherichia coli mastitis. Sci Rep 7:3441

Kehrli ME Jr, Goff P, Stevens MG, Boone TC (1991) Effects of granulocyte colony stimulating factor administration to periparturient cows on neutrophils and bacterial shedding. J Dairy Sci 74:2448

Kornalijnslijper JE, Daemen AJ, van Werven T, Niewold TA, Rutten VP, Noordhuizen-Stassen EN (2004) Bacterial growth during the early phase of infection determines the severity of experimental Escherichia coli mastitis in dairy cows. Vet Microbiol 101(3):177–186. https://doi.org/10.1016/j.vetmic.2004.04.005

Lee JW, O'Brien CN, Guidry AJ, Paape MJ, Shafer Weaver KA, Zhao X (2005) Effect of a trivalent vaccine against Staphylococcus aureus mastitis lymphocyte subpopulations, anti body production, and neutrophil phagocytosis. Can J Vet Res 69:11–18

Lendeckel U, Venz S, Wolke C (2022) Macrophages: shapes and functions. ChemTexts 8:12. https://doi.org/10.1007/s40828-022-00163-4

Lin J, Hogan JS, Smith KL (1999) Growth responses of coli form bacteria to purified immunoglobulin G from cows immunized with ferric enterobactin receptor FepA. J Dairy Sci 82:86–92

McClure AM, Christopher EE, Wolff WA, Fales WH, Krause GF, Miramonti J (1994) Effect of Re-17 mutant Salmo nella typhimurium bacterin toxoid on clinical coliform mastitis. J Dairy Sci 77:2272–2280

Mueller R, Carroll EJ, Panico L (1983) Hemolytic complement titers and complement C3 levels in endotoxin- induced mastitis. Am J Vet Res 44(8):1442–1445

Mukhopadhyay S, Plüddemann A, Gordon S (2009) Macrophage pattern recognition receptors in immunity, homeostasis and self tolerance. Adv Exp Med Biol 653:1–14. https://doi.org/10.1007/978-1-4419-0901-5_1

Nickerson SC, Owens WE, Watts JL (1989) Effects of recombinant granulocyte colony-stimulating factor on *Staphylococcus aureus* mastitis in lactating dairy cows. J Dairy Sci 72:3286

Pankey JW, Boddie NT, Watts JL, Nickerson SC (1985) Evaluation of protein A and a commercial bacterin as vaccines against *Staphylococcus aureus* mastitis by experimental challenge. J Dairy Sci 68:726–731

Rainard P, Poutrel B (1995) Deposition of complement components on *Streptococcus agalactiae* in bovine milk in the absence of inflammation. Infect Immun 63:3422–3427

Rainard P, Poutrel B (2000) Generation of complement fragment C5a in milk is variable among cows. J Dairy Sci 83:945–951

Rainard P, Sarradin P, Paape MJ, Poutrel B (1998) Quantification of C5a/C5a(desArg) in bovine plasma, serum and milk. Vet Res 29:73–88

Rainard P, Gilbert FB, Germon P (2022) Immune defenses of the mammary gland epithelium of dairy ruminants. Front Immunol 13:1031785. https://doi.org/10.3389/fimmu.2022.1031785

Schukken YH, Bronzo V, Locatelli C, Pollera C, Rota N, Ca sula A, Testa F, Scaccabarozzi L, March R, Zalduendo D, Guix R, Moroni P (2014) Efficacy of vaccination on Staphylococcus aureus and coagulase-negative staphylococci intramammary infection dynamics in 2 dairy herds. J Dairy Sci 97:5250–5264

Shuster DE, Kehrli ME Jr, Rainard P, Paape M (1997) Complement fragment C5a and inflammatory cytokines in neutrophil recruitment during intramammary infection with Escherichia coli. Infect Immun 65:3286–3292

Sordillo LM, Babiuk LA (1991) Controlling acute Escherichia coli mastitis during the periparturient period with recombinant bovine interferon-gamma. Vet Microbiol 28:189

Ster C, Beaudoin F, Diarra MS, Jacques M, Malouin F, Lacasse P (2010) Evaluation of some Staphylococcus aureus iron-reg ulated proteins as vaccine targets. Vet Immunol Immunopathol 136:311–318

Takemura K, Hogan JS, Lin J, Smith KL (2002) Efficacy of immunization with ferric citrate receptor FecA from Escherichia coli on induced coliform mastitis. J Dairy Sci 85:774–781

Taylor PR, Martinez-Pomares L, Stacey M, Lin H-H, Brown GD, Gordon S (2005) Macrophage receptors and immune recognition. Annu Rev Immunol 23:901–944

Tian SZ, Chang CJ, Chiang CC, Peh HC, Huang MC, Lee J-W, Zhao X (2005) Comparison of morphology, viability, and function between blood and milk neutrophils from peak lactating goats. Canadian J. Vet Res 69:39–45

Tomazi T, Tomazi ACCH, Silva JCC, Bringhenti L, Bravo MLMC, Rodrigues MX, Bicalho RC (2021) Immuni zation with a novel recombinant protein (YidR) reduced the risk of clinical mastitis caused by Klebsiella spp. and decreased milk losses and culling risk after Escherichia coli infections. J Dairy Sci 104:4787–4802

Trapani JA (1995) Target cell apoptosis induced by cytotoxic T-cells and natural killer cells involves synergy between the pore-forming protein, perforin, and the serine protease, granzyrne B. Aust NZ J Med 25:793–799

Watson DL (1992) Vaccination against experimental staphylococ cal mastitis in dairy heifers. Res Vet Sci 53:346–353

Development of the Mammary Gland

5

Contents

Abstract

The mammary gland undergoes a series of structural and functional growth and differentiation depending on the reproductive stages of animals. The secretory tissue of the mammary gland is developed from ectoderm but associated connective tissues, adipose tissues, and smooth muscles are derived from mesoderm.

J. Mukherjee et al., *Veterinary Lactation Physiology*,
https://doi.org/10.1007/978-3-032-21123-1_5

Mammary stem cells (MaSCs) are multipotent adult stem cells of epithelial origin that give rise to different cellular components of the mammary gland. The specification of the mammary line is governed by different molecular signaling pathways, which subsequently develop into the formation of placode and mammary bud. Prenatal mammogenesis is characterized by the development of basic mammary structures with partially formed connective tissue, blood vessels, and lymph vessels. A notable development of the mammary gland with lobuloalveolar growth occurs after puberty, with the influence of reproductive hormones. It was estimated that 48–94% of mammary growth occurs during gestation in cows, which mostly constitutes the growth of mammary parenchyma and duct system. Lactational mammogenesis is characterized by an increase in secretory tissues that constitute 10% of mammary growth. The development of the mammary gland is regulated by ovarian hormones (estrogen and progesterone) and hypophyseal hormones (prolactin and growth hormone), along with placental lactogen, glucocorticoids, and oxytocin. There are several growth factors required for mammogenesis like insulin-like growth factor (IGF), epidermal growth factor (EGF) family, platelet-derived growth factor (PDGF), and transforming growth factor-β (TGF-β).

Graphical Abstract

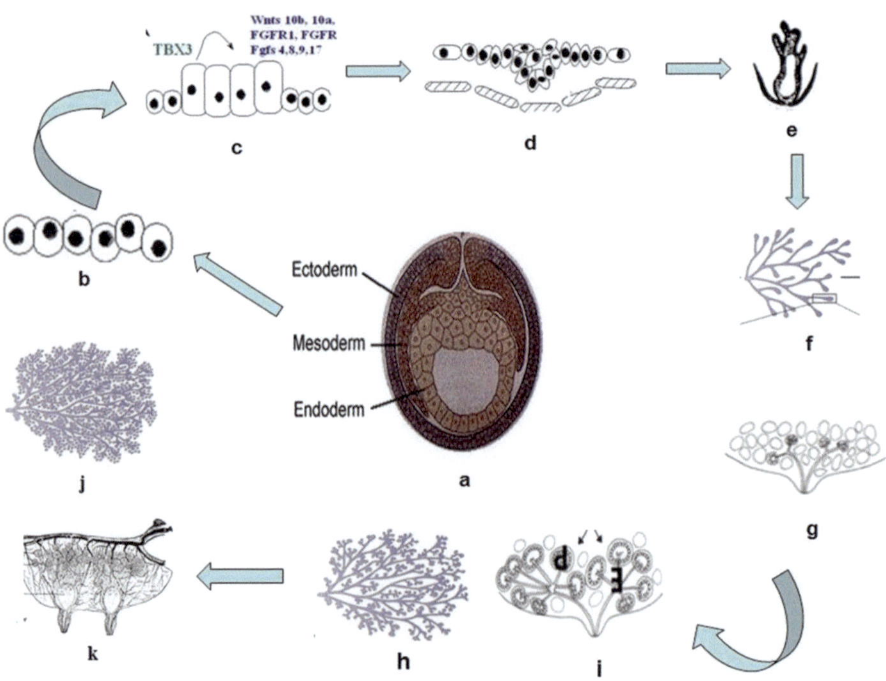

Description of the graphic: The mammary gland is developed from ectoderm (**a**) through a series of structural and functional growth and differentiation processes. Mammary stem cells (**b**) (MaSCs) give rise to different cellular components of the mammary gland through some molecular signaling pathway (**c**), which subsequently develop into placode and mammary bud (**d**). The mammary growth till birth is restricted up to canalization of secondary sprouts (**e**). Extensive growth and development of mammary ducts (**f**) is seen around puberty (**g**) under the influence of reproductive hormones. The mammary alveoli undergo budding morphogenesis (**h**) during the gestation (**i**). The proportion of secretory tissue (**j**) is increased around lactation (**k**)

Keywords

Growth factors · Hormones · Mammary stem cells · Mammogenesis

Inside the Chapter

- *Mammary stem cells (MaSCs)*
- *Embryonic mammogenesis*
- *Post-natal mammogenesis*
  - Mammogenesis from birth to puberty
  - Mammogenesis during the estrous cycle
  - Mammogenesis during gestation
  - Mammogenesis during Lactation
- *Hormones and growth factors in mammogenesis*

Learning Objectives

- Different stages of mammary gland development in cows, sheep, goats, pigs, and rats
- Mammary stem cells and their structural and functional growth and differentiation
- Molecular mechanisms controlling mammary growth and development
- Role of different hormones and growth factors in mammary gland development.

5.1 Introduction

The growth of the mammary gland is unique as the majority of mammary tissue grows postnatally. The growth and development of the mammary gland determine the milk production capacity of animals; hence, considerable research attention has been paid to exploring the underlying mechanism of mammary growth and its augmentation for better lactation performance. The mammary gland is derived from ectoderm, and associated connective tissues, adipose tissues, and smooth muscles are derived from mesoderm. The development of the mammary gland can be divided into five stages, namely prenatal, prepubertal, postpubertal, pregnancy, and lactation (Mukherjee and Das 2019). Prenatal mammogenesis is hormone-independent, whereas postnatal mammary gland development is entirely dependent on hormones. The mammary gland comprises parenchymal and stromal compartments (Mukherjee et al. 2023). The parenchyma is composed of inner luminal cells surrounding the central lumen and outer myoepithelial cells near the basement membrane (BM). The luminal cells are of two types, namely ductal and alveolar cells. The mammary stroma is composed of extracellular matrix and cellular components like mesenchymal cells, adipocytes, fibroblasts, leukocytes, and blood cells. All the cells of the mammary gland are derived from multipotent adult stem cells of epithelial origin called mammary stem cells (MaSCs). The first distinguishable feature of mammary gland development is a mammary band that appears as a single layer of flattened cuboidal cells on either side trunk from the upper limb to the lower limb, which undergoes ectodermal and mesenchymal modifications to form mammary line specification, placode, and mammary bud. The key molecular regulation of fetal mammogenesis is governed by Wingless-related integration site (WNT) and fibroblast growth factor (FGF) families of proteins that regulate several transcription factors expressed in endoderm and mesoderm such as Homeobox gene family (HOX), GATA-binding protein 3 (GATA3), and the T-box family (TBX). The postnatal is regulated by hormones (estrogen and progesterone, prolactin and growth hormone, placental lactogen, glucocorticoids, and oxytocin) and growth factors (IGF, EGF, PDGF, and TGF-β). In this chapter, the cow was used as a primary animal to discuss different aspects of mammary gland development, and the species-specific mammogenesis has been presented in a comparative manner.

5.2 Embryonic Development of the Mammary Gland

5.2.1 Mammary Stem Cells (MaSCs)

MaSCs are multipotent adult stem cells of epithelial origin that give rise to bipotent putative common progenitor cells from which unipotent luminal and basal progenitors are generated. The basal progenitor cells form ductal epithelium and myoepithelial cells, whereas luminal progenitors form secretory epithelial cells. The cell surface of markers of bovine MaSCs is a cluster of differentiation 24 (CD24) (heat-stable antigen) and CD49f (α6-integrin). The luminal progenitors are characterized by CD24 and CD49f (negative), whereas basal progenitors are characterized by cytokeratin (CK 24), smooth muscle alpha-actin (SMA), tumor protein (p63), and CD24 (negative). MaSCs undergo both symmetric and asymmetric divisions. Two daughter stem cells are generated through symmetric divisions, but asymmetric division gives rise to both stem cells and progenitor cells. Both MaSC and progenitor cells have self-renewal capacity, but the differential potential of progenitor cells is restricted compared to MaSC. Symmetric divisions of MaSC occur parallel to the basement membrane (BM), giving rise to ductal growth. In contrast, asymmetric division occurs in a perpendicular plane to generate progenitor cells apical to the MaSC. The differentiation of fetal MaSCs into unipotent luminal progenitor cells is mediated by Notch signaling (Fig. 5.1).

5.2.1.1 Mammary Band

The first distinguishable feature of fetal mammogenesis is the mammary band, which appears as a single layer of flattened cuboidal cells on either side trunk from the

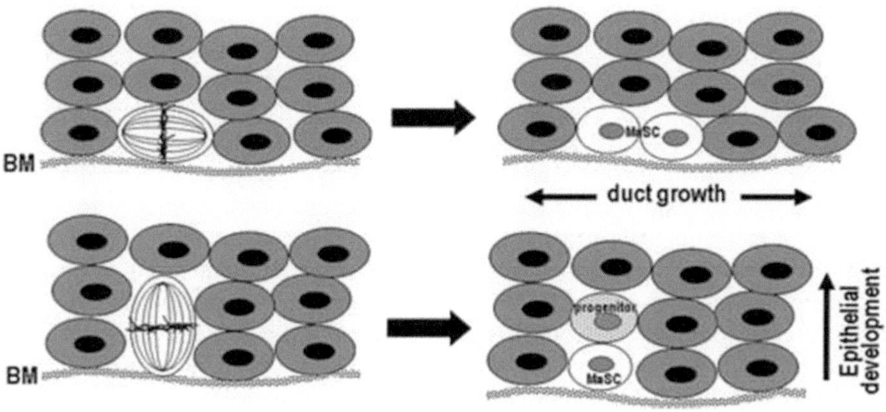

Fig. 5.1 Embryonic mammogenesis

upper limb to the lower limb. The mammary band can be appreciated in the bovine embryo as early as 32 days post-conception nearer to the time of placental attachment when the CRL of embryo is about 1.4 cm. These cuboidal cells originate from the ectoderm and their differentiation takes place in the mesoderm.

5.2.1.2 Mammary Streak

It can be appreciated in the bovine embryo at 34 days post-conception when the CRL of the embryo is 1.6 cm. It is characterized by further layering of ectodermal cells over the mammary band.

5.2.1.3 Mammary Lines

These are the transient structures that develop from the lower ectodermal layer (Malpighian or germinal layer) appreciated between fore and hind limbs posterior to umbilicus around 30, 34, and 10 days, respectively, in cows, buffaloes, and mice. The mammary lines disappear within a short span of time (35–42 days in cows) and minute lens-shaped mammary placodes are developed along the mammary lines.

The mammary placodes are developed as a result of the migration of cells that gives rise to multilayered columnar cell arrangement inside the mammary lines. There are one pair of mammary placode in humans and five pairs in mice.

5.2.1.4 Mammary Crest

The proliferation of the mesenchymal cell layer around the placodes leads to its condensation, and there is the formation of a cone-shaped mammary crest at 37 days of embryonic life in cows (CRL 1.9 cm).

5.2.1.5 Mammary Hillock

Rapid proliferation and inward growth of the ectodermal cells into the mesenchymal layer result in the formation of a dome of ectodermal cells into the mesenchyma in the form of the mammary hillock.

5.2.1.6 Mammary Bud

The continual invagination of the ectodermal layer into the mesenchymal layer and their concentric orientation result in the formation of knob-shaped mammary buds above the dermis. The ectodermal cells are then surrounded by fibroblast-like cells and sink within the collagen of the stroma with a small depression at the outer pole called the mammary pit. The underlying mesenchyme also undergoes dramatic changes characterized by condensation and elongation, which ultimately results in a sphere of epithelial cells arranged concentrically along with a stalk of epidermal-like cells that connect the skin. Two mammary buds are evident along the ventral midline of the embryo around the 41st and 43rd day post-conception in cows and buffaloes, respectively. The mammary buds give rise to the fore and rear quarters of the udder. Up to the mammary bud stage, embryonic mammogenesis is identical in both males and females. In males, mammary buds are spherical in contrast to ovoid in females. This sexual dimorphism occurs due to the interaction of testosterone with its receptor at myoepithelial cells that results in apoptosis of myoepithelial cells. The mammary gland development in females becomes faster than in males after the mammary bud stage.

Knowledge Corner...

Remarkably, male lactation has been scientifically documented in only a few species, most notably the Dayak fruit bat (*Dyacopterus spadiceus*) and the Bismarck masked flying fox (*Pteropus capistratus*). In these bats, the males have been observed to secrete milk from functional mammary glands, suggesting that under certain physiological or hormonal conditions, the male mammalian breast tissue can become sufficiently developed to support milk production. This rare occurrence provides valuable insight into the evolutionary and endocrine mechanisms underlying mammary gland function and sexual dimorphism in mammals.

5.2.1.7 Formation of Primary Sprout

The primary sprouts are formed when the solid core ectodermal cell layer invaginates deep into the mesenchymal layer. The formation of primary sprouts occurs at 56, 50, and 80 days of gestation in sheep, goats, and cattle. It gives rise to gland and teat cistern.

5.2.1.8 Formation of Secondary and Tertiary Sprouts

The secondary sprouts appear as the branches of the primary sprout. They are formed as a result of rapid growth and proliferation of ectodermal cells into the mesenchyme. Secondary sprouts are turned into tertiary sprouts due to the upward growth of secondary sprouts at various angles into the mesenchymal layer. Tertiary sprouts later convert into the duct system of the udder. The secondary sprouts are evident in sheep, goat, and cattle fetuses around 59, 60, and 90 days of gestation.

5.2.1.9 Canalization of Primary and Secondary Sprouts

The canalization of primary and secondary sprouts results in the degeneration of cells to form a lumen within the solid ectodermal core. The canalization of primary sprouts occurs in both directions, proximally toward the gland sinus and distally toward the apex of the teat. The canalization of secondary sprouts appears as irregularly shaped hollow sacks that ultimately give rise to the duct system of the mammary gland. The canalization of primary and secondary sprouts can be seen around 85 and 100 days of gestation in bovines.

5.2.1.10 Formation of Gland Cistern

Canalization of the primary sprout in the proximal direction gives rise to the formation of the gland cistern as the cell lining of primary sprouts is pushed back toward the glandular tissue. The initiation of gland cistern formation is seen around 80 days, 96 days, and 110 days in sheep, buffaloes, and cows, respectively. A fully developed gland cistern can be achieved around 181 days in buffaloes.

5.2.1.11 Formation of Teat Cistern

The downward canalization of the primary sprout results in the formation of teat cistern around 96 and 110 days of gestation in buffaloes and cattle, respectively. The tip of the mammary bud is opened. Initially, teat cistern appears like a duct, but horizontal movements of the cells increase the cavity of the teat cistern. At the distal end, streak canal is formed when the duct becomes narrow at its distal end. The Furstenberg Fürstenberg can be seen around 163 days in buffaloes near the streak canal. The keratin plug was seen around 176 days of gestation in buffaloes.

5.2.1.12 Formation of Mammary Gland-Supporting Structures

The dermis of the skin surrounding the udder is developed from the mesenchymal tissue. The epidermis and dermis layers of the skin can be observed between 74 and 115 days of gestation in bovines. The blood vessels can be appreciated at days 90, 80, and 50 of gestation, respectively, in bovines, ovines, and caprines. The nerves, along with small blood vessels, were evident around 110 days of gestation in bovine fetuses.

Fetal mammogenesis is completed within the first 6 months of gestation, and no further developments are seen thereafter before birth. At birth, the mammary gland shows the following characteristics.

- Teats are well formed.
- Canalization of secondary sprouts is partially completed and a solid core of cells is seen at the end.
- Few tertiary sprouts are present.
- Secretory or glandular parts are not well developed, and nonsecretory tissues like connective tissue, blood vessels, and lymph vessels are partially formed (Table 5.1).

Table 5.1 Features of the mammary gland during prenatal mammogenesis in different species

Stage of development	Cow		Buffalo		Pig		Sheep		Rat	
	Age of embryo (days)	Crown-rump length (mm)	Age of embryo (days)	Crown-rump length (mm)	Age of embryo (days)	Crown-rump length (mm)	Age of embryo (days)	Crown-rump length (mm)	Age of embryo (days)	Crown-rump length (mm)
Mammary band	32	14			21	10		10	11	6–10
Mammary streak	34	16			22	12				
Mammary lines	35	17	34	12	23	15			11–13	6–14
Mammary crest	37	19			25	18			12–14	12–17
Mammary hillock	40	21	37	17	26	20		20	13–15	17–18
Mammary bud	43	25	41	26	28	22	40		14–15	18–19
Early teat formation	65	80							15–18	19–30
Formation of primary sprout	80	120	57	67	40–60		60	150	14–18	18–32
Formation of secondary sprout	90	160							19	40
Canalization of primary and secondary sprouts	100	190	77	107	85		80		15–16	19–23
Formation of gland cistern	110	230	176	455						
Formation of teat cistern	130	300	181	478			140			
References	Schmidt (1971), Turner (1952)		Challana et al. (2024)		Hurley (2019), Turner (1952)		Jenkinson (2003)		Turner (1952)	

5.2.2 Molecular Basis of Embryonic Mammogenesis

During mammogenesis, the ectoderm contributes to the structural organization and mesenchyme controls the ectodermal modification during different stages of development such as mammary line specification, formation of placode, and mammary bud. The key regulators for mammary gland development are Wingless-related integration site (WNT) and fibroblast growth factor (FGF) families of proteins that regulate several transcription factors expressed in endoderm and mesoderm such as Homeobox gene family (HOX), GATA-binding protein 3 (GATA3), and the T-box family (TBX).

5.2.2.1 Specification of Mammary Line

The specification of the mammary line is governed by a mutual antagonism of the bone morphogenetic protein 4 (BMP4) and ventral site and transcription factor, TBX3, at the dorsal site. The overexpression of TBX3 results in the formation of mammary epithelium along the dorsoventral axis. In contrast, the overexpression of BMP4 inhibits TBX3 expression at the ventral site. The FGFs, namely FGF10, are released from somite tips, translocate toward the ectoderm, and interact with its receptor FGFR2b to upregulate TBX3 and WNT ligands.

TBX3 Signaling Pathway

TBX3 activates the nuclear factor kappa B (NFκB) pathway of cell cycle regulation. Tbx3 binds with NFκBIB, an inhibitor of the NFκB pathway, and blocks its action to regulate the cell cycle.

Wnt Signaling Pathway

It is also called Wnt (Tcf/Lef) signaling (Tcf: T-cell factor; Lef: lymphoid enhancer-binding factor). The Wnt signaling pathway is very crucial for almost all stages of mammogenesis. There are several Wnt ligands such as Wnt3 and Wnt6 that are present in the ectoderm Wnt5a and Wnt11 in the mesenchyme and Wnt10b in mammary placodes. The Wnt ligands are transcriptional and post-transcriptional regulating proteins that act in either canonical (β-catenin-dependent) or noncanonical (β-catenin-independent) pathways. In a canonical pathway, it is mediated through β-catenin, a crucial transcriptional factor that translocates to the nucleus and regulates the expression of target genes. In contrast, the noncanonical pathway involves the expression of target genes without β-catenin. During mammary gland development, the β-catenin-dependent Wnt signaling pathway is seen.

The β-catenin in the cytoplasm is destroyed by a "destruction complex" comprising Axin and adenomatous polyposis coli (APC) that act as scaffolds, glycogen synthase kinase-3β (GSK3β), and casein kinase 1 (CK1) that cause phosphorylation of β-catenin, followed by ubiquitination through beta-transducing repeat-containing protein (β-TrCP). Wnt proteins inhibit β-catenin destruction complex. Wnt proteins to the frizzled family of receptors on the cell surface prevent GSK3-mediated phosphorylation of β-catenin. The translocation of β-catenin to the nucleus activates target genes after binding with Tcf/Lef transcription factors. The important genes induced by β-catenin are LEF1 (lymphoid enhancer-binding factor 1), c-Myc (myelocytomatosis oncogene), T-cell factor (TCF-1), and cyclin D1 involved in cell cycle regulation and progression. LEF1 also induces the condensation of mesenchymes.

5.2.2.2 Placode Formation

The formation of mammary placode is induced by neuregulin 3 (Nrg3), a growth factor that acts through Erb-B2 receptor tyrosine kinase 4 (ErbB4) and promotes cell migration, proliferation, adhesion, and stratification. Nrg3 induces the migration of epithelial progenitor cells into the placode. However, Tbx2 and Wnt10b are also essential for the formation of placodes. TBX2 regulates the expression of cell adhesion molecules such as cadherins and integrins that facilitate epithelial cell migration during placode formation. The FGF4, FGF8, FGF9, and FGF17 are reported to be expressed in the mammary placode, and their disruption leads to impaired placode formation. Ectodysplasin (Eda), a tumor necrosis factor ligand expressed in mammary mesenchyme, is also involved in placode formation. The receptor of Eda (Edar) is identified in the epithelial cells of the mammary placode. The Edar signaling facilitates the positioning of the placode along the mammary line.

5.2.2.3 Formation of Mammary Buds

There are several signaling molecules identified in the mammary buds (Table 5.2), but the predominant regulator of mammary bud formation is parathyroid hormone-related peptide (PTHrP) secreted by the epithelial bud and acts in a paracrine manner within the mesenchyme. PTHrP interacts with its receptor, namely parathyroid hormone 1 receptor (PTHR1), in the mesenchyme and induces differentiation of mesenchyme. Eda-Edar-NFκB signaling upregulates the PTHrP mRNA within mammary buds. PTHrP-induced crosstalk between epithelial and mesenchymal tissue regulates the expression of BMPR1, LEF1, β-catenin, and MSX2. β-Catenin specifies mammary mesenchyme.

5.2.2.4 Ductal Morphogenesis, Sprout, and Lumen Formation

This stage of mammary gland development is mediated by Wnts, FGF10, Eda, and TGF-β pathways. The activation of Wnt signaling is mediated by Pygopus 2 (Pygo2), a histone methylation reader equipped for β-catenin binding. Lack of Pygo2 results in impaired elongation and branching of mammary sprouts. Branching of ducts also requires Eda and FGF10 for the development of ductal trees. Another important factor, namely latent TGFβ-binding proteins (LTBPs), also contributes to ductal morphogenesis, and it is considered an important marker for ductal luminal cells in the adult mammary gland.

Table 5.2 Signaling molecules identified in the mammary buds

Tissue	Signaling molecules	Functions	References
Epithelium	PTHrP	Induces differentiation of mesenchyme	Spina and Cowin (2021) Hens and Wysolmerski (2005)
	Wnts 10a, 10b, 6	Induction of epithelial patterning	Hens and Wysolmerski (2005) Wang et al. (2021)
	β-Catenin	Specifies mammary mesenchyme	Hens and Wysolmerski (2005) Wang et al. (2021)
	Axin2	Luminal lineage specification	Yu et al. (2016)
	LEF1	Induces the condensation of mesenchymes	Spina and Cowin (2021)
	FGFR2b, FGFR1b	Induces mammary bud formation through the activation of Tbx3 and Lef1	Pond et al. (2013)
	FGFS 4,8,9,17	Induces Tbx3 expression	Eblaghie et al. (2004)
	Sonic Hedgehog, Indian Hedgehog	Mitogenic effect on mammary stem cells Differentiation of mammary epithelial progenitors	Hui et al. (2013)
	Glioma-associated oncogene homolog (Gli2, Gli3) Patched-1 (Ptc1)	Regulates Hedgehog-associated transcriptional program. Gli2: Both activation and suppression Gli3: Suppression Ptc1: Receptor for Hedgehog (Hh) ligand	Hui et al. (2013)
	BMP2	Epithelial and mesenchymal communication	Forsman et al. (2013)
	Edar	Upregulates PTHrP mRNA within mammary buds	Spina and Cowin (2021)
	MSX1, MSX2	Branching morphogenesis	Satoh et al. (2004)
Mesenchyme	PTH1R	Receptor for PTHrP	Hens and Wysolmerski (2005)
	Eda-A1	Ductal morphogenesis through the upregulation of Wnt10a, Wnt10b, and PTHrP	Voutilainen et al. (2012)
	Wnt11, Wnt5a		

(continued)

Table 5.2 (continued)

Tissue	Signaling molecules	Functions	References
		Induces local accumulation of β-catenin (Wnt 11) Regulation of canonical Wnt signaling pathway (Wnt5a)	Yu et al. (2016)
	LEF1	Induces the condensation of mesenchymes	Spina and Cowin (2021)
	β-Catenin	Specifies mammary mesenchyme	Hens and Wysolmerski (2005) Wang et al. (2021)
	Homeobox genes (HOXA9, HOXB9, HOXC9)	Mesenchyme condensation Modulation of epithelial–mesenchymal interactions	Chen and Capecchi (1999)
	FGF7	Proliferative and morphogenic roles on both epithelial and myoepithelial cells	Palmieri et al. (2003)

5.3 Postnatal Mammogenesis

The postnatal mammogenesis can be broadly classified into four stages, namely prepubertal, postpubertal, pregnancy, and early lactation. Prepubertal mammogenesis is characterized by teat sphincter and smooth muscles that are not defined during prenatal growth. Significant mammary development in terms of ductal and lobuloalveolar growth occurs under the influence of ovarian hormones after puberty. During pregnancy, the growth of mammary parenchyma and duct system occurs. An increase in mammary secretory tissues is seen during early lactation.

5.3.1 Mammogenesis from Birth to Puberty

5.3.1.1 Cow

The prepubertal mammogenesis is characterized by the appearance of connective tissue and fat pads in the mammary gland with little growth of secretory tissue. At the initial phase of prepubertal development, the nonepithelial tissues of the mammary gland exhibit an isometric growth pattern where the mammary growth is proportionate to the body growth. The isometric growth lasts for 3 months in cows. The isometric phase of mammary growth is characterized by the growth of mammary fat pad and connective tissue, which increase the udder size. The growth of parenchyma and secretory alveoli can be appreciated during this phase. At birth, the mammary parenchyma appears like a threadlike mass and is barely palpable in heifers, which increases to 2.5 g, and the fat pad weighs around 80 g at 9 weeks of age. The mammary parenchyma grows to a tune of 60-fold from birth to 3 months of age. The isometric growth is followed by allometric growth in which mammary growth is three times faster than body growth. The allometric phase of growth lasts up to 9 months in cows. Allometric growth is characterized by extensive growth and development of mammary ducts invading the surrounding adipose tissue or mammary fat pad. The mammary tissues were reported to have 1.96 times more DNA compared to other body tissues. It was reported in heifers that the mammary gland weighed 2–3 kg after the allometric growth phase and the mammary parenchyma comprised connective tissue (40–50%), adipose tissue (30–40%), and epithelial cells (10–20%). The connective tissue within the mammary fat pad is arranged like a mesh-weave and later turns into collagenous fibrils, which will provide support to the pendulous udder. In this stage of mammary development, extensive branching of mammary ducts occurs and the distal branching of mammary ducts forms a structure called "terminal ductal unit" (TDU) analogous to the terminal ductal-lobular unit (TDLU) in the human breast. The proliferation of epithelial cells occurs progressively from the cisternal to the outer regions, and the cells at the interface of parenchyma and mammary fat pad show the highest proliferation rate. The myoepithelial cells were absent within the TDU in calves. The formation of the lumen in the TDU is facilitated by the loss of the epithelial cell junctions, and the epithelial cells are sloughed off into the lumen till the stabilization of epithelial cell layer. Cap cells of the TDLU are differentiated into myoepithelial cells. Mammogenesis from birth to 6 months of age is often used to predict milk production in mature animals.

5.3.1.2 Pigs

The mammary gland of newborn piglets comprises teat, fat pad, connective tissue, and two lactiferous ducts. The base of the teats has connective tissue support. The mammary parenchyma and fat pad show a slower growth rate till 90 days of age, which increases several folds after that. It was estimated that there was an increase in DNA per gland by fivefold after day 90 of age. The prepubertal mammogenesis in pigs is also characterized by the elongation of ducts and their canalization. The branching of primary and secondary ducts leads to the formation of several ductules that end with the terminal ductal lobular unit (TDLU) as human.

5.3.1.3 Sheep and Goat

Lambs exhibit positive allometric mammary growth between 4 and 12 weeks. A rapid growth of mammary parenchyma was seen in ewe lambs at the age of 8–16 weeks. It was recorded that there was a sixfold increase in live weight corresponding to the sixfold increase in mammary parenchyma and a fivefold increase in total mammary DNA between birth and 5 months of age. Development of mammary glands after this age is histomorphologically similar to cows.

5.3.1.4 Rodents

The mammary gland of rodents at birth appears like an epithelial rudiment that lies in the stromal environment and reaches adipose tissue. The isometric growth phase of mammary epithelial cells lasts for 22nd to 23rd day in rats. The terminal end buds (TEBs) formed at the ductal tips with epithelial cells. However, a group of newly formed epithelial cells undergo apoptosis to form a hollow luminal cavity in the TEB.

5.4 Molecular Regulation of Prepubertal Mammogenesis

At the initial phase of prepubertal mammary gland development, the proliferation of mammary epithelial cells is induced by IGF-I produced from the mammary fat pad. But the expansion of the mammary fat pad after allometric growth stimulates the synthesis of proinflammatory cytokines like tumor necrosis factor α (TNFα), interleukin (IL)-6, and IL-1b, which interferes in the insulin signaling, thus impairing the IGF-I-stimulated proliferation of epithelial cells. Other than these proinflammatory cytokines, there are several other inflammation-related proteins (IRP) like transforming growth factor β (TGFβ1), monocyte chemoattractant protein 1 (MCP-1), and plasminogen activator inhibitor-1 (PAI-1) that affect the growth of mammary parenchyma. TGFβ1 reduces the proliferation rate of epithelial cells. Being a chemoattractant molecule, MCP-1 helps in the recruitment of monocytes to the adipose tissue of the mammary fat pad. PAI-1 blocks the activity of tissue plasminogen activator together with the modulation of the activity of vitronectin and IGF-I-binding protein 5.

5.4.1 Mammogenesis During the Estrous Cycle

5.4.1.1 Cows

The mammary development during the estrous cycles in heifers is isometric. Within an estrous cycle, major mammary development is restricted at the follicular phase, particularly during estrus. The mammary DNA content is 8% higher during estrus compared to other phases. The mammary DNA content (mg/100 kg body weight) was reported to be 471 during estrus compared to 216 during diestrus. The mammary growth during the estrous cycle follows a branch-like growth pattern, along with the development of the duct system. In cows, the parenchymal growth of the mammary gland may increase up to 8% per estrous cycle, and the maximum growth occurs during the estrogenic phase of the estrous cycle. The alveolar lamina is shrunken and the epithelium turns from cuboidal to columnar during diestrus compared to estrous. There is higher collagen content in the mammary gland during estrus. In the first several estrous cycles, growth takes the form of duct lengthening, thickening, and branching. A differentiation of lobule and alveoli also occurs.

5.4.1.2 Pigs

In pigs, there is an increase in the parenchymal tissue mass by 51% and extraparenchymal tissue mass decreases by 16% during the estrous cycle compared to noncycling gilts. The ductal proliferation and elongation lead to the development of TDLU-2 from TDLU-1. Apart from the ductal proliferation, the mammary gland is characterized by a bulbous shape and undifferentiated cytology in and around the estrous cycle.

5.4.1.3 Sheep and Goat

Sheep reach puberty at 6–8 months old. The mammogenesis during the peripubertal period in goats was similar to heifers, and estrogen plays a pivotal role in mammary development during this period. A decrease in the epithelial cell proliferation rate and alteration of cell adhesion molecules were seen after ovariectomy in goats. In goat's milk, somatic cells were highest on the day of estrus, which decreased significantly during the luteal phase.

5.4.1.4 Rodents

The onset of puberty results in an allometric growth phase, along with the proliferation of ductal epithelium. The terminal end buds (TEBs) are filled with numerous epithelial cells. The proliferation of ductal epithelium leads to the formation of the branched ductal network in the mammary fat pad after several estrous cycles. There was an 8% higher DNA content in estrus compared to the luteal phase. However, the DNA synthesis in the mammary gland varies between species. It is higher in mice compared to rats during pro-estrus and estrus. A fully developed lobuloalveolar pattern is seen during diestrus with the highest rate of apoptosis.

5.5 Molecular Regulation of Mammogenesis During the Estrous Cycle

During puberty, estrogen, together with insulin-like growth factor-1 (IGF-1), regulates ductal morphogenesis and epithelial proliferation. Estrogen also acts in a paracrine fashion via the ESR1 receptor to stimulate the release of amphiregulin (AREG), which in turn induces the release of fibroblast growth factor (FGF) for luminal cell proliferation. Estrogen induces TGF-β1 signaling mechanisms to facilitate ductal bifurcation and lateral branching. Reelin (RELN) stimulates ductal elongation into the mammary fat pad. The expression of Slit2 and Netrin1 (NTN1) acts as adhesive cues to form tubular bilayers for ductal morphogenesis.

5.5.1 Mammogenesis During Gestation

5.5.1.1 Cattle

The growth of the mammary gland during gestation is allometric in nature. It was estimated that 48–94% growth of the mammary gland as a whole and 60–65% growth of mammary parenchyma occurred during gestation. The cell doubling time of the bovine mammary gland during gestation was reported as approximately 87 days, and total mammary DNA content remained unaltered after parturition in heifers. The mammary parenchyma grows extensively and replaces the adipose

Table 5.3 Summary of mammary development during pregnancy in cows

First trimester	Second trimester	Third trimester
Most of the duct growth Little increase in the secretory tissue	Growth of lobuloalveolar system Glandular proliferation increases near large ducts entering the gland cistern Further branching of small ducts Formation of end buds Secretory tissue replaces adipose tissue and forms small lobules Alveoli differentiate at the end of terminal ducts (smallest ducts)	A marked increase in the growth of duct secretory tissue, vascular system, and lymphatic system Alveoli initiated some secretory activity Epithelial cells become distended Fat droplets are present in the lumen of alveoli

tissue. The proportion of secretory tissue increases through the branching of ducts and terminal end buds by the fourth month of gestation. The secretory tissue forms the lobules, which in turn join together to form lobes. The lateral branching of the duct system occurs during early pregnancy, which leads to a connection between alveoli and primary milk-collecting ducts. The volume of the gland cistern is increased during the fifth–sixth months of gestation. The proliferation of epithelial cells decreased during mid-gestation, and these cells enter the differentiation phase during this period. The length of ducts increases up to 3 cm and appears with two layers of lining, but the ductules have a single layer of lining only. The mammary alveoli are lined by a single layer of cuboidal secretory epithelia, which become distended with granular cytoplasm and intracellular fat droplets around the ninth month of gestation prior to starting their secretory activity. There is extensive remodeling of stromal connective tissue between the lobules and lobes. The blood capillaries are seen formed around the third trimester of pregnancy. The complete development of the bovine mammary gland is seen in the term.

The development of the mammary glands in cows during pregnancy is summarized in Table 5.3.

5.5.1.2 Pigs

In swine, mammary growth is insignificant during the early gestation period except for duct development as the mammary DNA content remains unaltered during the second estrous cycle and early lactation period. The pregnancy-induced growth of the mammary gland is evident from day 74 of pregnancy with notable lobuloalveolar development. The mammary glands undergo extensive epithelial expansion and extensive lobulation and alveologenesis that lead to the formation of TDLU-3 morphotype form TDLU-2. The middle glands (3, 4, and 5) show the highest morphogenesis and become the largest, followed by the anterior (1 and 2) and posterior glands (6, 7, and 8). The massive development of mammary parenchyma was seen around the third semester (d75–d90), indicated by the threefold increase in the total DNA content. The parenchymal tissue exhibited the highest growth (200%) rates, with an increase in parenchymal DNA by ninefold between d75 and d105 of gestation. The total parenchymal cross-sectional area is increased by fourfold between d80 and d100 of gestation, which is decreased by 30% between days 100 and 110. In contrast, there is a decrease in parenchymal lipids by 70% during this period. Extraparenchymal tissue growth is reported to be 170% during 75–105 days of gestation. The mammary alveoli are lined with a single layer of epithelial cells characterized by irregular nuclei and microvilli at the apical surface during d90 of gestation. The lipid droplets are also evident at the basal surface. The cellular differentiation leads to the formation of cuboidal epithelium in the alveoli, along with an increase in lipid droplet size by d105. During this phase, the Golgi apparatus translocates to the supranuclear position. The lipid droplets occupy the majority of the cytoplasm, along with nuclear condensation. Prior to parturition, the microvilli are elongated and epithelial RNA is increased.

5.5.1.3 Sheep and Goat

In sheep and goats, the allometric growth pattern during gestation is evident around 80–115 days and 70–80 days, respectively. During this time, the mammary alveoli become engorged. The DNA doubling times of mammary tissue during gestation were 36 and 63 days, respectively, for goat and sheep. The highest proportion of epithelial tissue is seen around the 115th day of lactation in sheep. The other notable changes during this period are increased epithelial cell size, initiation of lactose synthesis, and elevation of RNA to DNA ratio. Increased number of mammary alveoli, epithelial cells, and parenchymal tissues, together with a reduction in stromal tissue, are the characteristic features of late gestation mammary growth in goats. The mammary growth during gestation was proportional to the litter size in sheep and goats.

5.5.1.4 Rodents

In rats, 20.9% of total mammary growth occurs during the first 10 days of pregnancy and 59.3% during the 20th day of pregnancy. In rabbits, 67% of mammary growth occurs during gestation, and the majority of mammary growth during gestation is seen around days 16–26. The DNA doubling time during gestation is estimated to be 7.8 and 6.7 days, respectively, for rats and mice. The weight of the mammary gland is increased from day 12 of pregnancy in mice, and the mammary DNA is doubled between days 12 and 19 of pregnancy. There is an accumulation of Golgi vesicles within the mammary secretory epithelium just before the parturition.

5.6 Molecular Regulation of Mammogenesis During Gestation

The branching morphogenesis of the mammary gland during gestation is dependent on the extracellular matrix (ECM). The ECM-receptors, ECM-degrading enzymes [matrix metalloproteinases (MMPs) and tissue inhibitors of metalloproteinases (TIMPs)] play a pivotal role in branching morphogenesis. The ECM/integrin profile varies considerably between different areas of the mammary gland depending on their morphogenic pattern. The TEBs and side branching that require proliferation, invasion, and low adhesion have different ECM/integrin profiles compared to dormant areas like primary ducts and noninvasive end buds. The MMP-3 facilitates second- and third-degree lateral branching by initiating a proteolytic cascade in the extracellular matrix (ECM). In mammary epithelial cells (MEC), MMP-3 facilitates higher expression of vimentin and lower expression of E-cadherin and β-catenin. The epithelial integrity is maintained by the E-cadherin/β-catenin complex; thus, lower expression of E-cadherin and β-catenin breaks epithelial integrity and facilitates MEC movement. MMP14 in TEB initiates the branching process.

5.6.1 Mammogenesis During Lactation

5.6.1.1 Cattle

The bovine mammary gland during lactation consists of 40–50% epithelial cells and 40% connective tissue. The lumen of the alveoli occupies 15–20% of the alveolar size. Approximately 10% of the mammary tissue growth occurs during lactation, and this growth is characterized by an increase in secretory tissues due to mitotic proliferation of cells both before and after parturition. Mammary DNA is thought to rise by about 65% during the 10 days prior to parturition and the 10 days following calving and is found at its maximum during peak lactation. Very little cell division takes place after peak lactation, and the lost cells are not replaced by newly created cells. The total mammary DNA contents (g) during early, peak, and late lactation in Holstein cattle are 96.4, 68.9, and 58.1, respectively.

5.6.1.2 Sheep and Goat

The udder growth is restricted between the last 30 days of pregnancy and the first 10 days of lactation. The udder volume is decreased during mid-lactation, and the degree of the reduction is increased with higher parities. The increase in mammary DNA in goats immediately after calving is reported to be insignificant. But there is a substantial increase in mammary DNA by 25% during the first three weeks of lactation in goats. At the onset of lactation, epithelial cells appear as columnar shapes surrounded by fibroblasts and capillaries. The number of secretory alveoli, epithelial cells, and parenchymal tissue, along with secretion in alveoli and ductules, is evident during early and mid-lactation. The stromal tissue is reduced during this period. The late lactation is characterized by reduced proliferation of alveoli and epithelial cells. The stromal tissue is increased and parenchymal tissue is reduced during late gestation.

5.6.1.3 Pigs

The mammary glands exhibit substantial growth during lactation. The total DNA in the mammary glands is increased to the tune of 82% at 21 days of lactation compared to the day of farrowing, which facilitates hypertrophy and hyperplasia of the secretory cells. The growth of the individual gland depends on the suckling intensity as the piglets have a strong teat preference. Glands 1, 6, and 7 have the least DNA content, and these glands are the smallest at day 5 of suckling. Glands 2 and 3 have intermediate DNA content, and the largest glands with the highest DNA content are 4 and 5 at day 5 of suckling. The suckling-induced mammary growth in sows continues till peak lactation. The mammary development during lactation in pigs is associated with parity, and the highest growth (70%) was seen in the first parity, which declined by 20–30% during the second and fourth parity.

5.6.1.4 Rodents

The mammary gland achieves its 98.3% of its growth by the third day of lactation in rats. The mammary DNA content is increased by 113% around peak lactation compared to late gestation probably due to suckling-induced prolactin release. If there is no suckling in rats, guinea pigs, and rabbits, then increase in mammary DNA will not occur. The declining cell numbers were reported in rats and mice during late gestation. In rabbits, 60–70% of mammary growth occurs during lactation, but, based on mammary DNA content, the growth is reported to be around 33% during lactation. The mammary gland histomorphology revealed binucleated luminal epithelial cells in mammary alveoli along with dilated milk ducts during lactation in rabbits.

5.7 Hormones and Growth Factors in Mammogenesis

The development of the mammary gland is regulated by hormones and growth factors, with their cell surface receptors in the mammary gland. The hormones important for mammary growth are ovarian hormones (estrogen and progesterone) and hypophyseal hormones (prolactin and growth hormone), along with placental lactogen, glucocorticoids, and oxytocin. Apart from these endocrine factors, there are several positive and negative growth regulators secreted from adipocytes, fibroblasts, and immune effector cells and exert local autocrine and paracrine signals to regulate mammary growth through epithelial–stromal interactions. The growth factors required for mammogenesis are insulin-like growth factor (IGF), epidermal growth factor (EGF) family, platelet-derived growth factor (PDGF), and transforming growth factor-β (TGF-β). Different histomorphological developments of the mammary gland are directed by different hormones and growth factors. The ductal elongation is mediated by estrogen, growth hormone, insulin-like growth factor-I, and epidermal growth factor, whereas progesterone, prolactin, and thyroid hormone influence ductal branching and alveolar budding. The role of hormones and growth factors during mammary gland development is also species-specific as the epithelial–stromal interactions differ between species.

5.7.1 Estrogen

Postnatal mammary ductal growth is induced by estrogen. Around 30–50% of mammary epithelial cells express estrogen and progesterone receptors. Estrogen receptors have two subtypes, namely ERα and ERβ. The expression of ERβ is

1000-fold lower compared to ERα. The location of two ER subtypes varies between species. In cattle, ERα expression is restricted to luminal epithelial cells, adipocytes, and fibroblast cells, but in other animals such as humans, monkeys, and mice, its expression is limited to epithelial cells only. Though the expression of ERβ can be seen in epithelial, myoepithelial, stromal, and fibroblast cells, their quantity is lower in bovines compared to the other species. The expression of ER also depends on the physiological state of animals. The highest expression of ERα was reported in nonpregnant heifers that gradually declined during lactation and the first 4 weeks of involution. The expression of ERβ, on the other hand, had a stable expression, except a significant increase only 2–4 weeks post milking. The action of estrogen on mammary tissue is mediated by ER in the stromal and luminal epithelial cells. The estrogen directly binds with ERα in the stromal cells and induces the release of IGF-1 that binds with IGF-1 receptors in luminal epithelial cells to induce their proliferation. Estrogen, in another way, binds to its receptor on luminal epithelial cells to induce the release of amphiregulin (AREG), an epidermal growth factor family protein that binds with its stromal cell receptors to induce the release of FGFs that bind with luminal cell receptor to stimulate the proliferation of luminal cells. In sheep, the allometric growth of the mammary gland for the first 13 weeks is independent of ovarian activity in contrast to goats.

5.7.2 Progesterone

Progesterone facilitates lobuloalveolar growth of the mammary gland in combination with estrogen. The receptors of progesterone are localized in epithelial and stromal cells, adipocytes of the mammary fat pad, and vascular tissues in cows. However, in other species (mice, monkeys, and humans), the receptors are mostly expressed in luminal epithelial cells. There are three isoforms of the progesterone receptors in heifers, namely A, B, and C. The B isoform of progesterone receptor is exclusively found in mammary epithelial cells and is thought to be the main mediator of alveologenesis. The ratio of these isoforms varies with the species and physiological state of the animals. In mice and bovines, the ratio of A and B isoforms is 3:1. During lactation and involution, only B isoforms are expressed in the mammary glands of cows. Progesterone induces the synthesis of tumor necrosis factor ligand superfamily, member 11 (TNFSF11), also known as RANKL (receptor activator of NFKB1 ligand), to induce alveologenesis. RANKL also acts in a paracrine manner to the neighboring cells to induce proliferation. RANKL is also involved in the synthesis of beta-casein (Csnb) and whey acidic protein (Wap) genes during alveolar differentiation. Progesterone induces lobular development and branching of ducts during recurrent estrous cycles in coordination with estrogen. There is also a synergistic relationship between estrogen and progesterone. Estrogen induces the expression of progesterone receptors in the epithelial cells. The mammogenic effects of progesterone are also modulated by prolactin and growth hormones.

5.7.3 Prolactin

Prolactin regulates the mammary lobuloalveolar growth, organogenesis, and functional differentiation of the mammary gland. Apart from the anterior pituitary, prolactin can also be synthesized from nonhypophyseal peripheral cell types like mammary epithelial cells. Hypophyseal prolactin acts over the mammary gland through classical endocrine pathways, whereas locally synthesized prolactin acts in a paracrine or autocrine fashion. Prolactin mediates both direct and indirect actions on the mammary gland. In the direct mechanism, prolactin binds with its specific receptors (PRLR) on the mammary gland epithelium and induces signal transduction via Janus kinase 2 (JAK2) and signal transducers and activators of transcription (STAT). The major mediator of prolactin in the mammary gland is STAT5a, which facilitates lobuloalveolar development during pregnancy. Indirectly, prolactin synthesizes some mammotropic factors from other organs to induce ductal branching and regression of the terminal end bud. Prolactin-induced mammotropic factors are IGF-1, EGF, Wnt gene products, keratinocyte growth factor (KGF), neuregulin (NRG), and hepatocyte growth factor (HGF) that facilitate epithelial–stromal crosstalk to induce growth and morphogenesis of mammary epithelium. Prolactin also stimulates the secretion of progesterone from the corpus luteum, which also induces lobuloalveolar growth of the mammary gland. The role of prolactin in the mammogenesis of cattle is questionable. According to some authors, prolactin induces positive allometric mammary growth in cattle during the peripubertal period. However, some authors reported a strong negative correlation between parenchymal growth and serum prolactin levels in prepubertal heifers. In pigs, prolactin alone fails to induce mammary growth. But prolactin in combination with estrogen can induce considerable mammary growth in this species. Gestational mammogenesis is mediated by prolactin in pigs from 90 to 109 days of gestation. In small ruminants, complete lobuloalveolar development requires prolactin, together with estrogen and progesterone. The histomorphogenic changes from TDLU-2 to TDLU-3 are mediated by prolactin and estrogen in sheep. Prolactin has a little role in mammary development during late pregnancy in sheep and goats, but the lactogenic differentiation of the mammary gland requires prolactin for optimal milk secretion. The mammogenic effects of prolactin on laboratory animals are well documented. In these species, prolactin stimulates lobuloalveolar growth during pregnancy.

Knowledge Corner...

Gynecomastia refers to the benign enlargement of the mammary glands in males, resulting from an elevated estrogen-to-androgen ratio. This condition has been observed in several species, including rams, bulls, dogs, rabbits, and goats. Hormonal imbalance may occur due to increased concentrations of free estrogens, reduced levels of free androgens, or abnormalities in androgen receptor function. Additionally, single-nucleotide polymorphisms (SNPs) in the prolactin gene have been associated with the occurrence of gynecomastia in goats.

5.7.4 Growth Hormone

The mammogenic role of growth hormone (GH) has been established for a long time in hypophysectomized, adrenalectomized, and ovariectomized rats. In heifers, exogenous growth hormone administration facilitates mammary parenchymal growth. The GH receptor is structurally similar to the prolactin receptor and composed of a single transmembrane domain and acts through Janus tyrosine kinases (JAK), which induces phosphorylation of a transcription factor(s), namely signal transducer and activator of transcription (STAT). The effect of GH on the mammary gland is either direct or indirect. The direct action of GH on the mammary tissue facilitates the growth and proliferation of mammary parenchyma. Indirectly, GH induces the secretion of IGF-1 and IGF-binding proteins (IGFBP) in the stromal cells, adipocytes, and hepatocytes that act via autocrine, endocrine, and paracrine mechanisms to facilitate mammary growth and development. In mice, stimulation of mammary growth by GH is potentiated by induced expression of stromal ER. Exogenous administration of GH in prepubertal heifers induces mammary development, but, in cattle, GH decreases the number of IGF-I-binding sites throughout pregnancy and the IGF-I binding affinity increases with advancing lactation. In pre- and postpubertal ewe, GH induces parenchymal development. GH facilitates ductal development, along with increasing the volume and mass of the udder in goats. Lactation stage-specific action of GH was reported in goats. GH has a little role in mammary cell proliferation during early lactation, but it induces a total volume of secretory tissue when administered during mid-lactation.

5.7.5 Glucocorticoids

The effect of glucocorticoids on growth and differentiation is controversial. Some authors suggested that they are essential for mammary growth and differentiation while others have designated glucocorticoids as synergistic hormones, not essential for mammogenesis. The expression of mammary glucocorticoid receptors (GRs) varies with the reproductive state of the animals. They gradually increase during gestation, stabilize around late pregnancy, and peak around parturition. The level of GR during lactation is similar to prepartum but drops suddenly during involution. These changes correlate with the stage-specific growth and differentiation of the mammary gland. Cortisol is reported to be involved in the epithelial cell proliferation and lobuloalveolar growth of mammary glands in mice and cows, respectively. The differentiation of mammary epithelium by cortisol facilitates prolactin to induce the synthesis of milk proteins. Upon receptor binding, cortisol exerts its effect through glucocorticoid response elements (GREs) that bind with DNA to induce transcription or via a DNA binding-independent protein–protein interaction. The epithelial proliferation is dependent on a DNA binding-dependent mechanism, but synthesis of milk protein is induced upon a DNA binding-independent protein–protein interaction. The differentiations induced by cortisol include modification of the ultrastructure of the mammary gland such as the development of rough endoplasmic reticulum and sealing of tight junctions required for copious milk secretion. Cortisol also regulates ECM to maintain the viability of mammary secretory epithelium.

5.7.6 Insulin

Insulin acts as a mitogenic hormone to induce a permissive effect on mammary growth and development. Insulin is unable to initiate the proliferation of new cells; rather, it helps to complete the divisional cycles that are already initiated. Earlier studies hypothesized that the action of insulin may mimic the action of IGF-1 as insulin exerts its effect through IGF-1 receptors. But recently it was found that insulin receptor B isoform (IRB) was only stimulated by insulin, not IGF-1 or IGF-2, as tyrosine phosphorylation of IRB protein is induced only by insulin. The expression of IRB was increased threefold at lactation day 1 in the murine mammary gland. Insulin induces differentiation of the mammary gland during late pregnancy to early lactation in the mouse mammary gland. The notable effects of insulin include expansion of the alveolar lumen, hyperplasia of mammary epithelium, and increased cytoplasmic droplets in the acini.

5.7.7 Placental Lactogen

Placental lactogen is mammogenic in rodents, where it helps in the expansion of the lobuloalveolar system by lobular budding during pregnancy and lactational differentiation during milk synthesis. However, the mammogenic effect of placental lactogen in cows remained doubtable as long as the concentration of placental lactogen was lower and the exogenous administration of placental lactogen had little effect on metabolism in lactating cows. Further, it was challenging to distinguish the mammogenic effects of prolactin and placental lactogen as both of the hormones act through prolactin receptors in the mammary gland. But exogenous administration of recombinantly derived bovine placental lactogen stimulates mammogenesis and lactogenesis in steroid-primed dairy heifers treated with bromocriptine (a prolactin antagonist). This study also confirmed that the mammogenic effect of placental lactogen is not mediated via prolactin receptors. The exogenous administration of bovine placental lactogen increased mammary parenchyma by 46–62% in heifers primed with estrogen and progesterone. In small ruminants, placental lactogen plays a notable role in mammary epithelial cell proliferations because in these species there is a positive correlation between the number of litters and milk yield. In ewe, the concentration of placental lactogen increased from day 50 of pregnancy and reached a peak prior to parturition. In guinea pigs, the concentration of placental lactogen is positively correlated with total mammary gland DNA and the wet weight of the mammary gland. The exact mechanism of the mammogenic effect of prolactin is yet to be resolved, but it was assumed that it stimulates mammary growth via locally produced growth factors like somatomedins and their binding proteins (IGFBPs).

5.8 Growth Factors

5.8.1 Insulin-Like Growth Factors (IGFs)

The mammogenic actions of IGF are regulated by the complex interactions between IGF ligands (IGF-I, IGF-II, and insulin), their receptors (IGF-IR, IGF-IIR, and insulin R), and IGF-binding proteins (IGFBP 2, 3, 4, and 5). IGF is mainly produced in the liver, but it is also produced in local tissues like the uterus and mammary gland. In the mammary gland, IGF is produced from stromal cells and mammary epithelial cells under the influence of growth hormone. Both IGF-I and II regulate cell growth, cell differentiation, and prevention of apoptosis in a endocrine, autocrine, or paracrine fashion in many species, including cattle, sheep, goats, pigs, and mice. IGF also facilitates cellular communication and cell–extracellular matrix (ECM) crosstalk. The primary receptor for IGF-I is IGF-IR that are expressed throughout mammary epithelium during all stages of postnatal mammary development. In addition, IGF-IR is also expressed in mammary stroma during pubertal, postpubertal, and gestational mammary growth in humans. In bovines, IGF-IIR is predominant, but its precise role is unknown. It is hypothesized that IGF-IIR is involved in the removal of IGF. Upon receptor binding, IGF-I initiates a downstream signaling cascade through the phosphorylation of tyrosine residues of an adaptor protein called insulin receptor substrate I (IRS-I), which activates phosphatidylinositol 3′kinase (PI3K) and serine-threonine kinase (Akt). This Akt promotes cell survival by inactivating the proapoptotic protein BAD, which causes cell death through phosphorylation. The IRS-I also induces RAS proteins and phosphorylation of β-catenin. Both RAS and β-catenin promote cell proliferation by stimulating cyclin D1. IGF-I induces TEB formation and ductal elongation in rodents through paracrine action. In mouse mammary glands, stroma-derived IGF-I acts as a local effector of growth hormone in combination with estrogen. In ewe, the highest expression of IGF-I mRNA in the mammary epithelial cells was reported around 4 weeks of postnatal age to promote allometric mammary growth before puberty and then gradually declined in adults. In cows, decreased IGF-I receptors were noted during pregnancy and lactation.

5.8.2 Epidermal Growth Factor (EGF) Family

The epidermal growth factor family comprises nearly 10 members, including EGF, transforming growth factor α (TGFα), heparin-binding EGF, neuregulins (four subtypes), amphiregulin, and several heregulins. All factors act through type I receptor tyrosine kinases or the ErbB. This receptor is a transmembrane glycoprotein having a molecular weight of 170 kDa and comprises an external domain for binding with ligands and an internal cytoplasmic domain with tyrosine kinase activity. Based on the binding of ErbB receptors, EGF ligands can be grouped into three categories. EGF, TGFα, and AREG are specific for only ErbB 1. Epiregulin (EREG), betacellulin (BTC), and heparin-binding EGF (HBEGF) can bind with both ErbB 1 and 4. Among the neuregulins (NRG), NRG1 and NRG2 are specific ligands for ErbB3 and ErbB4, whereas NRG3 and NRG4 can only bind with ErbB4. The actions of EGF families of proteins depend upon the phosphorylation of cytoplasmic substrates.

5.8.2.1 Epidermal Growth Factors (EGFs)

EGF has an important role in mammary gland growth and differentiation in different species, including rodents. EGFs act through ErbB-1 receptors found in mammary ducts and surrounding stromal cells. The higher expression of ErbB-1 receptors was reported during mid-pregnancy compared to late pregnancy and lactation in cows. Both in vitro and in vivo studies have demonstrated that EGF induces DNA synthesis in mammary tissues in cows and sheep. IGF acts as a mitogen for mammary epithelial cells and induces duct growth in mice. EGF is also involved in epithelial–stromal interactions in the mammary gland through autocrine and paracrine action. Estrogen-induced production of EGF facilitates stromal cell proliferation and TEB formation through paracrine action, but studies have reported that locally produced EGF alone can facilitate duct growth in ovariectomized mice. The maximum proliferation of mammary tissue in bovines can be achieved upon EGF treatment induced by estrogen and progesterone. EGFs have a dose-dependent response. In bovine mammary tissue culture, EGF can induce DNA synthesis at a concentration of 10 nM, whereas a high dose of EGF was reported to inhibit the growth of TEB in mice.

5.8.2.2 Transforming Growth Factor (TGF)

Transforming growth factor-α (TGFα) is reported to be a potent mitogen for mammary epithelial cells in rats, humans, and cows. It induces lobuloalveolar growth of mammary glands in virgin mice with higher potency than EGF. The localization of TGFα mRNA in mammary ductal and alveolar cells increased to a tune of two to threefold during pregnancy and lactation in rats and humans. Fifteen percent of stromal cells also express TGFα mRNA during pregnancy. The effect of TGFα is potentiated by estrogen as the TGF gene contains estrogen-responsive elements.

TGFβ, in contrast, inhibits epithelial cell proliferation, regulates remodeling of extracellular matrix (ECM), controls epithelial–mesenchymal interaction, and stimulates apoptosis. The expression of TGFβ mRNA is restricted in end buds, duct epithelium, and stromal cells. The expression of TGFβ is highest in heifers during mammogenesis and involution. The lower level of TGFβ expression is seen during lactogenesis and galactopoiesis. TGFβ induces the synthesis of ECM proteins like laminin, fibronectin, and collagen IV, along with inhibition of ECM proteases such as type IV collagenase, plasminogen activator inhibitor 1 (PAI-1), and urokinase type plasminogen activator (uPA) to modulate ECM structure during involution. There are three receptors of TGFβ, namely TGF-βR1, TGF-βR2, and betaglycan. TGF-βR1 and TGF-βR2 are abundant in ductal epithelium and alveoli in heifers.

5.8.2.3 Neuregulins (NRGs)

Neuregulins play a pivotal role in the embryonic development of the mammary gland. They are expressed in mesenchyme and epithelial tissue during pregnancy in mice. NRG has three isoforms, namely NRG 1, 2, 3, and 4, out of which NRG3 induces placode formation during embryonic development by aggregating epithelial cells during the middle of embryogenesis. NRG3 binds with its specific receptors ErbB4 to exert its action. The epithelial aggregation is stimulated by NRG3 as a mesenchymal paracrine signal during placode formation. NRG3 also promotes stem cell renewal and specification of mammary lineage along with their differentiation. Neuregulin also stimulates lobuloalveolar differentiation in vitro mammary cell culture and induces the expression of β-casein.

5.8.2.4 Amphiregulin (AREG)

AREG is the most abundant EGF ligand in the mammary gland around puberty to regulate estrogen-primed ductal morphogenesis during puberty. AREG was identified in the luminal epithelium, myoepithelial cells, and stroma of the mammary gland. The transcription of AREG is regulated by estrogen. The binding of estrogen with its receptor (ERα) in the mammary gland activated transcriptional co-activator CITED1 to facilitate the synthesis of the inactive amphiregulin precursor. A disintegrin and metalloprotease 17 (ADAM17) cleaves inactive AREG to its active form in the epithelial cells. Active AREG then transverses into the cap cells of TEB, where it interacts with ErbB1 in the surface of stromal cells. Interaction of AREG with its receptors initiates downstream signaling pathways to produce growth factors like HGF or IGF-1 locally that induce the proliferation.

5.8.2.5 Heparin-Binding EGF (HB-EGF)

It is so named due to the presence of a heparin-binding domain at the amino-terminal end. HBEGF acts through the EGF receptor to induce mitogenic response in mammary epithelial cells. It is expressed in the mammary gland of mice at the onset of pregnancy and exists till parturition. The expression is decreased during lactation and re-expression occurs during involution (Table 5.4).

Table 5.4 Species-specific EGF ligands and ErbB receptors during different stages of mammogenesis

Species	EGF ligands			ErbB receptors		
	Puberty	Gestation	Lactation /involution	Puberty	Gestation	Lactation/involution
Mice	Amphiregulin (AREG) (epithelium) TGFα (epithelium) Epiregulin (EREG) Heparin-binding EGF (HBEGF) (epithelium and adipocytes)	AREG, EREG, HBEGF and TGFα (onset of gestation) EREG and TGFα (downregulated at the end of gestation) NRG1 (peak at day 15 of gestation) EGF (progressivelyIncreases from mid-gestation	EGF (lactation) TGFA, HBEGF, and NRG1 (Involution)	ErbB1 (stroma), ErbB2 (MEC), and ErbB3	ErbB1 (ducts), ErbB2 (ducts), and ErbB3 (MEC)	ErbB1, ErbB2, and ErbB3 (all three receptors are decreased during lactation and re-expressed during involution)
Rats	TGFα (ductal and alveolar epithelium) AREG, EREG, HBEGF (adult virgin rats)	TGFα (MEC, stroma)	TGFα (MEC, stroma)	ErbB1 (TEB) ErbB2 (epithelial and stroma) ErbB3 (ducts and stroma) ErbB4 (TEBs, stroma, and ducts)	ErbB1, 2, and 3 (MEC, ducts, and stroma) ErbB1 (the alveoli)	ErbB1 (downregulated in all cell type)
Cow	EGF, TGFα	TGFα	TGFα (onset of the dry period)	ErbB1, ErbB2, ErbB3, and ErbB4	ErbB1	ErbB1
Sheep	AREG, EGF, and TGFα	AREG, EGF (goat)	AREG, EGF, TGFα	ErbB1	ErbB1	
Dogs						

(continued)

Table 5.4 (continued)

Species	EGF ligands			ErbB receptors		
	Puberty	Gestation	Lactation /involution	Puberty	Gestation	Lactation/involution
				ErbB1 (myoepithelial cells and the perilobular stroma in most normal and mammary tumors, upregulated during estrus) ErbB2 (epithelium, overexpressed during tumor)		
Cats				ErbB2 (lower expression in normal animals, overexpressed during mammary malignant tumor)		

Exercises

Objective Questions

1. Ductal growth of the mammary gland is mediated by ____________________________ hormone.
2. The secretory tissue of the mammary gland is developed from________________.
3. The first distinguishable feature of mammary gland development is_________________.
4. Extensive branching of mammary ducts occurs and the distal branching of mammary ducts forms a structure called___________________.
5. The cell surface of markers of bovine MaSCs are _____________, ___________, and __________.
6. In __________________ phase of growth, the mammary growth is proportionate with the body growth.
7. The lens-shaped minute structures developed as a result of the migration of cells that gives rise to multilayered columnar cell arrangement inside the mammary lines are called________________.

Subjective Questions

1. Briefly describe the molecular mechanism behind the specification of mammary lines.
2. Describe the role of prolactin in mammary growth.
3. How do ovarian hormones help in mammogenesis in cows?
4. Describe in brief the interactions between IGF ligands (IGF-I, IGF-II, and insulin) during mammogenesis.
5. Write in brief the functions of mammary epithelial cells.

Answers to Objective Questions

1. Estrogen
2. Ectoderm
3. Mammary band
4. Terminal ductal unit
5. CD24, heat-stable antigen, and CD49f
6. Isometric growth
7. Mammary placode

References

Books

Mukherjee J, Das PK (2019) Immune responses of mammary gland. In: Sar TK (ed) Mastitis: symptoms, triggers and treatment, 1st edn. Nova Science Publishers, Inc., New York, p 89

Mukherjee J, Das PK, Banerjee D (2023) Lactation physiology. In: Das PK, Sejian V, Mukherjee J, Banerjee D (eds) Textbook of veterinary physiology. Springer, Singapore. https://doi.org/10.1007/978-981-19-9410-4_25

Schmidt GH (1971) Biology of lactation. W. H. Freeman, San Francisco

Turner CW (1952) The mammary gland, 1st edn. Lucas Brothers, Publishers, Missouri, Columbia, p 383

Research Articles

Challana A, Gupta A, Bansal N, Uppal V (2024) Morphogenesis of Mammary Glands in Buffalo (*Bubalus bubalis*). Anat Res Int 2014:687936

Chen F, Capecchi MR (1999) Paralogous mouse Hox genes, Hoxa9, Hoxb9, and Hoxd9, function together to control development of the mammary gland in response to pregnancy. Proc Natl Acad Sci USA 96:541–546. https://doi.org/10.1073/pnas.96.2.541

Eblaghie MC, Song SJ, Kim JY, Akita K, Tickle C, Jung HS (2004) Interactions between FGF and Wnt signals and Tbx3 gene expression in mammary gland initiation in mouse embryos. J Anat 205(1):1–13. https://doi.org/10.1111/j.0021-8782.2004.00309.x

Forsman CL, Ng BC, Heinze RK, Kuo C, Sergi C, Gopalakrishnan R, Yee D, Graf D, Schwertfeger KL, Petryk A (2013) BMP-binding protein twisted gastrulation is required in mammary gland epithelium for normal ductal elongation and myoepithelial compartmentalization. Dev Biol 373(1):95–106

Hens JR, Wysolmerski JJ (2005) Molecular mechanisms involved in the formation of the embryonic mammary gland. Breast Cancer Res 7(5):220–224

Hui M, Cazet A, Nair R, Watkins DN, O'Toole SA, Swarbrick A (2013) The Hedgehog signalling pathway in breast development, carcinogenesis and cancer therapy. Breast Cancer Res 15:203. https://doi.org/10.1186/bcr3401

Hurley WL (2019) Mammary gland development in swine: embryo to early lactation. Animal 13 (S1):S11–S19

Jenkinson CMC (2003) The pattern and regulation of mammary gland during foetal life in the sheep [Ph.D. Dissertation], Massey University, Palmerston North, New Zealand, 2003

Palmieri C, Roberts-Clark D, Assadi-Sabet A, Coope RC, O'Hare M, Sunters A, Hanby A, Slade MJ, Gomm JJ, Lam EWF, Coombes RC (2003) Fibroblast growth factor 7, secreted by breast fibroblasts, is an interleukin-1beta-induced paracrine growth factor for human breast cells. J Endocrinol 177(1):65–81. https://doi.org/10.1677/joe.0.1770065

Pond AC, Bin X, Batts T, Roarty K, Hilsenbeck S, Rosen JM (2013) Fibroblast growth factor receptor signaling is essential for normal mammary gland development and stem cell function. Stem Cells 31(1). https://doi.org/10.1002/stem.1266

Satoh K, Ginsburg E, Vonderhaar BK (2004) Msx-1 and Msx-2 in mammary gland development. J Mammary Gland Biol Neoplasia 9(2):195–205

Spina E, Cowin P (2021) Embryonic mammary gland development. Semin Cell Dev Biol 114:83–92

Voutilainen M, Lindfors PH, Lefebvre S, Ahtiainen L, Fliniaux I, Rysti E, Murtoniemi M, Schneider P, Schmidt-Ullrich R, Mikkolaa ML (2012) Ectodysplasin regulates hormone-independent mammary ductal morphogenesis via NF-κB. Proc Natl Acad Sci 109(15):5744–5749

Wang J, Song W, Yang R, Li C, Wu T, Bing Dong X, Zhou B, Guo X, Chen J, Liu Z, Yu QC, Li W, Fu J, Zeng YA (2021) Endothelial Wnts control mammary epithelial patterning via fibroblast signaling. Cell Rep 34:108897. https://doi.org/10.1016/j.celrep.2021.108

Yu QC, Verheyen EM, Zeng YA (2016) Mammary development and breast cancer: a Wnt perspective. Cancer 8(7):65. https://doi.org/10.3390/cancers8070065

Lactogenesis

6

Contents

Abstract

Lactogenesis refers to the onset of milk secretion, marked by enzymatic and structural differentiation of the mammary alveolar cells. This functional transformation of the mammary gland in preparation for milk synthesis is driven by hormonal changes during pregnancy and early lactation. These hormonal shifts lead to the up- and downregulation of genes responsible for secretory differentiation and activation. Throughout this process, the alveolar cells exhibit ultrastructural changes such as an increase in DNA content, a higher presence of mitochondria, Golgi apparatus, and secretory vesicles. Additionally, microvilli

J. Mukherjee et al., *Veterinary Lactation Physiology*,
https://doi.org/10.1007/978-3-032-21123-1_6

begin to appear and the tight junctions between cells close, signaling further maturation. As secretory activation begins, key enzymes involved in glycolysis, the pentose phosphate pathway, and the synthesis of milk components like fat, protein, and lactose are activated to support the metabolic needs of milk production. This heightened metabolic demand during early lactation places dairy cows under significant metabolic stress, often resulting in a state of negative energy balance (NEB). To adapt, the body prioritizes nutrient allocation through homeostatic and homeorhetic mechanisms. One major adjustment is the development of insulin resistance, which helps redirect glucose toward the mammary glands by boosting liver gluconeogenesis and minimizing glucose use by other tissues. Enhanced fat breakdown (lipolysis) and reduced fat storage (lipogenesis) allow fatty acids to serve as key energy sources and contribute to milk fat synthesis. Concurrently, muscle protein is broken down to supply amino acids for glucose production via gluconeogenesis. Various body systems realign to support these metabolic shifts. The skeletal system undergoes increased bone demineralization to supply minerals needed for milk production. Digestive and renal systems adapt to improve nutrient absorption and retention. Cardiovascular activity also increases, ensuring greater blood supply to the mammary glands. However, elevated glucocorticoid levels and changes in blood metabolites can significantly suppress the immune system, making cows more vulnerable to diseases during this critical period of lactation.

Graphical Abstract

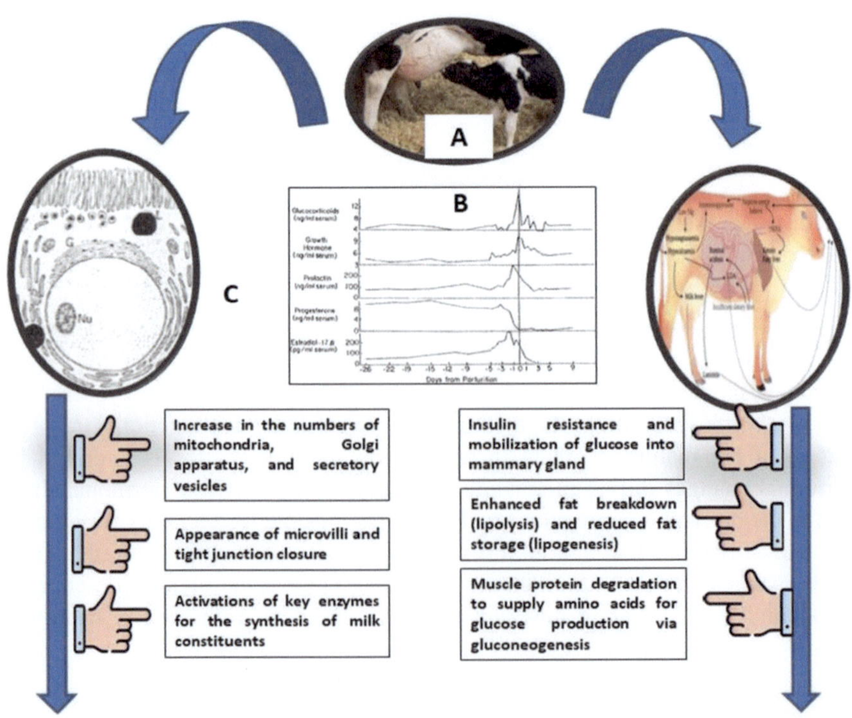

Description of the graphic: Lactogenesis, or the initiation of milk secretion (**A**), is regulated by hormonal changes occurring during pregnancy and early lactation (**B**). These hormonal shifts promote both enzymatic activity and structural changes in the mammary alveolar cells (**C**), marked by an increase in mitochondria, Golgi apparatus, and secretory vesicles, along with the formation of microvilli and the sealing of tight junctions. The process of secretory activation involves the activation of key enzymes necessary for producing milk components. During this time, the body undergoes metabolic adaptations (**D**) that prioritize directing nutrients to the mammary gland for milk production. These changes include the development of insulin resistance and increased glucose transport to the mammary tissue, enhanced breakdown of fat (lipolysis) and reduced fat synthesis (lipogenesis) for generating milk fat, as well as muscle protein breakdown to provide amino acids for gluconeogenesis and milk protein synthesis

Keywords

Lactogenesis · Secretory differentiation · Secretory activation · Metabolic adaptation · Homeorhesis

Inside the Chapter

- *Key lactation factors for the initiation of lactation*
  - Endocrine factors
  - Molecular factors
- *Secretory differentiation of mammary gland*
- *Secretory activation of mammary gland*
- *Metabolic adaptations during the initiation of lactation*
  - Feed intake and digestion
  - Glucose metabolism
  - Lipid metabolism
  - Protein metabolism
  - Mineral Metabolism
- *Adaptive changes in other organs during the initiation of lactation*
  - Digestive system
  - Excretory system
  - Cardiovascular system Muscular system
  - Skeletal system
  - Immune system

Learning Objectives

- Secretory differentiation and activation of mammary epithelial cells at the initiation of milk secretion
- Metabolic adaptations during the initiation of lactation to cope up negative energy balance
- Alterations in the different body systems to support metabolic adaptations during lactogenesis

Lactogenesis refers to the initiation of milk production, marking the beginning of secretory activity in the mammary gland characterized by the enzymatic and cytological differentiation of mammary alveolar cells. The mammary gland undergoes progressive structural changes that lead to the onset of abundant milk secretion either in late pregnancy or around the time of birth. The timing of lactogenesis differs across species. In ruminants, significant mammary gland secretory activity occurs during the latter half of pregnancy. Conversely, in species like rats, mice, and pigs, this activity typically begins in the final stages of pregnancy. In primates, however, lactogenesis is triggered after the placenta is expelled at birth. Historically, lactogenesis was thought to occur in two distinct stages. The first stage, known as lactogenesis I, involved limited milk secretion during late pregnancy, while the second stage, lactogenesis II, was marked by a substantial increase in milk production following childbirth. These stages were later redefined as secretory differentiation and secretory activation, respectively. Secretory differentiation involves the transformation of mammary epithelial cells into lactocytes—specialized cells capable of producing milk components such as lactose, casein, α-lactalbumin, and fatty acids. Secretory activation refers to the onset of copious milk secretion.

6.1 Key Lactation Factors for the Initiation of Lactation

6.1.1 Endocrine Factors

The functional differentiation of the mammary gland for the preparation of milk production is affected by the alteration of endocrine milieu during pregnancy and lactation (Table 6.1). The term "lactogenic complex" was used to denote a group of hormones of pituitary, ovarian, and placental origin. Studies in rats showed that the secretory differentiation was initiated after the addition of progesterone and prolactin in the rats treated with estrogen, growth hormone, and deoxycorticosterone acetate. In contrast, estrogen and progesterone withdrawal favors secretory activation. In most of the mammals, studies to date have shown that estrogen, progesterone, and prolactin, together with glucocorticoids and insulin, are required for secretory differentiation. Growth hormone has a permissive action on the initiation of lactation. The endocrine profile around parturition is characterized by decreasing levels of progesterone and placental lactogen and increasing levels of prolactin, estrogen, prostaglandin F2α, oxytocin, and adrenal steroids.

6.1.1.1 Progesterone

Progesterone is one of the major factors of inhibition of lactation during pregnancy in all eutherian mammals. The inhibition of lactation by progesterone is mediated through two pathways. Firstly, it inhibits the action of prolactin by blocking the prolactin receptors, and secondly, it inhibits the formation of α-lactalbumin, an important component of enzyme lactose synthetase. Therefore, the withdrawal of

Table 6.1 Endocrine alterations and their responsiveness in different tissues during late pregnancy and lactation in ruminants

Hormones		Late pregnancy	Early lactation/ lactogenesis	Mid-lactation
Potential homeorhetic hormones	Progesterone	↓	↓	↑
	Placental lactogen	↑	↓	–
	Estrogens	↑	↓	–
	Prolactin	↓	↑	No significant change
	Somatotropin	↓	↑	No significant change
	Leptin	Unknown	Unknown	Unknown
Homeostatic hormones	Insulin	↑	↓	–
	Glucagon	No significant change	No significant change	No significant change
	CCK and Somatostatin	Unknown	Unknown	Unknown

Ingvartsen and Andersen (2000), Mukherjee et al. (2023)

progesterone after parturition is one of the potent stimuli for the initiation of lactation. Progesterone competes with glucocorticoids for their receptors. Hence, the withdrawal of progesterone promotes the lactogenic action of glucocorticoids. Progesterone withdrawal also stimulates triglyceride uptake from plasma and increase in the mammary blood flow.

6.1.1.2 Estrogen

The concentration of estrogen increased during peripartum, and it was thought that increasing estrogen levels triggers the lactation initiation by stimulating prolactin release. Estrogen triggers the transcription of prolactin gene and favors its secretion. Estrogen also has mitogenic roles in the mammary gland after binding with its receptor in epithelial and stromal cells. Estrogen also has an influence on other hormones required for lactogenesis. Estrogen stimulates the release of uterine PGF2α from the sheep.

6.1.1.3 Adrenal Corticoids

Adrenal corticoids are required to induce lactation in the hypophysectomized rat, mouse, and goat but not in rabbits. The role of adrenal corticoids on lactogenesis is effective after the withdrawal of progesterone as progesterone competes with glucocorticoid receptors. Adrenal corticoids promote the differentiation of rough endoplasmic reticulum and Golgi complex. They also favor milk protein synthesis induced by prolactin.

Prostaglandin $F_{2\alpha}$ (PGF2α)

The PGF2α is involved in the luteolysis and normal termination of pregnancy; hence, it is postulated that PGF2α has some role in the lactogenesis. PGF2α is an important mediator of prolactin action. It also stimulates the release of other lactogenic hormones such as prolactin, growth hormone, and glucocorticoids.

6.1.1.4 Prolactin

Prolactin plays a pivotal role in the lactogenesis in several species of mammals. Prolactin plays a crucial role in the differentiation of milk initiation and galactopoiesis. Prolactin binds with prolactin receptors to activate Janus kinase (JAK2)/signal transducer and activator of transcription 5 (STAT5) signaling pathway, which augment milk protein genes. The declining concentration of progesterone at the end of pregnancy triggers α-lactalbumin synthesis and activation of lactose synthetase for the synthesis of milk sugar. Prolactin also controls water and electrolyte transport and the synthesis of immunoglobulins.

The lactogenesis in ruminants is triggered mainly by prolactin and glucocorticoids. However, for the maximum action of these hormones, declining level of progesterone is essential. Other hormones like thyroid hormones act in conjugation with prolactin for the synthesis of α-lactalbumin.

6.1.2 Molecular Factors

The altered endocrine milieu around parturition is associated with transcriptional switch that leads to up- and downregulation of certain genes associated with secretory differentiation and activation.

6.1.2.1 Cattle

In cattle, the major changes in the expression pattern of genes are associated with cellular (40%) and physiological (37%) processes. More than 10 genes associated with the transport of amino acids (SLC7A5, SLC1A4, SLC1A5, and SLC6A), glucose (SLC2A1), electrolytes (SLC39A12, SLC34A2, and SLCO1A2), and other nutrients (SLC25A21 and VLDL-R2) are upregulated during the initiation of lactation. Around 18 genes associated with metabolism of glucose, lipid, protein, and nucleic acid are upregulated during lactogenesis. The upregulated genes are associated with glucose transport are 6-phosphofructo-2-kinase, pyruvate dehydrogenase kinase 4, and carbonic anhydrase VI. Genes are associated with lipid metabolism such as lipoprotein lipase, acetyl-CoA synthetase 2, long-chain acyl-CoA synthetase homolog 1, and aldo-keto reductase family 1. The other upregulated genes are cell signaling factors [STAT5, protein p8, Rab18, sterol regulatory element-binding transcription factor 1 (SREBP1)], cytokines, and growth factors (IGF-I). STAT5 mediates the functions of several hormones such as prolactin, somatotropin, and interleukins 3 and 5. STAT5 phosphorylates are also essential for the differentiation of mammary epithelial cells. SREBP1 regulates fat synthesis by PUFAs. Among the upregulated genes, lactoperoxidase and parathyroid hormone-like hormone showed maximum increase to the tune of 80- and 30-folds, respectively, from late gestation to early lactation. The downregulated genes during lactogenesis are associated with cell proliferation (cyclins, cell division cycle-associated proteins), DNA replication (centromere proteins, minichromosome maintenance proteins, histone), microtubule-associated protein (tau, kinesin, tubulins), and RNA degradation proteins (RNA-binding motif protein, proteasome, proteasome activator).

6.1.2.2 Goats

In goats, the major genes upregulated during lactation in goats are mainly associated with lipid and protein metabolism. Aldehyde dehydrogenase 2 (ALDH2), acetyl-CoA acetyltransferase (ACAT), and long-chain acyl-CoA synthetase isoform 1 (ACSL1) are the top three expressed genes in the fatty acid metabolism pathway during 100 and 310 days postpartum. The genes associated with lactose synthesis such as lactose synthase B protein (LALBA), beta-1, 4-galactosyltransferase I (B4GT1), and UTP–glucose-1-phosphate uridylyltransferase (UGPA) were also expressed during the initiation of lactation. The genes encoding milk proteins such as beta-lactoglobulin (BLG) and alpha-lactalbumin (LALBA) and casein (CSN1S1, CSN1S2, CSN2, and CSN3) are significantly upregulated during the first 100 days postpartum, but the expression of genes such as CSN1S1, CSN1S2, and LALBA is decreased at 310 days postpartum.

6.1.2.3 Pigs

The lactogenesis in sow are associated with the upregulation of certain differentially expressed genes associated with secretory activation of mammary epithelial cells. The most upregulated genes are associated with colostrogenesis. These changes are induced by endocrine factors with the activation of transcription factors such as SREBP1 and XBP1. The upregulated genes during colostrogenesis in sows are casein alpha-S2 (CSN1S2), LALBA, whey acidic protein (WAP), serum amyloid A2 (SAA2), and butyrophilin subfamily 1 member A1 (BTN1A1).

6.1.2.4 Sheep

The transciptome analysis of sheep mammary gland during lactation has revealed that there was a substantial increase in the genes associated with protein synthetic machinery. The top 10 genes upregulated during lactation are genes associated with milk protein synthesis (*CSN2*, *LGB*, *LALBA*, *CSN1S1*, *CSN1S2*, *CSN3*) and eukaryotic translation elongation factor 1 alpha 1 (*EEF1A1*), glycosylation-dependent cell adhesion molecule 1 (*GLYCAM1*), fatty acid synthase (*FASN*), and ribosomal protein S29 (*RPS29*). The most expressed gene was β-casein gene (CSN2). The *GLYCAM1* gene encodes milk fat globule glycoprotein.

6.2 Secretory Differentiation of the Mammary Gland

The secretory differentiation is required to develop biochemical and cytological machinery to synthesize milk. The potential milk secretory epithelial cells undergo differentiation during the peri-parturient period in response to different endocrine factors. Several studies have confirmed that the proliferation of mammary epithelium (hyperplasia) occurs during gestation, whereas the cell differentiation (hypertrophy) is the characteristic feature during lactation.

Rodents

In rodents, the differentiation of mammary gland alveoli occurs with the formation of lobuloalveolar structures under the influence of prolactin. Prolactin induces insulin-like growth factor (IGF-2), which facilitates the transcription of Wnt4, RankL, and cyclin D1 associated with the proliferation of mammary epithelial cells. The changes that occur around pregnancy are an increase in ductal branching and alveolar bud formation with a concomitant increase in mammary DNA content. In the latter half of gestation, the alveolar buds form lobuloalveolar units, which subsequently give rise to pre-secretory alveolar unit, and the size of epithelial compartment is increased. The luminal space is occupied by some proteinaceous substance during the late pregnancy, which may contain immunoglobulin, lactoferrin, and Muc1. The secretory alveolar compartment becomes more prominent after the parturition with the expansion of the luminal compartment. The mammary gland starts secreting copious amounts of milk by the ninth day of lactation in mice.

Ruminants

The proliferation of mammary epithelium occurs during pregnancy in cows and decreased after parturition. In contrast, mammary growth continues till early lactation in dairy goats, with a maximum during day 5 of lactation. The mammary DNA is increased by nearly 65% during 10 days prior to pre-calving and found to be maximum during peak lactation. In pregnant mammary gland, the areas of stroma, epithelium, and lumen were 33%, 34%, and 32%, respectively. The number and volume of secretory alveoli are increased between day 280 of gestation and 50th day of lactation, which is indicated by a decrease in the stromal tissue. The percentage of active epithelium is increased and nonactive epithelium is decreased progressively from 15 days prepartum to the day of calving. Around the 15th day precarving, the nuclear area increased significantly, with a decrease in the percentage of rough endoplasmic reticulum, Golgi complex, and mitochondria. The number of vacuoles and cytoplasmic fat droplets was appreciated in higher numbers. There were abundant lysosomes in the cytoplasm. The percentage of mitochondria, Golgi, and secretory vesicles started increasing from the seventh day prepartum, along with an increase in the cytoplasm to nucleus ratio. The secretory activity of the epithelium is indicated by the appearance of fat droplets and casein-containing vesicles under the apical plasma membrane. The appearance of microvilli can also be appreciated 1 week prior to calving. The epithelial cells become cuboidal and flat with the accumulation of fat and protein granules. Around calving, the Golgi and secretory vesicle increased with a decrease in fat and nuclei. The mammary secretory epithelium becomes polarized with abundant rough endoplasmic reticulum, Golgi bodies, mitochondria, and secretory vesicles containing casein. The microvilli at the apical surface are protruded into the lumen of the alveoli. The nuclei become oval and located at the basal surface, and there is an increase in the cytoplasm to nucleus ratio.

Another important aspect of secretory differentiation of the mammary gland is the tight junction closure. During pregnancy, the tight junctions are leaky and closed during the time of parturition. During lactation, the complete closure of tight junctions occurs. The closing of tight junction is regulated by local factors (intramammary pressure and TGF-β) and systemic factors (progesterone, glucocorticoids, and progesterone). The decrease in the permeability of tight junctions is associated with increased milk secretion rate.

In goats, the growth of mammary gland is highest on day 5 of lactation, reached a plateau, and decreased slight on the 30th day of lactation. The total mammary gland DNA content of virgin goats was 196 ± 52 mg, which increased almost ninefold (962 ± 150 mg) during 1 day prepartum and reached exponentially up to 3958 ± 681 mg on the fifth day of lactation. The decreased growth of the mammary gland from the 5th to 30th day coincides with the reduced DNA content during this period. The total RNA content is also increased tenfold from 62 ± 22 mg in virgin goats to 627 ± 146 mg, 3651 ± 1293 mg, and 5553 ± 456 mg, respectively, during mid-pregnancy, parturition, and first 2 days of lactation.

Knowledge Corner...
Certain marsupials, such as the tammar wallaby, can simultaneously produce two distinct types of milk from separate teats—one providing nutrient-dense milk for the older young-at-foot, and the other delivering a more dilute milk suited for the newborn in the pouch.

6.3 Secretory Activation of the Mammary Gland

In cows, milk constituents are synthesized before the parturition, which indicates that the onset of secretory activation starts parallel with structural differentiation of the mammary gland. In contrast, the enzymatic activation of the mammary gland occurs immediately after the parturition in rats and guinea pigs. Another important difference related to lactogenesis between these two species is that in cows there are no significant alterations in the availability of mammary gland metabolites during early lactation unlike in rats.

The secretory activation of the mammary gland is characterized by the development of enzymatic machinery in newly differentiated secretory cells for the synthesis of milk. The increase in the enzymatic activities was seen in rats during the first 3 days of lactation and no further increase in the activities was seen till the 15th day of lactation. The important enzymes that are activated during the initiation of lactation are depicted in Table 6.2.

Rodents

In rats, the lactose starts synthesizing in the mammary gland before parturition, and the amount of lactose synthesized on the 29th day of pregnancy is two-thirds of normal milk. The accumulation of lactose was correlated with the increased activities of lactose synthetase and α-lactalbumin. In guinea pigs, the concentration of milk lactose and proteins is reported to increase during the time of pregnancy and early lactation (Table 6.3), which indicates the initiation of the secretory activities during late pregnancy and early lactation. The maximum activities of the enzymes were recorded during the second and third days of lactation in guinea pigs.

Table 6.2 Important enzymes activated during the initiation of lactation

Metabolic pathways	Enzymes involved
Glycolysis	Hexokinase, glucose-6-P isomerase, fructose-1,6-di phosphate aldolase, glyceraldehyde-3-P dehydrogenase
Hexose monophosphate pathway	Glucose-6-P dehydrogenase, P-gluconate dehydrogenase
Milk fat synthesis	α-Glycerol-P dehydrogenase, fatty acid synthetase, citrate cleavage enzyme
Milk lactose synthesis	UDP glucose-4-epimerase, UDPG pyrophosphorylase, glucose phosphomutase
Amino acid metabolism and protein synthesis	Aspartate aminotransferase
Mitochondrial activity	Succinate debydrogenase, butyryl-CoA dehydrogenase
General metabolic status	Isocitrate dehydrogenase, extramitochondrial malate dehydrogenase

Table 6.3 Changes in guinea pig mammary glands during pregnancy and lactation

Stage		Tissue weight (gm)	Lactose (mg)/gram sample	Protein (mg)/gram sample	RNA (mg)/ gram sample	DNA (mg)/ gram sample
Pregnant						
	40 days	5.3	2.8	43	1.3	2.6
	60 days	5.9	4.4	44	1.0	3.1
Lactating						
	0–6 h	7.0	10.9	50	1.3	5.9
	2 days	12.7	10.6	55	3.3	10.0
	3 days	14.1	12.3	64	3.8	9.1
	5 days	10.1	10.5	47	4.0	7.5
	10 days	16.4	8.5	49	2.9	5.8
	15 days	9.8	7.4	43	2.1	4.5

Baldwin (1966)

Table 6.4 Ratios of enzyme activities between late pregnancy and early lactation in guinea pigs

Enzyme	Ratios of enzyme activities	
	Pregnant 65 days	Lactating 3 days
G]ucose-6-P dehydrogenase	1	1
6-P-Gluconate dehydrogenase	0.39	0.17
Fructose-l,6-di P aldolase	1	1
Glyceraldehyde-3-P dehydrogenase	2.7	2.3
Glucose-6-P isomerase	14.5	9.8
Fatty acid synthetase	1	1
Citrate cleavage enzyme	1.4	1.3
Glycerol-P dehydrogenase	2.8	0.5
UDP ghcose-4-epimerase	1.6	1.4
Succinic dehydrogenase	0.02	0.02

Baldwin (1966)

The activities of enzymes during late pregnancy are different from the initiation of lactation, and very little changes occurred thereafter (Tables 6.4 and 6.5).

Ruminants

Similar to rodents, the synthesis of milk constituents starts before parturition in cows, but the activities of enzymes change a little. It has been reported that the concentration of lactose increases from 8 to 10 days prepartum and reaches about half of the concentration of normal milk just before the partition (Table 6.6). The concentration of glucose is low around 2 days prepartum and increased during lactation. The amount of casein is also increased before prepartum and decreased gradually on the second day postpartum. The noncasein proteins are decreased concomitantly with increased lactose concentration.

The enzymatic alterations in the mammary gland of cows during late gestation and early lactation are different from rodents. No changes in the enzymatic activities between late gestation and early lactation were reported (Table 6.7), which was consistent with the constant level of proteins and DNA in the mammary tissue during this period. These findings have confirmed that ruminants do not suddenly achieve enzymatic potential.

Pigs

In sow, the mammary growth during lactation is characterized by a 55% increase in tissue mass and a 100% increase in DNA per gland during 5 and 21 days of lactation. The presecretory activation of mammary gland in sows is indicated by the alteration in the mammary gland metabolites. The concentrations of different metabolites in sow mammary gland during 6–11 days postpartum are depicted in Table 6.8.

The concentrations of glucose, lactose, G6P, UDP, and Pi are increased, whereas the concentrations of G1P, galactose, and fructose are decreased from parturition to

Table 6.5 Alterations in the enzyme activities (units/gm of tissue) in the mammary gland of guinea pigs during pregnancy and lactation

Enzymes	Stages				
	Pregnant (40 days)	Pregnant (60 days)	Lactating (0–6 hrs)	Lactating (2 days)	Lactating (5 days)
Hexokinase	0.3 ± 0.14	0.42 ± 0.08	0.93 ± 0.40	2.08 ± 0.56	1.52 ± 0.72
Glucose-6-P mutase	1.79 ± 0.18	2.59 ± 0.65	4.10 ± 1.17	7.02 ± 3.41	9.01 ± 4.80
Glucose-6-P isomerase	11.5 ± 2.76	14.5 ± 6.34	23.4 ± 8.43	35.1 ± 5.32	48.3 ± 24.2
Fructose-l,6-diP aldolase	1.03 ± 0.58	1.00 ± 0.29	2.73 ± 1.27	4.54 ± 0.88	4.49 ± 1.96
Glyceraldehyde-3-P dehydrogenase	1.46 ± 0.35	2.70 ± 1.37	7.5 ± 2.27	7.00 ± 1.22	10.2 ± 4.74
Isocitrate dehydrogenase	3.32 ± 0.88	4.42 ± 1.30	11.1 ± 4.15	14.7 ± 2.70	17.3 ± 2.70
Succinate dehydrogenase	0.007 ± 0.003	0.018 ± 0.008	0.034 ± 0.0017	0.049 ± 0.028	0.055 ± 0.040
Butyryl-CoA dehydrogenase	0.009 ± 0.004	0.028 ± 0.016	0.040 ± 0.019	0.105 ± 0.026	0.118 ± 0.027
Aspartate aminotransferase	5.14 ± 0.73	6.16 ± 1.33	7.30 ± 2.67	14.1 ± 1.82	13.7 ± 0.76
Glucose-6-P dehydrogenase	2.91 ± 1.29	3.2 ± 0.80	8.04 ± 3.32	20.4 ± 5.26	20.3 ± 6.56
P-gluconate dehydrogenase	0.62 ± 0.14	1.27 ± 0.72	2.33 ± 1.14	4.98 ± 2.06	4.51 ± 0.62
UDP g]ucose-4- epimerase	0.80 ± 0.192	1.61 ± 0.370	2.04 ± 0.69	6.58 ± 0.942	4.62 ± 1.71
UDPG pyrophosphorylase	8.84 ± 1.76	17.2 ± 2.23	23.9 ± 6.94	70.3 ± 27.3	54.2 ± 18.3
Malate dehydrogenase	9.15 ± 2.97	9.1 ± 1.79	12.3 ± 8.29	37.5 ± 14.0	34.4 ± 10.4
Citrate cleavage enzyme	0.23 ± 0.06	0.17 ± 0.07	0.31 ± 0.27	1.06 ± 0.35	1.27 ± 0.23
Fatty acid synthetase	0.10 ± 0.03	0.12 ± 0.04	0.16 ± 0.04	0.9 ± 0.11	1.32 ± 0.71
α-Glycerol-P dehydrogenase	0.12 ± 0.02	0.34 ± 0.13	0.42 ± 0.16	0.52 ± 0.16	0.35 ± 0.27

Baldwin (1966)

Table 6.6 Concentration of milk constituents during prepartum in cows

Stage	Milk constituents				
	Lactose (g/100 g)	Glucose (mg/100 g)	Casein (g/100 g)	Noncasein (g/100 g)	Fat (g/100 g)
45 days prepartum	0.05 ± 0.03	1.1 ± 0.2	0.24 ± 0.007	37 ± 3.8	0.5 ± 0.24
5 days prepartum	1.7 ± 0.13	2.6 ± 0.8	4.8 + 0.15	13 ± 0.7	4.3 ± 0.2

Hartmann (1973)

day 5 lactation. The concentrations of UDPgal, UDPglc, AMP, cAMP, ADP, and UMP are decreased between parturition and 1–2 days of lactation. There was a striking difference between the concentrations of different metabolites in sow mammary gland during early lactation between suckled and unsuckled mammary gland. In unsuckled mammary gland, the concentrations of the aforesaid metabolites remain unchanged between parturition and 2 days postpartum. The activities of enzymes in the mammary tissue of sow during 30 days postpartum were studied (Table 6.9), and it was found that there was a linear relationship between the ratios of lactose to fat and the ratios of the activities of the UDP glucose-4-epimerase and fatty acid synthetase.

6.4 Metabolic Adaptations During the Initiation of Lactation

The high metabolic priority for milk production during the initiation of lactation imposes tremendous metabolic challenges in dairy cows, which results in a negative energy balance (NEB). In high-yielding cattle, 80% of net energy intake and 85% of circulating glucose are utilized for milk production. The fundamental consequence of NEB is the partitioning of nutrients toward the mammary gland to favor the lactation. There are two types of regulations involved in the partitioning of nutrients, namely homeostasis and homeorhesis. The term homeostasis refers to the ability of the body to maintain constant physiological equilibrium. Homeorhesis, on the other hand, refers to the alterations in the metabolism of body tissues to support a physiological state. The classic example of homeorhesis is the metabolic change occurring during the initiation of lactation (Table 6.10). The major metabolic changes happen in homeorhesis and include an insulin-resistant state in which the sensitivity and responsiveness to insulin are decreased in many peripheral tissues (Table 6.11). A significant decrease in insulin concentration was also reported after calving. This decreased insulin status favors transporting glucose to tissues that are less dependent on insulin such as the mammary gland. The magnitude of insulin sensitivity in dairy cows is measured using the euglycemic–hyperinsulinemic clamp test. In this test, insulin is infused at a constant rate to elevate plasma insulin level along with simultaneous glucose administration at different rates to maintain euglycemic state (normal blood glucose). Stimulation of somatotropic axis during the initiation of lactation causes high-circulation somatotropin (bST). Reduced insulin and high bST promote lipolysis and mobilization of fatty acids to the

Table 6.7 Alterations in the enzyme activities (units/gm of tissue) in the mammary gland of cows during pregnancy and lactation

Enzymes	Stages				
	14 days prepartum	Lactating (0–10 hrs)	Lactating (3 days)	Lactating (10 days)	Lactating (40 days)
Hexokinase	0.205 ± 0.086	0.178 ± 0.038	0.19 ± 0.072	0.23 ± 0.107	0.495 ± 0.209
Glucose-6-P mutase	1.30 ± 0.36	2.88 ± 0.931	2.85 ± 1.25	1.98 ± 0.634	2.32 ± 0.424
Glucose-6-P isomerase	6.21 ± 2.82	5.81 ± 1.51	8.03 ± 2.20	8.02 ± 2.99	7.06 ± 5.47
Fructose-l,6-diP aldolase	1.26 ± 0.691	1.21 ± 0.447	1.37 ± 0.53	0.714 ± 0.174	0.896 ± 0.285
Glyceraldehyde-3-P dehydrogenase	0.754 ± 0.288	1.23 ± 0.633	1.23 ± 0.38	0.871 ± 0.506	2.26 ± 2.13
Isocitrate dehydrogenase	16.9 ± 6.43	28.6 ± 9.54	14.1 ± 10.4	13.6 ± 6.44	58.8 ± 12.9
Succinate dehydrogenase	0.048 ± 0.013	0.059 ± 0.013	0.333 ± 0.018	0.049 ± 0.029	0.066 ± 0.042
Butyryl-CoA dehydrogenase	0.174 ± 0.026	0.128 ± 0.064	0.155 ± 0.031	0.145 ± 0.062	0.211 ± 0.110
Aspartate aminotransferase	3.96 ± 0.774	4.25 ± 1.06	3.41 ± 0.88	3.58 ± 1.66	4.56 ± 0.989
Glucose-6-P dehydrogenase	2.06 ± 0.517	1.7 ± 0.373	1.32 ± 0.519	1.21 ± 0.922	1.30 ± 0.463
P-gluconate dehydrogenase	0.895 ± 0.895	0.968 ± 0.315	0.891 ± 0.165	0.786 ± 0.297	1.11 ± 0.380
UDP g]ucose-4- epimerase	0.878 ± 0.195	1.24 ± 0.446	0.836 ± 0.515	1.04 ± 0.657	1.70 ± 1.26
UDPG pyrophosphorylase	5.8 ± 1.64	5.43 ± 1.83	10.8 ± 5.25	7.35 ± 3.18	16.5 ± 9.77
Malate dehydrogenase	8.03 ± 1.42	7.9 ± 1.27	7.06 ± 2.41	5.8 ± 1.59	9.66 ± 3.26
Citrate cleavage enzyme	0.182 ± 0.066	0.812 ± 0.166	0.816 ± 0.115	0.167 ± 0.080	0.211 ± 0.105
Fatty acid synthetase	0.484 ± 0.16	0.462 ± 0.027	0.367 ± 0.145	0.322 ± 0.244	0.599 ± 0.257
α-Glycerol-P dehydrogenase	0.147 ± 0.038	0.162 ± 0.066	0.247 ± 0.079	0.266 ± 0.110	0.523 ± 0.230

Baldwin (1966)

Table 6.8 The concentrations of different metabolites in sow mammary gland during 6–11 days postpartum

Mammary gland metabolites	Concentration between 6 and 11 days postpartum
Glucose	669 μM (220–1367)
Glucose 6-phosphate (G6P)	63·0 μM (27·6–101·4)
Glucose 1-phosphate (G1P)	18·3 μM (13·1–24·8)
UDP glucose (UDPglc)	296 μM (170–494)
UDPgalactose (UDPgal)	635 μM (230–945)
Lactose	162 mM (124–187)
UDP	105 μM (85–130)
UMP	1760 μM (1326–2587)
Inorganic phosphate	135 mM (1·4–29·3)
ATP	<0·5 μM
ADP	53·6 μM (10·5–171·25)
AMP	215 μM (61·6–491·6)
cAMP	22·3 μM (3·5–61·6)
Galactose	198 μM (118–474)
Fructose	226 μM (172–283)

Atwood and Hartmann (1995)

Table 6.9 Alterations in the enzyme activities (units/gm of tissue) in the mammary gland of sows during 30 days postpartum

Enzymes	Enzyme activities in the mammary gland 30 days postpartum
Hexokinase	0.436 ± 0.096
Glucose-6-P mutase	7.75 ± 2.03
Glucose-6-P isomerase	14.1 ± 3.78
Fructose-l,6-diP aldolase	1.44 ± 0.482
Glyceraldehyde-3-P dehydrogenase	3.03 ± 0.728
Isocitrate dehydrogenase	6.27 ± 0.689
Succinate dehydrogenase	0.189 ± 0.048
Butyryl-CoA dehydrogenase	0.510 ± 0.263
Aspartate aminotransferase	19.4 ± 10.2
Glucose-6-P dehydrogenase	25.3 ± 14.2
P-gluconate dehydrogenase	1.62 ± 0.570
UDP g]ucose-4- epimerase	3.92 ± 0.819
UDPG pyrophosphorylase	40.8 ± 21.0
Malate dehydrogenase	26.0 ± 13.7
Citrate cleavage enzyme	2.16 ± 0.856
Fatty acid synthetase	3.59 ± 1.56
α-Glycerol-P dehydrogenase	0.303 ± 0.104

Baldwin (1966)

Table 6.10 The major metabolic adaptations during the state of NEB

Function	Metabolic changes	Tissues involved
Feed intake and digestion	Increase in food and water intake	CNS
	Hypertrophy of digestive tract	All segments of GI tract
	Increased nutrient absorption	
Lipid metabolism	Increased lipolysis Decreased lipogenesis	Adipose tissue
Glucose metabolism	Increased gluconeogenesis and glycogenolysis	Liver
	Utilization of acetate for energy (ruminanta)	Mammary gland
Protein metabolism	Mobilization of protein reserve	Muscle and other body tissue
Mineral metabolism	Increased absorption and mobilization of reserve	Gut, bone, kidney, and liver
Water metabolism	Increased absorption and expansion of plasma volume	Gut, kidney, CNS

Bauman and Currie (1980)

mammary gland and gluconeogenesis in the liver for the synthesis of glucose. The major metabolic and physiological alterations at the initiation of lactation are summarized in Table 6.10.

6.4.1 Feed Intake and Digestion

Impairment in the feed intake has been reported in transition dairy cows. The voluntary dry matter intake (VDMI) in cows is reported to decrease from the 26th week of pregnancy to the tune of 0.17 kg/week till 3 weeks before calving. Nearly a 30% decrease in the dry matter intake (DMI) occurred during 5–6 days prepartum. The lowest VDMI was reported at calving and increased rapidly during the first 3 weeks of lactation and estimated increase by nearly 1.5–2.5 kg/weeks. The VDMI is 20% lower in primiparous cows than multiparous.

Regulation in the feed intake in animals is a complex process; many of the mechanisms are yet to be explored. The feed intake during the transition period is regulated by several factors such as hormones, neuropeptides, and blood metabolites. Other indirect regulators of feed intake are environmental factors and physical constraints.

The hepatic oxidations of metabolic fuels are the main regulator of feed intake in animals. The oxidation of fuels generates ATP, which controls the satiety center by altering the firing rate of the hepatic vagus nerve. Generation of higher ATP in hepatic oxidation decreases the firing rate and suppresses satiety, whereas lower ATP during decreased oxidation stimulates hunger by increasing the firing rate of the hepatic vagus nerve. The major metabolic fuels that are oxidized in the liver of ruminants are nonesterified fatty acids (NEFA), amino acids, glycerol, lactate, amino acids, and propionate. However, the NEFAs are the primary fuels. The NEFAs

Table 6.11 The tissue sensitivity and responsiveness to some homeorhetic and homeostatic hormones during late pregnancy and early lactation

Hormones		Late pregnancy	Early lactation/ lactogenesis	Mid-lactation
Tissue sensitivity	Insulin	↓	↓	↑
	Catecholamines	↑	↑	–
Tissue responsiveness	Insulin	↓	↓	–
	Catecholamines	↑	↑	↓
Liver	Gluconeogenesis	–	↑	–
	Ketogenesis	–	↑	–
Adipose tissue	Lipogenesis	↓	↓	↑
	FA esterification	↓	↓	↑
	Lipolysis	↑	↑	–
	Glucose utilization	↓	↓	–
Skeletal muscle	Protein synthesis	↓	↓	–
	Protein degradation	↑	↑	–
	Glucose utilization	↓	↓	–

Ingvartsen and Andersen (2000)

undergo oxidation to yield acetyl-CoA, which is further oxidized completely or generates ketone bodies. During the time of high lipid mobilization, the rate of NEFA oxidation becomes limited that increases ketone bodies in blood. The complete oxidation of fatty acids generates 14 ATPs. As the ATP is the main driver of satiety and hunger, the feed intake in ruminants is mainly controlled by the circulating NEFA concentration. During the immediate peripartum period, the NEFA concentration remains elevated due to increased fat mobilization in response to decreased insulin sensitivity. The hepatic oxidation of NEFA generates more ATP, which decreases feed intake during this period. The propionate stimulates the oxidation of acetyl-CoA. Therefore, the diet containing high starch during this period can increase propionate and further diminishes feed intake. As the lactation advances, the concentration of insulin, growth hormone, and blood glucose increases (Table 6.12).

In response to increased plasma insulin and glucose along with decreased GH, the lipolysis decreases and NEFA concentration in blood is lowered. Studies have shown that NEFA concentration was the highest on the day of calving and 3 days postpartum but rapidly declined on days 14 and 21 postpartum (Garverick et al. 2013). Decreased NEFA in blood limits the ATP generation through oxidation, which decreases satiety signals and feed intake increases.

Hormone insulin, leptin, and ghrelin control feeding behavior in cows by stimulating certain neuropeptides and neurotransmitters such as proopiomelanocortin, α-melanocyte-stimulating hormone, and agouti-related

Table 6.12 The concentrations of insulin, growth hormone, and blood glucose during different days of postpartum period in cows

Parameters	Days postpartum		
	1–20	21–40	41–56
Insulin (μU/mL)	8.8 ± 0.5	10.3 ± 0.4	11.9 ± 0.6
GH (ng/mL)	19.3 ± 1.0	16.4 ± 1.2	13.6 ± 1.1
Glucose (mg/100 mL)	37.3 ± 0.7	40.6 ± 0.8	43.3 ± 0.8

Smith et al. (1976)

Table 6.13 The concentrations of leptin, ghrelin, and NEFA during different days of postpartum period in cows

Weeks relative to peripartum	Ghrelin (Pg/mL)	Leptin (ng/mL)	NEFA (mmol/L)
−3	5.50 ± 8.66	5.99 ± 0.11	0.20 ± 0.04
−2	44.70 ± 7.32	6.01 ± 0.09	0.20 ± 0.03
−1	44.85 ± 6.96	5.57 ± 0.17	0.21 ± 0.04
0	65.40 ± 5.30	5.22 ± 0.06	0.28 ± 0.02
1	70.85 ± 4.92	3.69 ± 0.09	0.35 ± 0.04
2	74.55 ± 6.84	3.23 ± 0.15	0.35 ± 0.04
3	74.90 ± 4.49	3.20 ± 0.04	0.45 ± 0.11
4	74.95 ± 4.50	3.01 ± 0.05	0.34 ± 0.03
5	70.45 ± 2.89	3.11 ± 0.10	0.33 ± 0.03
6	65.45 ± 6.97	3.10 ± 0.09	0.34 ± 0.02

Nowroozi-Asl et al. (2016)

proteins within the central nervous system. Decreased insulin concentration during calving and immediate postpartum period inhibits proopiomelanocortin and α-melanocyte-stimulating hormone that activate anorexic pathways and decreased feed intake during this period.

Leptin is secreted from the white adipose tissue in ruminants and is involved in energy homeostasis. Higher concentration of leptin causes diminished feed intake and increased energy expenditure, whereas low concentration of leptin induces feed intake by modulating the activity of the neurons located in the arcuate, ventromedial, and dorsomedial hypothalamic nuclei. The state of negative energy balance is associated with reduced plasma leptin level that induces feed intake and depletion of lipid reserve. The secretion of leptin is regulated by insulin and GH secretion. Decreased level of insulin and increased level of GH induce leptin release. The leptin concentration is reported to increase during the postpartum period (Table 6.13). When the cow is under positive energy balance, insulin becomes a positive regulator of leptin secretion.

Another important regulator of feed intake during the initiation of lactation is ghrelin secreted from the stomach in animals. It is also an indicator of negative energy balance and strongest peripheral stimulator for the food intake. Increased concentration of ghrelin during the postpartum period (Table 6.10) increases the demand for feed during lactation.

Spexin (SPX) is a neuropeptide expressed by neurons in the hypothalamus. The expression of SPX was also found in the stomach, small intestine, and colon of cows and reported to control feed intake during the transition period in cows. The concentration of spexin is negatively correlated with NEFA and ghrelin concentration. It is also inversely related to progesterone and blood metabolites. Spexin inhibits appetite in mammals. It has been reported that spexin concentration decreased from 21 days prepartum to calving and increased during the 14th day of lactation.

6.4.2 Glucose Metabolism

It has been estimated that nearly 72 grams of glucose is required to produce 1 kg of milk. Therefore, the consumption of glucose in the mammary gland is tremendously increased during the initiation of lactation and nearly 50–85% of whole-body glucose is consumed by the mammary gland. The glucose demand is increased approximately 2.5-fold during the third week of lactation compared to the dry period. This increasing demand for glucose is fulfilled by the increased hepatic gluconeogenesis and decreased peripheral utilization of glucose. It has been estimated that gluconeogenesis increased from 1200 g/d at 21 days prepartum to 3 kg/d at 3 weeks postpartum. The hepatic glucose production is increased to a tune of 3600 g per day during peak lactation compared to the dry period. The characteristic changes in glucose metabolism are brought about by insulin resistance during this period. The glucose influx into the insulin-dependent tissues is zero to negative during the period of transition and early lactation. Moreover, total splanchnic output of glucose is increased to the tune of 267% from the gluconeogenesis during 9 days prepartum to 21 days postpartum. The substrates for hepatic gluconeogenesis are propionate, lactate, amino acids, and glycerol. Propionate produced during rumen fermentation is the main gluconeogenic precursor contributing 50–60% glucose production via gluconeogenesis. Lactate produced from Cori cycle constitutes 15–20% of glucose production. Amino acids generated during protein catabolism contribute 20–30% glucose production during the transition period. Glycerol produced through lipolysis generates 2–4% glucose through gluconeogenesis during the transition period.

In gluconeogenesis pathways, propionate is metabolized to succinyl CoA with the help of enzymes mitochondrial propionyl-CoA carboxylase (PCoAC) and methylmalonyl-CoA mutase (MMUT). The succinyl CoA then enters the TCA cycle to become oxaloacetate. Lactate and glucogenic amino acid (mostly alanine) are converted into pyruvate, which is carboxylated to oxaloacetate by the enzyme pyruvate carboxylase (PC) in the mitochondria. Oxaloacetate is in turn metabolized either to phosphoenolpyruvate (PEP) by the enzyme phosphoenolpyruvate carboxykinase (PEPCK) or used as an acetyl-CoA acceptor in the tricarboxylic acid (TCA) cycle. There are two isoforms of PEPCK, namely PEPCK-C (cytosol) and PEPCK-M (mitochondria).

PEPCK-C is required for the gluconeogenesis from amino acid precursors, whereas PEPCK-M is responsible for gluconeogenesis from lactate. Therefore, the major regulators of gluconeogenesis are PC and PEPCK-M in case of lactate precursors, PC and PEPCK-C in case of amino acid precursor, and PCoAC, MCM, and PEPCK-C in case of propionate precursors. The gluconeogenesis from the propionate precursor can also be modified through vitamin B12 as it acts as the coenzyme for MCM. Another important feature of gluconeogenesis control is that when the feed intake is reduced during transition periods, expression of PC controls the gluconeogenesis, and when the feed intake is optimum, PEPCK-C controls the gluconeogenesis.

6.4.2.1 Endocrine Control of Glucose Metabolism During the Period of Lactogenesis

The glucose homeostasis in ruminants during the transition period is controlled by insulin, glucagon, catecholamines, and glucocorticoids. The control of gluconeogenesis by insulin and glucagon is mediated through the regulation of PEPCK. The expression of PC is increased around caving in response to a reduced insulin/glucagon ratio. Glucocorticoids increase the availability of gluconeogenic precursors, but their efficacy is questionable. The glucogeogenesis is allosterically active by acetyl-CoA, which increases the expression of PC. Acetyl-CoA inhibits the expression of pyruvate kinase. One of the major allosteric regulators of gluconeogenesis is fructose 2,6 bisphosphate that activates phosphofructokinase-1 (PFK-1) to induce glycolysis and inhibits fructose 1,6-bisphosphatase (FBPase-1) to decrease gluconeogenesis.

Epinephrine favors the release of glucose by increasing hepatic gluconeogenesis. Both adrenaline and noradrenaline concentrations, along with the expression of β-adrenergic receptors (β-AR), are increased after calving till 2 months postpartum.

6.4.2.2 Molecular Control of Glucose Metabolism During the Period of Lactogenesis

In nonruminants, the control of gluconeogenesis occurs through the alterations in the expression patterns of PEPCK and pyruvate kinase (PK) genes. The expression of PEPCK. is suppressed by insulin through transcriptional regulation. In contrast, glucagon and glucocorticoids induce the activity of PEPCK. The control of gluconeogenesis for lactate precursor is regulated through the expression of PC and PEPCK. Studies have shown that glucocorticoids have little effect on pyruvate kinase; hence, the control of gluconeogenesis from lactate by the glucocorticoids is restricted to the actions of PC and PEPCK.

The control of gluconeogenesis in ruminants, on the other hand, is regulated by the expression of PC. At the time of feed deprivation or greater nutritional demands, the expression of PC is increased, whereas the expression of PEPCK is not consistent with the aforesaid physiological status. In cows, the expression of PC increased tremendously during the period of transition to lactation, whereas the expression of PEPCK remained unchanged during this period.

The insulin-dependent inhibition of gluconeogenesis is mediated by protein kinase B-forkhead box transcription factor 1 pathway. The FOXO family of transcription factors promotes the expression of PEPCK and glucose 6 phosphatase (G6PC) expression. Insulin phosphorylates FOXO1 to promote its exclusion from the nucleus and the transcription activity is inhibited. During the early lactation period, the expression of G6PC and PEPCK is high, which coincides with decreased insulin sensitivity.

Another important transcriptional regulator of ruminant gluconeogenesis is adenosine 5′-monophosphate-activated protein kinase (AMPK), which acts as the intracellular "energy sensor" of cells. The AMPK is activated by metabolic stress and restores intracellular energy by activating ATP-generating pathways and decreasing ATP-consuming pathways.

The AMPK inhibits hepatic gluconeogenesis by decreasing the activity of cAMP-response element-binding protein (CREB). AMPK inhibits CREB-regulated transcription coactivator 2 (CRTC2) by phosphorylation and prevents its trans-nuclear migration. This leads to decreased activity of CREB and inhibits G6PC and PEPCK.

6.4.3 Lipid Metabolism

The period of transition from pregnancy to lactation is characterized by increased lipolysis and reduced lipogenesis. The reduced glucose concentration during the state of negative energy balance causes mobilization of triglycerides to generate nonesterified fatty acids (NEFA), which are oxidized in the liver for energy production. A high amount of NEFA production sometimes exceeds the hepatic oxidizing capacity and leads to the production of ketone bodies such as acetoacetate, β-hydroxybutyrate (BHB), and acetone. The alternated endocrine milieu during the transition period is instrumental for lipid metabolism. The lipolysis is of two types: basal lipolysis and demand lipolysis. The basal lipolysis depends on the adipocyte stores and increases throughout lactation. The demand for lipolysis is regulated in response to energy demands and induced by endocrine responses. During the lipolysis, the triglycerides are broken down by lipases such as hormone-sensitive lipase (HSL), adipose triglyceride lipase (ATGL), and monoglyceride lipase (MGL). HSL and MGL play a major role in demand lipolysis. The control of lipolysis is therefore dependent on the expression of these enzymes and their activators.

6.4.3.1 Regulations of Lipolysis During the Period of Lactogenesis

Endocrine Factors

Catecholamines

The catecholamines and insulin are the most important activators of lipolysis in cattle. The metabolic stress during the transition period induces the release of catecholamines (adrenaline and noradrenaline). The catecholamines act through adipocyte β-adrenergic receptors (βAR) and activate adenylate cyclase, which converts ATP to cAMP and subsequent activation of protein kinase. The protein kinase phosphorylates a lipid droplet-associated protein called perilipin 1. In the feeding state, perilipin 1 protects the lipid droplets by acting as a coat over it. The phosphorylation of perilipin 1 initiates the lipolysis pathway. The concentrations of adrenaline and noradrenaline are increased immediately before calving and decreased after calving till 2 months postpartum. The expression of βAR increases during 1 month postpartum. The perilipin 1 concentration decreases during the first 3 weeks after parturition compared to other periods.

Insulin

Insulin suppresses the lipolysis and stimulates lipogenesis. Binding of insulin with its receptor results in the phosphorylation of insulin receptor substrates 1 and 2 (IRS-1/IRS-2). This leads to subsequent activation of phosphatidylinositol 3-kinase (PI3K), phophoinositide-dependent kinase 1 (PDK1), and protein kinase B (AKT). The activation of ATK results in the inhibition of PKA-induced phosphorylation of perilipin 1 to decrease lipolysis.

Growth Hormone

The growth hormone (GH) also induces lipolysis by increasing the response of adipocytes to adrenergic stimuli. Studies have shown that administration of GH leads to two to sixfold increase in the adipose tissue response to adrenergic stimulation. GH also inhibits the sympathetic effect on adipose tissue through adenosine.

Leptin

Leptin reduces lipogenesis and increases lipolysis and fatty acid oxidation. The concentration of leptin is increased during the dry period and declines during the first week of lactation.

Adipokines and Other Proteins

Adipokines are secreted from the adipose tissue and act in an autocrine, paracrine, and endocrine manner to modulate the lipolysis during the period of transition.

Angiopoietin-like 4 (ANGPTL4): It is also known as a fasting-induced adipose factor that inhibits the uptake of fatty acids by the adipocytes for esterification. ANGPTL4 is secreted during the period of negative energy balance and enhances lipolysis by increasing cAMP and the phosphorylation of PKA.

Adiponectin (Acrp30): It promotes lipogenesis in adipocytes and enhances insulin sensitivity. It also induces β-oxidation of fatty acids. The expression of adiponectin is decreased after calving compared to the dry period. The concentration of adiponectin reaches peak between 40 and 70 days of the lactation cycle.

Resistin: It is a peptide hormone synthesized by the adipose tissue that increases lipolysis by inducing the transcription of ATGL and HSL. The concentration of resistin is increased after calving and returns to the prepartum state by 6 weeks of lactation.

Retinol-binding protein 4 (RBP4): It inhibits lipogenesis and glucose uptake by the adipose tissue. The concentration of RBP4 is decreased after day 1 of parturition and returns to the precalving state by the second week of lactation.

α/β hydrolase domain-containing protein 5 (ABHD5/CGI-58): It is activated in response to the phosphorylation of perilipin 1. This ABHD5 activates ATGL and facilitates lipolysis. The expression of ABHD5 is decreased after calving.

Lipases: The expression of ATGL is reported to decrease during the late gestation and early lactation period compared to the dry periods in cows. Similarly, the expression of HSL and MGL is decreased during the 3 weeks postpartum compared to the dry period.

Knowledge Corner...
Whale milk has a fat content of up to 50%, giving it a paste- or toothpaste-like consistency. This prevents the milk from dispersing in the water when it is ejected into the calf's mouth.

6.4.4 Protein Metabolism

The increasing demands for the amino acids (AAs) to synthesize milk protein are met by a decrease in the amino acid utilization in the tissue other than the mammary gland to support mammary uptake of amino acids. The amino acid availability is fulfilled by increased amino acid mobilization from the tissue proteins. It has been estimated that the total mobilization of body protein may exceed 20 kg in dairy cows during early lactation. The major tissues involved in amino acid mobilization are skeletal muscle through increased proteolysis. The amino acids thus released from tissue protein are used by the mammary gland either for milk protein synthesis or by the hepatocytes for gluconeogenesis. The concentration of essential amino acids is decreased by 20% from the first to third week postpartum; in contrast, the nonessential protein and nonprotein AA are increased linearly during postpartum (Table 6.14). The concentrations of methionine and lysine are decreased by 22.0% and 24.5%, respectively, after calving. The muscle proteins lack several amino acids, particularly branched-chain amino acids (BCAAs) relative to milk protein (Table 6.15), so the mammary gland is dependent on dietary and microbial amino acids for milk protein synthesis.

6.4.4.1 Endocrine Regulation of Protein Metabolism During the Period of Lactogenesis

Increased lipolysis and decreased protein synthesis are regulated by a decreased level of insulin and insulin-like growth factor (IGF)-I. Though the level of growth hormone is elevated during early lactation, the concentration of IGF-I is decreased from 2 weeks prepartum due to the lack of feedback control of growth hormone by IGF-I. This decrease is consistent with a decreased level of IGF-binding protein-3

Table 6.14 Concentrations of different amino acids in the plasma of dairy cows during different days peripartum

Amino acids (μmol/L)	Days peripartum									
	−21	−14	−7	1	7	10	14	17	21	28
Ala	237.49	242.83	206.79	139.24	180.05	171.23	197.10	214.33	219.66	233.94
Gly	187.98	218.27	256.33	394.75	602.86	520.11	557.45	497.57	499.07	413.09
Leu	163.93	157.64	136.15	97.33	176.97	194.35	160.78	173.05	175.43	189.96
Pro	75.36	74.79	65.05	48.36	82.24	74.84	77.58	87.86	84.10	84.81
Ser	80.66	89.01	91.81	88.76	94.85	91.08	120.06	121.22	107.14	101.22
Phe	50.55	49.98	46.54	38.41	52.45	56.25	49.64	47.39	45.02	49.60
Asp	6.98	5.93	5.29	3.42	6.47	5.90	7.25	7.66	8.36	7.65
Cys	107.04	103.58	91.95	57.15	74.07	71.82	70.87	77.26	77.79	80.78
Glu	105.65	98.23	80.72	67.99	79.16	77.56	79.26	90.03	85.68	95.22
Tyr	52.55	50.16	43.27	24.46	36.25	41.22	41.48	50.55	47.79	50.51
Trp	44.24	40.34	29.13	12.96	37.78	40.78	41.79	43.67	43.46	46.50
Essential amino acids	922.62	895.33	760.39	562.50	962.85	1007.73	884.34	941.15	935.72	1018.51
BCAA	548.76	531.59	453.69	309.54	607.90	656.76	542.34	579.48	586.92	643.24

Zhou et al. (2016)

Table 6.15 Ratios of essential AA in skeletal muscle and milk protein in dairy cattle

Amino acid	Ratios of muscle AA / milk AA
Arginine	2.15
Histidine	0.99
Isoleucine	0.54
Leucine	0.81
Lysine	0.92
Methionine	0.81
Phenylalanine	0.82
Threonine	1.13
Tryptophan	0.53
Valine	0.75

Doepel et al. (2004), Waghorn and Baldwin (1984)

Table 6.16 Plasma concentrations of calcium, phosphorus, and magnesium during the peripartum period in cows

Plasma minerals	Weeks in peripartum				
	−3 weeks	−1 week	Calving	1 week	3 weeks
Total calcium (mg/dL)	8.09 ± 0.71	8.07 ± 0.86	7.99 ± 0.73	8.12 ± 0.72	8.24 ± 0.74
Phosphorus (mg/dL)	4.14 ± 1.37	3.94 ± 1.24	3.84 ± 1.23	3.92 ± 1.26	4.06 ± 1.29
Magnesium (mg/dL)	1.96 ± 0.68	1.97 ± 0.71	1.73 ± 0.71	1.91 ± 0.73	2.19 ± 0.62

Enculescu (2019)

and increased level of IGF-binding protein-2. Reduced IGF-I, along with decreased insulin level, leads to the suppression of protein synthesis and promotes proteolysis. The uptake of amino acids in the peripheral tissues is also inhibited and leads to direct amino acids in noninsulin-dependent tissues like the mammary gland.

6.4.5 Mineral Metabolism

The transition from pregnancy to lactation is characterized by altered mineral concentrations in the blood, particularly calcium, phosphorus, and magnesium, to support the milk production (Table 6.16). The imbalance in mineral concentration around the peripartum period is associated with the incidence of diseases, decreased milk production, and reduced reproductive efficiency.

6.4.5.1 Calcium

Hypocalcemia is a serious threat to the dairy farmers and occurs during the transition period. The normal calcium level in the dairy cows ranges from 2.2 to 2.5 mM, out of which 48–52% remains as a biologically active form (ionized calcium), 40–45% is present as a bound form with albumin, and the remaining portions are bound with bicarbonate, phosphate, citrate, or lactate. There is a huge drainage of calcium through colostrum and milk during the initiation of lactation. Colostrum contains approximately 2.0–3.0 g/L of calcium. It has been estimated that nearly 20–40 grams of calcium are secreted by the mammary gland in Holstein cows during the first day postpartum. Therefore, the need for calcium increases tremendously during the period of lactogenesis and the mobilization of calcium to the mammary gland starts before the parturition, which is reflected by the reducing calcium concentration from 9 days prepartum in dairy cows. If the cows failed to meet this increasing calcium demand, hypocalcemia (<2.0 mM) developed in 45% in multiparous cows and 25% in primiparous cows during 48 h after calving.

To support the adequate calcium level during this period, the immediate homeostatic mechanism ensures increased intestinal reabsorption of calcium and bone resorption, decreased urinary excretion by increasing renal reabsorption, salivary recycling, and reduced fecal excretion. Parathyroid hormone and 1,25-dihydroxyvitamin D conserve calcium pool in the blood by increasing intestinal absorption and renal reabsorption of calcium together with bone resorption of calcium and phosphorus. Parathyroid hormone-related peptide (PTH-related peptide) also plays a significant role in calcium metabolism during the transition period. Serotonin regulates calcium homeostasis through their action on the PTH-related peptide. 1,25-Dihydroxyvitamin D3 also favors the transport of calcium in the enterocyte by inducing the expression of calcium channel proteins and intracellular calcium-binding proteins. Calcitonin, on the other hand, decreases intestinal absorption and increases urinary excretion during the state of hypercalcemia.

The renal excretion of calcium in ruminants is very less (0.5–2 g per day), and the renal loss of calcium is already restricted during late gestation. Therefore, decreasing the renal loss of calcium may not be an effective mechanism to compensate calcium pool. In addition to this, the bone calcium contributing to the calcium pool is estimated at nearly 6–10 g. So, the main regulatory mechanism is restricted only to increase calcium reabsorption in the digestive tract.

Less incidence of hypocalcemia in primiparous cows may be due to the fact that their bones contain more osteoclasts for the bone resorption and parathyroid hormone only needs to activate them. But, in older cows, parathyroid hormone needs to induce osteoclasts production followed by their activation to mobilize bone calcium. The intestinal receptors for 1,25-dihydroxyvitamin D are also reduced with the age.

A calcium-sensing receptor has been identified in the mammary gland of humans that acts as a feedback regulator of calcium balance. When the calcium influx inside the mammary gland is decreased, the expression of calcium-sensing receptor also decreased, which leads to increased secretion of parathyroid hormone-related protein secretion and improves blood calcium level through calcium mobilization from bones.

6.4.5.2 Phosphorus

The majority of phosphorus (80–85%) present in the animal body is in the form of insoluble salts in the skeleton. The remaining 15–20% are present as a phosphorus pool in the body fluids and soft tissues in the form of inorganic (HPO_4^{2-}, $H_2PO_4^{-}$)

or organic form (bound with carbon compounds). In the nonskeletal phosphorus pool, the majority (>99%) of phosphorus remains as intracellular with an estimated concentration of 100 mmol/L. The concentration of phosphorus in the plasma in dairy cows is nearly 1.5 mmol/L. The concentration of phosphorus in the milk ranges from 0.7 to 1.2 gm/kg of milk and 50% of this phosphorus exists in casein micelles. The phosphorus concentration in the colostrum is higher than milk.

The dairy cows are in negative phosphorus balance (−4 to −14 g/d) during the early lactation period. This negative balance is not only due to loss of phosphorus in milk as the same reduction was reported in mastectomized cows. Reduced feed intake during late gestation may also contribute to the negative phosphorus balance during early lactation. The dietary supplementation of phosphorus did not improve milk production during early lactation, which proved that the cows mobilize calcium from bone to maintain the calcium balance rather than dietary intake.

Reduced bone mineralization during early lactation is the natural homeostatic process to restore body calcium pool. Decreased bone strength during early lactation has been reported in several species such as rats, sheep, pigs, and cows. Parathyroid hormone (PTH) and 1,25-dihydroxyvitamin D3 are reported to be involved in the bone metabolism. Hypocalcemia-induced stimulation of PTH secretion causes activation of vitamin D (calcitriol) in kidneys. Both PTH and calcitriol stimulate bone resorption to facilitate mobilization of phosphorus from bones. Higher secretion of prolactin during early lactation also potentiates the bone resorption during the early lactation period. Parathyroid hormone-related protein (PTHrP) is also involved in the regulation of phosphorus metabolism during early lactation. The concentration of PTHrP is lower in serum during the early lactation period in cows. Estradiol is reported to prevent bone resorption in dairy cows. The declining level of estradiol during calving also accelerate the bone resorption process.

6.4.5.3 Magnesium

The plasma concentration of magnesium is 1.8–2.4 mg/dL. Nearly 60–70% of the total magnesium in the body is present in the skeleton in the form of hydroxy apatite crystals and 30% is present in the intracellular space. It has been estimated that nearly 1–5% of intracellular magnesium is in ionized form. In the plasma, a substantial portion (20–40%) of magnesium is bound to albumin and globulin and nearly 10% of magnesium forms complexes with bicarbonate, phosphate, and citrate. The magnesium concentration in the colostrum is threefold higher than milk. The magnesium concentration in the milk varies with the stage of lactation cycle and is estimated to be 16–21 mg/1dL, 12 mg/dL, and 18 mg/dL during early, mid, and late lactation in cows. The initiation of lactation results in severe drainage of extracellular magnesium to cause hypomagnesemia. Magnesium deficiency during the peripartum period results in severe complications and affects the production performance. The magnesium homeostasis during the initiation of lactation is maintained by an increased absorption from the rumen and reticulum into the extracellular space. The drainage of magnesium from bones is unlikely as the ratio between calcium:magnesium is 42:1 and magnesium drainage may result in impaired calcium homeostasis. Magnesium helps to induce the functions of insulin and increases insulin sensitivity in adipose tissue to reduce lipolysis. The hypomagnesemia results in a decreased insulin responsiveness and stimulates lipolysis in sheep, and magnesium supplementation during the peripartum period restores glucose metabolism and insulin function in ewes.

6.5 Adaptive Changes in Other Organs During the Initiation of Lactation

In order to support the metabolic adaptation during the initiation of lactation, different organ systems of the body orient themselves that enables the body to meet the increased energy demands of milk production. The skeletal system undergoes excessive bone de-mineralization to provide adequate mineral supplementation during the initiation of lactation. The gastrointestinal and renal systems are also modified to increase the absorption and reabsorption to meet the nutrient requirement.

6.5.1 Digestive System

The transition from the gestation to lactation is characterized by the changes in the size, morphology, and functionality of the stomach to support increased nutrient absorption. There is an increase in the rumen mass by nearly 5% between 7 days prepartum and 10 days postpartum without changing the rumen volume, and this increase is continued till 4 months postcalving. The small intestine mass is also increased progressively and reaches peak at 90 days postpartum in cows. The functional histological alterations in the rumen during the initiation of lactation include increased differentiation and desquamation, along with an increase in the size of rumen papillae and surface area. The studies in rats also showed increased length and weight of the intestine with increased villi length in duodenum, ileum, and jejunum.

6.5.2 Excretory System

The major regulatory role of the excretory system is to conserve the ions during the early lactation period. In cows, no significant alterations in glomerular filtration rate were reported during the onset of lactation. However, the urine volume is reported to be increased during 3 weeks postpartum in cows. The reabsorption of Na^+, K^+, and $C1^-$ ions is increased during early lactation in order to conserve these ions. The creatinine concentration decreased from 10.5 mM to 5.0 mM from 2 weeks prepartum to 3 weeks postpartum. A significant decrease in the urine to plasma ratio was also reported from 2 weeks prepartum to 3 weeks postpartum. The filtration rate of urea in the kidney is increased by nearly twofold from 2 weeks prepartum to 3 weeks postpartum in cows along with urea reabsorption. The urea concentration in the urine is increased by twofold from prepartum to lactation. The increased urinary urea concentration is associated with an equivalent decrease of nonurea solutes in urine and increase urine volume. The urinary excretion of Na^+ decreases from 156 mM to 90 mM from 2 weeks prepartum to 3 weeks postpartum. A significant drop in urine K^+ concentration was also reported from 2 weeks prepartum (227 mM) to 3 weeks postpartum (142 mM). The urinary $C1^-$ concentration was also reduced from 193 mM to 74 mM from 2 weeks prepartum to 3 weeks postpartum. The urinary calcium excretion is decreased during lactation to accommodate the large calcium demand for milk production. In cows, the calcium reabsorption mainly occurs at proximal tubules (70%) and thick ascending limb of the loop of Henle (20%). The reabsorption of calcium is facilitated by transport proteins such as transient receptor potential vanilloid type 5 (TRPV5), calbindin-D28K ($CaBP_{D28K}$), and sodium/Ca exchanger type 1 (NCX1). Higher expressions of these proteins are increased in lactating mice. In contrast, the expression of TRPV5 protein is decreased during lactation in goats and no changes are observed in sheep.

6.5.3 Cardiovascular System

The blood flow to the mammary gland is directly proportional to the milk production. The partitioning of nutrients between milk and body tissue is regulated by the blood perfusion rate in the mammary gland. It has been estimated that the lactating mammary gland of a Jersey cow weighing 350 Kg and producing 16 kg of milk is perfused with blood at the rate of 7 liters/min, which is nearly 15.6% of cardiac output. Therefore, the cardiovascular adjustments play a pivotal role to meet the lactation challenges. No significant alterations in the cardiac morphology have been reported in goats between pregnancy and lactation, but the cardiac output is increased during pregnancy and lactation. The heart rate is increased during the early lactation period in cows compared to the dry period. The cardiac output and cardiac index are also increased during early lactation in cows. A significant increase in the left ventricular volume in diastole (LVVd) and left ventricular diameter in diastole (LVDd) was reported during the early lactation period in cows, which are indicative of increased cardiac size. No alterations in the ejection fractions were reported during lactation in cows. The cardiac parameters also differ between high- and low-yielding cows. In high-producing cows, left ventricular volume in systole is significantly higher and ventricular fractional shortening and ejection fraction are lowered compared to low-producing cows.

6.5.4 Muscular System

The skeletal and adipose tissue reserves are depleted during the transition from pregnancy to lactation to meet the increasing nutrient demand. The dynamics of change in skeletal muscle and adipose tissue is dependent on the stages of lactation. The early lactation is characterized by the negative energy balance as the feed intake is not sufficient to meet the energy demands. This leads to mobilization of body tissue, particularly body fat and skeletal muscle. It has been estimated that there are nearly 30–100 kg differences in the adipose tissue and 2.3–21 kg differences in the muscle mass from prepartum to peak lactation in dairy cows. The amino acids derived from muscles are utilized as gluconeogenic substrates for glucose production. The muscle mobilization starts from 7 days prepartum to 30 days postpartum in dairy cows. After the peak lactation period, increased energy and protein intake lead to positive energy balance and insulin sensitivity, which reduces the tissue depletion. Little or no alterations in the muscle mass have been reported from 30 to 60 days postpartum.

6.5.5 Skeletal System

The mineral content in bones is decreased during early lactation to support increasing demands for calcium and phosphorus. The decrease in the bone strength has been reported in rats during early lactation, which was subsequently restored after weaning. The bone mineralization is decreased in sheep and cows during early lactation, which increases again after mid-lactation. The bone mineralization and resorption are mediated by two types of cells osteoblasts or bone-forming cells and osteoclasts or bone-destroying cells. Osteoclasts absorb the bone by acidification of extracellular matrix with the help of enzyme cathepsin K. During bone resorption, different collagen products such as C-terminal crosslinking telopeptide of type I collagen (CTX-I) are released into the bloodstream, which acts as a bone demineralization marker. Osteoblasts deposit organic matrix in the bone called osteoid and facilitate the mineralization of bone. A non-collagenous protein called osteocalcin is secreted by osteoblasts and is considered another marker for osteoblast function. The carboxylation of osteocalcin at 3 glutamate residues during post-translational modification increases the affinity of osteocalcin for calcium ions in the bones. It is stored in the bone matrix and helps in bone mineralization. Uncarboxylated osteocalcin, on the other hand, has no affinity for calcium, and it is released into the bloodstream to facilitate β-cell proliferation, insulin, and adiponectin production. Osteopontin-induced insulin secretion inhibits osteoblast activity and favors bone resorption. In recent years, the role of cytokines in the regulation of osteoplastic and osteoclastic activities has been demonstrated in transition cows. The cytokines that increase the activities of osteoclasts are interleukins (IL-1, IL-6, IL-8), tumor necrosis factor-α (TNF-α), and macrophage inflammatory protein-1α (MIP-1α). The osteoclast activity is inhibited by IL-4, IL-10, and interferon-γ (IFN-γ). The differentiation of osteoblasts is induced by IL-10 and IFN-γ, whereas IL-4 and TNF-α inhibit osteoblasts differentiation. In transition cows, plasma IL-6 levels increased during late pregnancy, whereas concentrations of IFN-γ and IL-4 were increased during late lactation. The plasma level of CTX-I increased in late pregnancy and early lactation, whereas higher levels of osteocalcin are reported during mid-lactation. The reversal of bone resorption starts immediately after weaning. In mice and rats, the bone mineral content is recovered within 2–4 weeks and 4–8 weeks, respectively.

6.5.6 Immune System

The period around calving and early lactation is characterized by immune suppression due to altered activities of the immune cells involved in innate and adaptive immune responses. The functional activities of neutrophils such as chemotaxis, phagocytosis, and oxidative burst are decreased during immediate postcalving and early lactation period. The numbers and proliferative capabilities of lymphocytes are also decreased during this period. The major factor contributing to this immune suppression is the circulating glucocorticoids, which are increased around calving. The glucocorticoids cause downregulation of L-selectin and CD18 adhesion molecules that are required for the activation and migration of neutrophils at the site of infection. The concentration of glucocorticoids remains elevated only for 24 h around calving, but the immune suppression continues till the first 3 weeks of lactation. Therefore, some factors other than glucocorticoids may contribute to the immune suppression. Altered metabolic profiles and circulating metabolites such as glucose, NEFA, and β-hydroxy butyric acid are reported to affect the immune system. Glucose is the main metabolic fuel for the immune cells and has stimulatory effects on the immune system by inducing the neutrophil chemotaxis and proliferation of lymphocytes. The reduced glucose concentration during early lactation may be a contributing factor to immune suppression during early lactation. The higher concentrations of ketone bodies such as β-hydroxy butyric acid during early lactation also have a negative impact on chemotaxis and phagocytosis of neutrophils and lymphocyte proliferation response. High NEFA concentration reduces mitogenesis of mononuclear cells and reduces the secretion of IFN-γ and IgM. Some immune mediators are released from the adipose tissue during the transition period, which may also affect the immune system in an autocrine and paracrine manner. These compounds include TNF-α, IL-6, adiponectin, leptin, resistin, visfatin, and lipid adipokines (endocannabinoids and steroids). These molecules are increased with lipid mobilization and affect the adaptive immune system. Adiponectin reduces the secretion of TNF-α and other pro-inflammatory cytokines to modulate the activities of macrophages. Adiponectin also helps in modulating adaptive immune system through dendritic cell activation and T-cell polarization. Leptin promotes shifting of lymphocyte form type 1 (pro-inflammatory) to a T2 helper and favors the maturation of dendritic cells. Leptin is also involved in the activation of Toll-like receptor and phagocytosis in polymorphonuclear cells. The concentration of leptin is lowest during the first week postpartum, which may contribute to immune suppression. Resistin is an adiponectin that has pro-inflammatory roles. The concentration of resistin is increased during the first week postpartum in dairy cows.

Exercises

Objective Questions

1. The withdrawal of ____________________ and __________________ hormones favors secretory activation in ruminants.
2. In high-yielding cattle, _____________ of net energy intake and __________ of circulating glucose are utilized for milk production.
3. The metabolic changes occur during the initiation of lactation is a classic example of ____________________ mechanism.
4. The magnitude of insulin sensitivity in dairy cows is measured by _______________ test.
5. The volatile fatty acid that acts as predominant gluconeogenic precursor in ruminants is __________________.
6. The growth hormone (GH) also induces lipolysis. (True/False).
7. ______________________ are called bone-forming cells and __________________ are called bone-destroying cells.
8. The hormone decreases calcium in blood is __________________.
9. _________________ hormone plays a predominant role in peripartum immune suppression.
10. Blood metabolite that plays significant role in feed intake __________________.

Subjective Questions

1. Briefly describe the endocrine alterations during the initiation of lactation and their roles in nutrient partitioning.
2. Write down the differences between homeostasis and homeorhesis with suitable examples.
3. How is the secretory activation in ruminants different from rodents?
4. Describe the details of the molecular regulation of glucose metabolism during lactogenesis in ruminants.
5. Describe in brief the regulation of feed intake by adipocytes during the transition period.
6. What are the predisposing factors for peripartum immune suppression?

Answers to Objective Questions

1. Estrogen, progesterone
2. 80%, 85%
3. Homeorhesis
4. Euglycemic–hyperinsulinemic clamp test
5. Propionate

6. True
7. Osteoblasts, osteoclasts
8. Calcitonin
9. Glucocorticoids
10. NEFA

References

Books

Mukherjee J, Das PK, Banerjee D (2023) Lactation physiology. In: Das PK, Sejian V, Mukherjee J, Banerjee D (eds) Textbook of veterinary physiology. Springer, Singapore. https://doi.org/10.1007/978-981-19-9410-4_25

Research Articles

Atwood CS, Hartmann PE (1995) Assessment of mammary gland metabolism in the sow: I. Development of methods for the measurement of cellular metabolites in milk and colostrum. J Dairy Res 62(2):189–206. https://doi.org/10.1017/S0022029900030910

Baldwin RL (1966) Enzymic activities in mammary glands of several species. J Dairy Sei 49:1533–1542

Bauman DE, Currie WB (1980) Partitioning of nutrients during pregnancy and lactation: a review of mechanisms involving homeostasis and homeorhesis. J Dairy Sci 63:1514–1529

Doepel LD, Pacheco JJ, Kennelly MD, Hanigan IFL, Lapierre H (2004) Milk protein synthesis as a function of amino acids. J Dairy Sci 87:1279–1297

Enculescu M (2019) The evolution of the blood serum indicators during the transition period in dairy cows. Anim Sci LXII(1):2019

Garverick HA, Harris MN, Vogel-Bluel R, Sampson JD, Bader J, Lamberson WR, Spain JN, Lucy MC, Youngquist RS (2013) Concentrations of non-esterified fatty acids and glucose in blood of peri-parturient dairy cows are indicative of pregnancy success at first insemination. J Dairy Sci 96:181–188

Hartmann PE (1973) Changes in the composition and yield of the mammary secretion of cows during the initiation of lactation. J Endocrinol 59:231–247

Ingvartsen KL, Andersen JB (2000) Integration of metabolism and intake regulation: a review focusing on periparturient animals. J Dairy Sci 83:1573–1597

Nowroozi-Asl A, Aarabi N, Rowshan-Ghasrodashti A (2016) Ghrelin and its correlation with leptin, energy related metabolites and thyroidal hormones in dairy cows in transitional period. Pol J Vet Sci 19(1):197–204

Smith RD, Hansel W, Coppock CE (1976) Plasma growth hormone and insulin during early lactation in cows fed silage based diets. J Dairy Sci 59(2):248–254

Waghorn GC, Baldwin RL (1984) Model of metabolite flux within mammary gland of the lactating cow. J Dairy Sci 67:531–544

Zhou Z, Loor JJ, Piccioli-Cappelli F, Librandi F, Lobley GE, Trevisi E (2016) Circulating amino acids in blood plasma during the peripartal period in dairy cows with different liver functionality index. J Dairy Sci 99(3):2257–2267

Biosynthesis of Milk Constituents

7

Contents

J. Mukherjee et al., *Veterinary Lactation Physiology*,
https://doi.org/10.1007/978-3-032-21123-1_7

Abstract

The synthesis of milk constituents in the mammary epithelial cells involves several complex and coordinated biochemical and metabolic pathways. The precursors of milk constituents are transported from blood to milk via transcellular and paracellular routes with the help of transport proteins at the apical and basolateral membranes. Glucose is the main energy source in the mammary gland. The mammary gland utilizes glucose in three ways: synthesis of lactose, synthesis of NADPH and milk fat, and nucleic acid synthesis and energy production. The mammary gland is considered the most efficient tissue to produce lipids. Dietary fatty acids are transported from the intestine to the mammary gland in the form of chylomicron, but mammary gland can also synthesize fatty acids either from acetate (ruminants) or glucose (nonruminants). These fatty acids are esterified with glycerol to form milk triglycerides. Milk proteins are synthesized from amino acids in the ribosome followed by post-translational modification in the Golgi complex. Lactose and milk proteins are packaged into secretory vesicles and released in milk by exocytosis. Milk fat globules are extruded from the apex of the secretory cell surrounded by milk fat globule membrane. RNA and pyridine nucleotides are synthesized from ribose. Immunoglobulins are transported directly into the milk through the process of transcytosis. There is notable diversity in the metabolism of the mammary gland between species that leads to species-specific milk composition.

Graphical Abstract

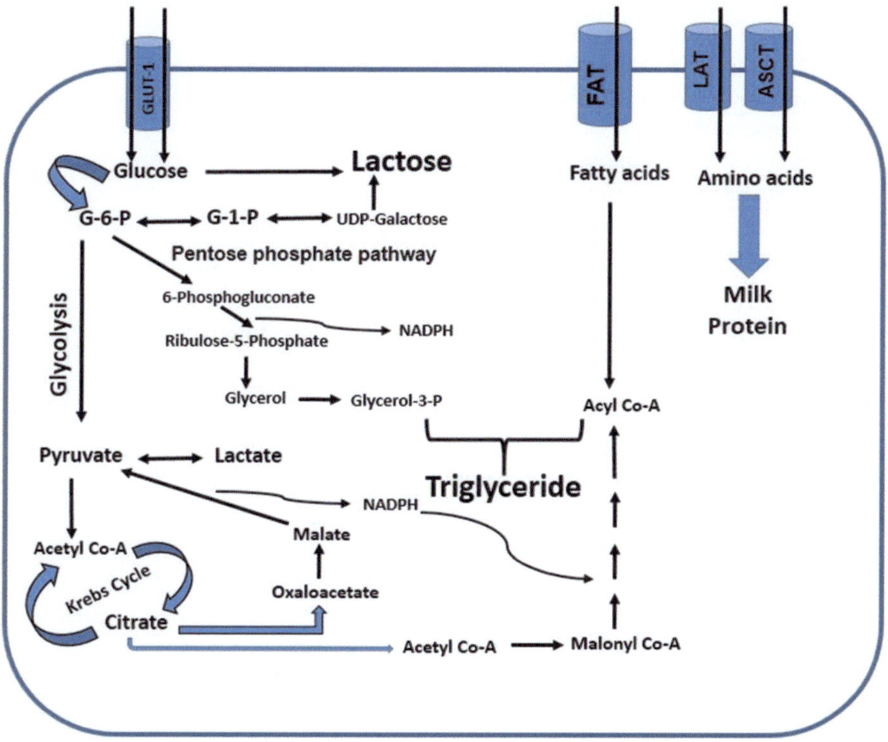

Description of the graphic: The mammary gland is a metabolically active organ that transforms basic blood metabolites into fat, lactose, and protein. Glucose enters the mammary gland via facilitative glucose transporters (GLUT) and is phosphorylated to glucose-6-phosphate (G6P). G6P is then converted into glucose-1-phosphate (G1P) and further into uridine diphosphate glucose (UDP-glucose), which is essential for lactose synthesis. G6P can also undergo glycolysis to produce pyruvate or enter the pentose phosphate pathway after being converted into 6-phosphogluconate. This pathway produces NADPH, a crucial coenzyme for fatty acid synthesis. Pyruvate enters the tricarboxylic acid (TCA) cycle to generate ATP, while the TCA intermediate citrate produces acetyl-CoA and malonyl-CoA, which are precursors for the de novo synthesis of fatty acids. In addition to synthesizing fatty acids, the mammary gland also imports them from the bloodstream via fatty acid translocase (FAT). Glycerol, required for forming triglycerides, is derived from triose phosphate during glycolysis and through glycerol phosphorylation. Milk triglycerides are formed when fatty acids and glycerol undergo esterification. The gland also absorbs amino acids using L-type amino acid transporters (LAT) and alanine–serine–cysteine transporters (ASCT), which are then used in milk protein synthesis

Keywords

Mammary gland · Metabolism · Nutrient uptake · Biosynthesis · Lactose · Protein · Lipids · Water and electrolytes

Inside the Chapter

- *Glucose metabolism in the mammary gland*
  - Sources of glucose
  - Glucose uptake by the mammary gland
  - Regulation of Glucose Transport in the Mammary Gland
  - Utilization of glucose by the mammary gland
  - Lactose synthesis
  - Glycolysis and pentose phosphate pathway
  - Glucose sparing action in the mammary gland of ruminants
- *Lipid metabolism in the mammary gland*
  - Transport of circulating lipids into the mammary gland
  - De novo fatty acid synthesis
  - Production of acetyl-CoA
  - Formation of malonyl CoA
  - Production of NADPH
  - Reactions of Fatty acid synthase complex
  - Fatty acid desaturation
  - Synthesis of glycerol and glycerides
  - Triglyceride synthesis
  - Synthesis of phospholipid
  - Milk cholesterol synthesis
  - Secretion of milk lipids
  - Regulation of milk fat synthesis
- *Protein metabolism of the mammary gland*
  - Amino acid uptake by the mammary gland
  - Utilization of amino acids
  - Milk protein synthesis
  - Post-translational modifications of milk proteins
  - Secretion of milk Proteins
  - Metabolism of amino acids in the mammary gland
  - Transcytosis of milk proteins
  - Transport of water and electrolytes across mammary gland

Learning Objectives

- Metabolism of the mammary gland
- Nutrient uptake and utilization by the mammary gland
- Biosynthesis of milk constituents
- Molecular mechanisms controlling mammary gland metabolism

Mammary gland is a unique exocrine gland that secretes milk, a complex mixture containing fat droplets, casein micelles, carbohydrate, ions, and other soluble factors in the aqueous phase. Some of these components are either derived directly from blood or synthesized de novo within the mammary gland from plasma precursors. The mammary gland is thus a highly metabolically active organ of the body that converts simple metabolites of the blood (glucose, acetate, ß-hydroxybutyrate, amino acids, and fatty acids) for the synthesis of fat, lactose, and protein. There is huge variability in the availability and utilization of these precursors to form milk constituents that leads to species-specific changes in milk composition (Mukherjee et al. 2023). The uptake of nutrients and the secretion of milk precursors occur through transcellular and paracellular routes. The transcellular routes are further classified into the membrane route, Golgi route, milk fat route, and transcytosis. Milk lactose is synthesized from glucose in the Golgi complex and secreted as secretory vesicles. Milk proteins are synthesized from amino acids in the ribosome and modified post-transcriptionally at the Golgi bodies and secreted by exocytosis of secretory vesicles. For fatty acid synthesis, the required precursor and co-factors are acetyl-CoA and NADPH, respectively. Milk lipids are secreted in the form of milk fat droplets. α-Glycerol phosphate and α-keto acids are required for the synthesis of triglyceride and nonessential amino acid. RNA and pyridine nucleotides are synthesized from ribose. Immunoglobulins are transported directly into the milk through the process of transcytosis.

7.1 Glucose Metabolism in the Mammary Gland

Glucose is the main energy source for the lactating mammary gland, whereas 60% of total glucose in ruminants is utilized for lactose synthesis. This is confirmed by the fact that, in lactating sows, 54% of mammary CO_2 originates from the oxidation of glucose, which is nearly 8% in lactating goats.

In lactating cows, there is a huge demand for glucose for the production of milk. It is estimated that the total daily glucose requirement during lactation is about 1140 g, out of which 700 g appears in the milk, which constitutes nearly 60% of total glucose requirement. The glucose turnover rate is also very high, amounting to 1440 g/day (60 g/h) in cows and 144 g/day (6 g/h) in ewes during lactation. In lactating goats, 75% of total glucose taken up by the mammary gland is used for lactose synthesis, 4.5% is utilized for milk triacylglycerol synthesis, and nearly 8% of glucose is completely metabolized in the pentose phosphate shunt, which yields 34% of the NADPH required for milk fatty acid synthesis.

Similarly in nonruminant animals, the majority of glucose entering the mammary gland is used for milk lactose and fat synthesis. In lactation sows, 40% of the glycerol and 59% of the lactose are synthesized from plasma glucose. In lactating women, 98% of the glucose and 68% of the galactose for lactose synthesis are derived from blood glucose. In nonruminant animals, milk fatty acids are exclusively synthesized from blood glucose.

The mammary gland is unable to synthesize glucose from other precursors due to the lack of glucose-6-phosphatase enzyme.

Hence, the mammary gland is principally a glucose-utilizing tissue where the majority of glucose is oxidized and little is synthesized.

7.1.1 Sources of Glucose

The proportion of digestible carbohydrate (glucose, starch) in the ruminant diet is very less. They escape rumen fermentation; hence, very little portion of these carbohydrates is available for utilization. The major dietary carbohydrates in ruminant diet are structural polysaccharides such as cellulose, hemicellulose, and lignin. They undergo fermentation in the rumen and yield volatile fatty acids (VFAs). The major volatile fatty acids are acetate, propionate, and butyrate found in the blood after absorption to the proportion of 65:20:10, respectively.

Acetate is not glucogenic and is mainly utilized for the production of energy and milk fat. The major glycogenic volatile fatty acid in the mammary gland is propionate. Two moles of propionate molecules synthesize one mole glucose (1 gm of propionate can generate 1.23 g glucose). The butyrate does not contribute directly to glucose synthesis, but it stimulates glucose production by increasing phosphorylases and gluconeogenesis. Butyrate also produces acetyl-CoA by β-oxidation, which activates pyruvate carboxylase, a key gluconeogenic enzyme.

The ruminal lactic acid also contributes to glucose synthesis indirectly. The lactic acid is produced in the mammary gland by fermentation. The lactate in blood produces blood glucose via the lactic acid cycle.

7.1.2 Glucose Uptake by the Mammary Gland

The mammary gland receives 60–85% of the total circulatory in ruminants during lactation. In bovines, it was estimated that 72 g of glucose is taken up by the mammary gland for 1 kg of milk production. The average glucose uptake in the mammary gland of lactating Holstein cow is nearly 300 mmol/h to support the production of milk at the rate of 0.6 kg/h. The rate was 9 mg/min/100 g of mammary tissue in lactating goats and sows.

Transport of glucose through biological membrane requires special transporter proteins and specific mechanisms because glucose is unable to pass through the phospholipid bilayer biological membrane as it is a polar and hydrophilic molecule.

The entry of glucose in the mammary epithelial cells is mediated by two different mechanisms: Na^+-dependent transport and facilitated transport. In Na^+-dependent transport, the entry of glucose is coupled with Na^+ ions. Glucose enters the cells against their concentration gradient utilizing Na+/K+/ATP pumps that push Na^+ ions into the cells against their electrochemical gradient. This type of transport mechanism is mediated by Na^+/glucose co-transporters (SGLT).

In facilitated diffusion, bidirectional transport of glucose occurs due to concentration gradient at the basolateral surface of mammary epithelial cells and mediated by facilitative glucose transporters (GLUTs). A new class of glucose transporter, SWEETs, has been identified that is structurally different from the GLUT or SGLT family of transporters, having seven transmembrane domains. The arterial glucose concentration is 3–5 mM, 9–11 mM, and 4–8 mM, respectively, in cows/goats, rodents, and humans. The intracellular concentration of glucose in mammary epithelial cells is estimated as 0.1–0.5 mM in cows, goats, and rats and 1.3 mM in humans. Therefore, a concentration gradient of glucose is achieved at the basolateral membrane of mammary epithelial cells.

Glucose enters the mammary epithelial cells through three transporter proteins, namely GLUT1, GLUT8, SGLT1, and SWEETs. In the Golgi apparatus, GLUT1, GLUT8, and SGLT1 facilitate glucose transport between the cytoplasm and Golgi apparatus. GLUT8, GLUT12, and SGLT1 help to maintain glucose equilibrium between the glucose in MEC and the glucose in milk. The trafficking of GLUT occurs between the plasma membrane and intracellular pool. Similarly, in bovine mammary gland, GLUT1 trafficking also occurs between the plasma membrane and the Golgi membrane.

A high abundance of GLUT1 is reported in the mammary gland of cows, goats, sows, rats, mice, and humans. Bovine mammary epithelial cells express a low level of GLUT3–5. In goats, the expression GLUT12 was also reported during pregnancy and lactation. In porcine mammary gland, SGLT1 was also expressed from gestation to peak lactation.

After the entry of glucose in the mammary gland, it is phosphorylated by hexokinase to convert into glucose-6-phosphate (G6P). The phosphorylation of glucose prevents its back diffusion from the mammary gland. On the other hand, the activity of glucose glucose-6-phosphatase that catalyzes the conversion of G6P to glucose is extremely low in the mammary gland.

Studies have shown that both hexokinase-1 (HK1) and 2 (HK2) are expressed in the mammary glands of rats and sows. But HK1 is expressed both in lactating and nonlactating mammary glands, whereas HK2 is only expressed during lactation. The activity of HK is increased with the glucose availability in lactating bovine mammary epithelial cells.

Knowledge Corner...
Ruminant mammary glands receive relatively less glucose compared to nonruminants because much of the dietary carbohydrate is fermented into VFAs in the rumen. The liver produces most of the glucose that does reach the mammary gland.

7.1.3 Regulation of Glucose Transport in the Mammary Gland

The utilization of glucose for milk lactose synthesis is the metabolic priority in lactating animals, which is maintained by coordinated actions of several factors.

7.1.3.1 Physiological State of Animals

The changes in the expression pattern of glucose transporters during different physiological stages have been reported in several animals. In rodents, glucose transports in the mammary gland increase dramatically (up to 40-fold) from the virgin to mid-lactation stage. The expression of GLUT1 and GLUT8 progressively increases from pregnancy to early lactation in mice. Similarly, in cows, GLUT1, GLUT8, GLUT12, SGLT1, and 2 mRNA level is reported to increase from 40 days prepartum to 7 days postpartum. A notable decrease in the GLUT1 mRNA has been reported in cows after early lactation. The changes in the expression pattern of glucose transporters during different developmental stages are consistent with the changes in the cellular differentiation.

7.1.3.2 Endocrine Regulation

The transport of glucose into the mammary gland is influenced by lactogenic hormones. Studies in mice showed that prolactin and glucocorticoids increased glucose uptake by the mammary epithelial cells. But, in contrast, lactogenic hormones failed to stimulate glucose uptake by the bovine mammary epithelial cells. Administration of exogenous growth hormone increases glucose uptake without affecting plasma glucose concentration in cows and goats.

7.1.4 Utilization of Glucose by the Mammary Gland

The glucose is utilized in the mammary gland by three metabolic processes: synthesis of lactose, synthesis of NADPH and synthesis of milk fat, nucleic acid synthesis, and energy production. It is estimated that 50–60% of the glucose that is converted into glucose-6-phosphate is utilized for the synthesis of lactose. The remaining 30–40% is metabolized via the glycolytic and pentose phosphate pathway.

7.1.5 Synthesis of Lactose

In the lactose synthesis pathway, glucose is phosphorylated at its sixth position to form glucose-6-phosphate by enzyme hexokinase. In the next step, enzyme phosphoglucomutase transfers the phosphate group from position 6 to 1 to form glucose-1-phosphate. The enzyme UDP glucose pyrophosphorylase converts glucose-1-phosphate into uridine diphosphate glucose (UDP glucose) with the help of uridine triphosphate (UTP). In this reaction, one phosphate is liberated from UTP. The phosphoglucomutase then transfers the phosphate group from position 6 to 1 to form glucose-1-phosphate, which combines with uridine triphosphate to form uridine diphosphate glucose and liberates pyrophosphate catalyzed by the enzyme UDP glucose pyrophosphorylase. UDP glucose is converted into UDP-galactose by UDP-galactose 4-epimerase. UDP-galactose enters the Golgi complex by a solute carrier family of protein (SLC35A2 or SLC35B1). The glucose enters the Golgi complex with the help of glucose transporter 1 (GLUT1). Finally, UDP-galactose combines with glucose to form lactose in the Golgi complex with the help of lactose synthetase enzyme. Both glucose and UDP-galactose enter the Golgi vesicle and convert into lactose by the enzyme the lactose synthase. After the synthesis, lactose is encapsulated by the membrane of Golgi to become secretory vesicles, which are transported to the apical membrane and fused with it to discharge their content via exocytosis.

Glycerol is one of the alternate sources of carbon for the lactose synthesis. Glycerol is taken up by the mammary gland by aquaporin 3 (AQP3) and utilized for de novo synthesis of glucose and UDP-galactose. In humans, glycerol contributes 14–70% of the UDP-galactose. In this reaction, glycerol is phosphorylated by glycerokinase and subsequently converted to dihydroxy acetone phosphate by the enzyme glyceraldehyde-3-phosphate dehydrogenase (G3PD). The dihydroxyacetone phosphate then enters the triose isomerase reaction in the glycolytic pathway.

7.1.5.1 Lactose Synthase (LS)

The enzyme LS is an enzyme complex made of two different proteins, namely β-1,4-galactosyltransferase-1 (B4GALT1) and mammary-specific modifier protein α-lactalbumin (LALBA) in 1:1 stoichiometry. B4GALT1 transfers galactose from UDP-galactose and LALBA acts as an enzyme modifier.

B4GALT1 is a Mn-dependent enzyme that transfers D-galactose from UDP-galactose to N-acetylglucosamine. The N-terminal domain of B4GALT1 is attached to the Golgi membrane and acts as a nucleotide donor (UDP-galactose) and C-terminal domain acts as a glucose acceptor. The active site is present between these two domains. Apart from this, B4GALT1 has two ion-binding sites (sites 1 and 2). Manganese (Mn) is required for the optimal activity of B4GALT1 that binds at site 1 and site 2 has a low affinity for Mn or Ca.

During the process of lactose synthesis, inactive B4GALT1 in the Golgi becomes activated when UDP-galactose binds at the N-terminal end. Activation of B4GALT1 leads to its conformational change that allows binding of LALBA to B4GALT1. It has been reported that binding of LALBA with B4GALT1 increases its activity by 1000-fold. B4GALT1 transfers D-galactose to the OH-4 position of glucose for the synthesis of lactose. After the synthesis, lactose and LALBA dissociate from B4GALT1 and the enzyme becomes inactive.

7.1.6 Glycolysis and Pentose Phosphate Pathway

G6P can be converted to fructose-6-phosphate by phosphoglucoisomerase that enter the glycolytic pathway (Embden–Meyerhof pathway) to generate triose phosphate and pyruvate. The triose phosphate is utilized for the synthesis of α-glycerol-phosphate that provides backbone for the biosynthesis of major lipid triglycerol. The pyruvate enters the tricarboxylic acid cycle (TCA) to produce ATP. Citrate, produced in the TCA cycle, enters the mitochondria to generate acetyl-CoA by ATP citrate lyase enzyme. This acetyl-CoA is used for fatty acid elongation. The pyruvate and other TCA cycle intermediates can produce amino acids such as alanine and glutamine, which are used for milk protein synthesis. G6P enters the pentose phosphate pathway after converting into 6-phosphogluconate. The pentose

Table 7.1 Activities of citrate cleavage enzymes (nmoles/mg cytosol protein/minute) in different species

Enzymes	Enzymatic reaction	Species					
		Mouse	Rat	Rabbit	Sow	Cow	Sheep
ATP-citrate lyase	Conversion of citrate to acetyl-CoA	49	70	40	29	3	<1
NAD-malate dehydrogenase	Oxidation of malate to oxaloacetate using the reduction of NAD + to NADH	–	2870	2700	1871	1822	2460
NADP-malate dehydrogenase	Conversion of malate to oxaloacetate with the help of $NAPD^+$	139	218	0	1	1	<1

phosphate pathway generates pyridine nucleotide in the form of NADPH, which is required for fatty acid synthesis.

7.1.7 Glucose-Sparing Action in the Mammary Gland of Ruminants

The major portion of mammary glucose is utilized for lactose synthesis, and a very little amount is available for milk fat synthesis. Ruminants have a well-developed glucose-sparing mechanism in the mammary gland that prevents the use of glucose in the synthesis of milk fatty acids. This is mediated by the low activities of key enzymes such as adenosine triphosphate (ATP)-citrate lyase, nicotinamide adenine dinucleotide phosphate (NADP)-malate dehydrogenase, and pyruvate carboxylase required for the citrate cleavage pathway for the generation of extra-mitochondrial acetyl-CoA (Table 7.1).

7.2 Lipid Metabolism in the Mammary Gland

The mammary gland has a remarkable ability to synthesize lipids. It was estimated that a cow produces 1.5 kg of milk fat/day at the production potential of 30 kg of milk/day at peak lactation and mobilizes nearly 1 kg of adipose tissue lipid/day. The mammary gland is considered the most efficient tissue to produce lipids (Table 7.2).

The predominant milk fats are triglycerides (95%). The remaining portion comprises small diacylglycerol, phospholipids, and free fatty acids, such as conjugated linoleic acid, sphingomyelin, and butyric acid. The fatty acids of these triglyceride components come from two sources: circulating blood lipids and lipids synthesized within the mammary gland (de novo synthesis). The amount of fatty acids synthesized de novo in the mammary gland is estimated to be 40% by weight. Fatty acids of milk fat comprising carbon chains from C4-C14 and a part of C16 are derived from de novo synthesis in cows and goats.

Table 7.2 Rate of fatty acid synthesis in the adipose tissue and mammary gland during lactation in different species

Species	Rate of fatty acid synthesis μmol/h/animal			References
	Nonlactating	Peak lactation		
	Adipose tissue	Adipose tissue	Mammary gland	
Cow	278,000	800	630,000	Vernon (1988)
Sheep	33,000	250	65,000	Vernon (1988)
Rat	345	39	2950	Agius et al. (1979), Kanto and Clawson (1980)
Mouse	44	7	423	Romsos et al. (1978)

7.2.1 Transport of Circulating Lipids into the Mammary Gland

Dietary fatty acids are transported from the intestine to the mammary gland in the form of chylomicron. These chylomicrons consist of triglyceride core and small amounts of cholesteryl ester. They appear as spherical particles enclosed by a monolayer surface made of phospholipid lecithin, diglyceride, cholesterol, protein, monoglyceride, and fatty acids. The chylomicrons are synthesized in the intestinal epithelium after absorbing the dietary lipids. The chylomicrons are transported via the lymph. First, they enter the intestinal lymphatic vessels through the thoracic duct and then the blood for their transportation into the mammary gland.

A small amount of triglycerides is also carried in the form of very-low-density lipoproteins (VLDLs). VLDLs are synthesized in the liver and their size is smaller than chylomicron.

7.2.1.1 Fatty Acid Uptake by the Mammary Gland from Plasma

The chylomicron and VLDL are large molecules, and their trans-endothelial migration and tissue uptake require additional machinery. It has been established that triglycerides present in chylomicrons and VLDL are hydrolyzed before tissue uptake, and this reaction is catalyzed by lipoprotein lipase (LPL). Lipoprotein lipase cleaves fatty acid from these lipoprotein triacylglycerol and then they are taken up by the cells. The activity of LPL in rat is increased before the parturition and remained elevated till the suckling continues. It has also been reported that prolactin augments the activity of LPL.

Before transportation into the cells, fatty acids are released from their carrier proteins and subsequently enter the external plasma membrane. Then they are transported across the membrane bilayer, followed by the dissociation from external membrane.

There are different transporter proteins available for the transport of fatty acids into the cells. Two important fatty acid transporters are fatty acid translocase (FAT) or CD36 and fatty acid transport proteins/solute carrier 27 (FATP/SLC27A) and acyl-CoA synthetase (ACSL) families of proteins.

FAT/CD36 is a scavenger receptor protein expressed in the immune cells, platelets, adipocytes, enterocytes, myocytes, and retinal and mammary epithelial cells. Studies have shown that FAT/CD36 is highly upregulated in the bovine mammary gland during lactation. Structurally CD36 is present in the plasma membrane as rafts with a hairpin structure at the membrane bilayer and two cytoplasmic tails. When the ligand binds with CD36, it internalizes with the ligands and translocates to a lysosome. Other than fatty acids, FAT/CD36 recognizes lipoproteins and microbial lipids. Some nonlipid components such as collagen and thrombospondin 1 also have affinity for FAT/CD36. The CD36 controls the entry of long-chain fatty acids in collaboration with SLC27A and acyl-CoA synthetase (ACSL).

FATP/SLC27A and acyl-CoA synthetase (ACSL) families of proteins contain acyl-CoA synthetases. After internalization of fatty acids by CD36, ACSL converts these fatty acids into fatty acyl-CoA through coenzyme-A thioesters formation. This is called bioactivation of fatty acids that facilitates metabolic trapping of fatty acids entered into the mammary epithelial cells. These activated fatty acids are then transport into the endoplasmic reticulum by heart-type fatty acid-binding protein (FABP3).

7.2.2 De Novo Fatty Acid Synthesis

The substrate for de novo fatty acid synthesis in the ruminants is acetate. Butyrate can also contribute to the synthesis of the first four carbons of fatty acids. It was estimated that about 50% of the total fatty acids are synthesized from acetate. In contrast, glucose is the principal substrate for fatty acid synthesis in nonruminants. Fatty acid synthesis also requires NADPH as reducing equivalent, which is derived from pentose-phosphate cycle and the isocitrate cycle (ruminants) or from pentose-phosphate cycle and the malate transhydrogenation cycle (nonruminants). The other co-factors required for de novo synthesis of fatty acids are Mn^{+2}, biotin, and HCO_3^-. The de novo fatty acid synthesis occurs in the cytosol and basic building block is acetyl-CoA. The synthesis of fatty acids occurs in three steps:

1. Substrates for fatty acid synthesis are converted to acetyl-CoA and NADPH in the cytosol.
2. Acetyl-CoA is converted into malonyl-CoA.
3. Reactions of fatty acid synthase complex where primers of fatty acids (acetyl-CoA and/or butyryl-CoA) are added to form fatty acids, which are subsequently released from fatty acid synthase complex.

Knowledge Corner...

The unsaturated fatty acids from a ruminant's diet are mostly hydrogenated (saturated) by rumen microbes. The mammary gland then takes up these more saturated fatty acids from the blood to synthesize milk fat.

7.2.3 Production of Acetyl-CoA

7.2.3.1 Pathways of Acetyl-CoA Synthesis in Nonruminants

In nonruminants, glucose is the main source of carbon for fatty acid synthesis. At the initial step, glucose is converted into pyruvate in the cytoplasm. This pyruvate is then transported into the mitochondria where pyruvate undergoes oxidative decarboxylation to form acetyl-CoA, which is translocated into the cytosol where the final step of fatty acid synthesis occurs (Fig. 7.1).

The transport of acetyl-CoA from mitochondria to cytosol involves four possible mechanisms:

Simple diffusion: This mechanism stated that the transport of acetyl-CoA across mitochondrial membrane is mediated by simple diffusion and the CoA moiety is returned to mitochondria. But as CoA is relatively impermeable to mitochondria this mechanism is questionable.

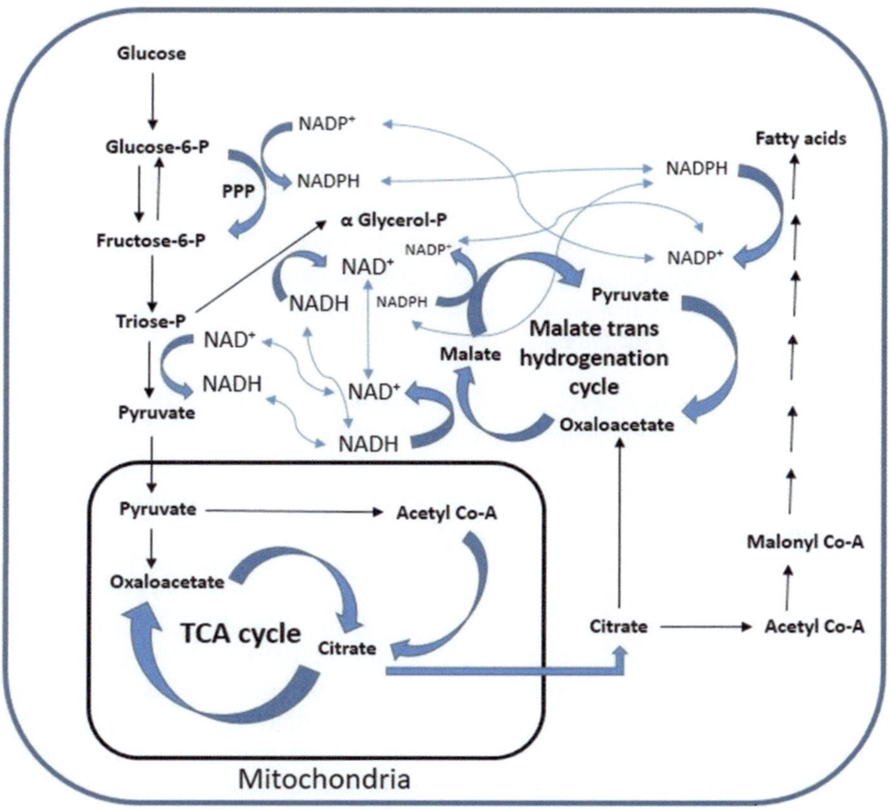

Fig. 7.1 Fatty acid synthesis in nonruminants. (Adapted from Bauman and Davis (1974))

Carnitine-mediated transfer: In this proposal, acetyl-CoA is converted into acetyl carnitine with the help of enzyme carnitine acetyltransferase present in both cytosol and mitochondria. This acetyl carnitine is translocated into the mitochondrial membrane. But localization of carnitine acetyltransferase and the carnitine availability is higher in energy-utilizing organ such as the liver rather than the lipogenic tissues such as the liver and adipose tissue. Cernitine-mediated transfer does not require any energy.

Direct diffusion of acetate: The acetyl-CoA undergoes hydrolysis by acetyl-CoA hydrolase into the mitochondria. The acetate thus generated diffuses in the mitochondrial membrane and transported into the cytoplasm. The enzyme acetylthiokinase present in the cytosol facilitates regeneration of acetyl-CoA. In this mechanism, one ATP is utilized per acetyl group. But low activity of hydrolase in mammary tissue puts this hypothesis in question.

Translocation via *citrate:* It is thought to be the major mechanism involved in the fatty acid translocation. This mechanism starts with the condensation of acetyl-CoA and oxaloacetate in the mitochondria by citrate synthetase to form citrate. The citrate is diffused through mitochondrial membrane and cleaved in the cytosol with the help of enzyme ATP-citrate lyase to form acetyl-CoA and oxaloacetate (citrate cleavage cycle). The acetyl-CoA is used for fatty acid synthesis, and the oxaloacetate is utilized to generate pyruvate by the enzyme malate dehydrogenases. This reaction yields NADPH, which is used as a cofactor during milk fat synthesis.

The enzyme citrate synthetase is exclusively found in the mitochondria and ATP-citrate lyase is found in the cytosol. In nonruminants, the activity of ATP-citrate lyase increases during the onset of lactation and decreases after weaning.

Two key enzymes of citrate cleavage pathway, namely ATP-citrate lyase and NADP-malate dehydrogenase, are absent in ruminants; hence, they are not able to utilize glucose carbon for fatty acid synthesis.

7.2.3.2 Pathways of Acetyl-CoA Synthesis in Ruminants

In ruminants, volatile fatty acids such as acetate and β-hydroxybutyrate (BHBA) are the main precursors or carbon for milk fat synthesis. These two VFAs have equal contribution for the first four carbons of fatty acids; however, the remaining carbons are supplied mainly by the acetate (Fig. 7.2).

The acetate is converted to acetyl-CoA in the cytosol and generates fatty acid via malonyl-CoA pathway. β-Hydroxybutyrate (BHBA) is oxidized into acetyl-CoA in the mitochondria through a series of biochemical reactions catalyzed by β-hydroxybutyrate dehydrogenase. The oxidation of BHB to acetyl-CoA occurs through a linear sequence of metabolic reactions in the mitochondria catalyzed by the enzymes β-hydroxybutyrate dehydrogenase (BDH1/2), succinyl CoA:3: oxoacid-CoA transferase (SCOT), and acetyl-CoA acetyltransferase (ACAT1/2) with the generation of one molecule of NADH and succinate and two molecules of acetyl-CoA. This acetyl-CoA then enters the TCA cycle.

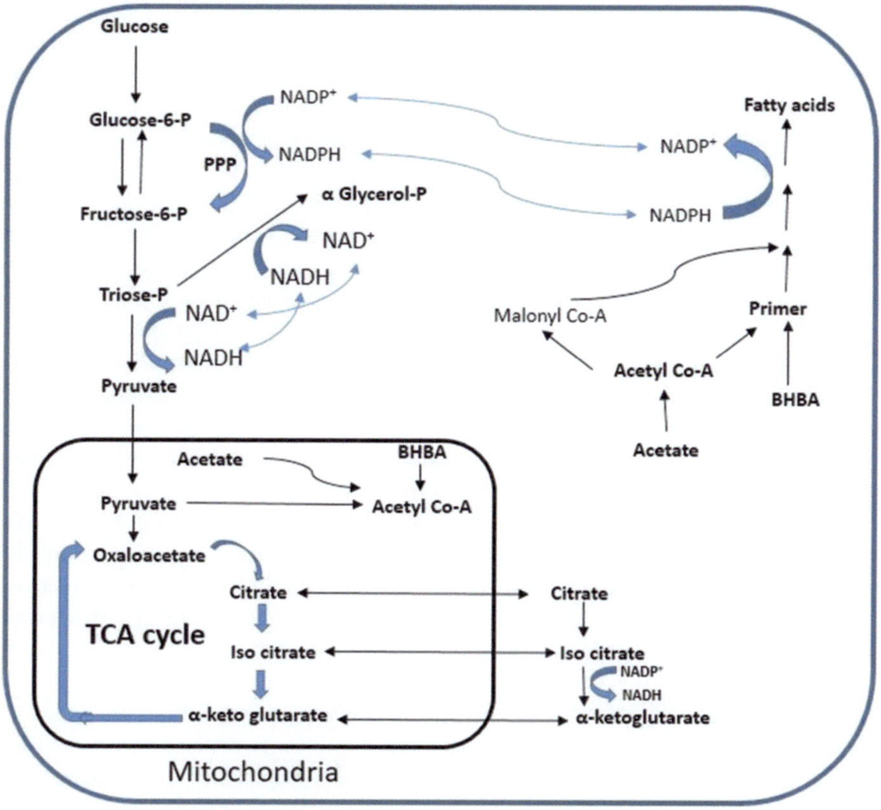

Fig. 7.2 Fatty acid synthesis in ruminants. (Adapted from Bauman and Davis (1974))

7.2.4 Formation of Malonyl-CoA

The enzyme acetyl-CoA carboxylase causes carboxylation of acetyl-CoA to malonyl-CoA. This reaction requires biotin as a co-factor for CO_2 fixation. It also requires ATP. The reaction occurs in the cytoplasm and mitochondrial outer membrane. This malonyl-CoA is used for chain elongation in the fatty acid synthesis.

7.2.5 Production of NADPH

NADPH acts as the source of reducing equivalents during the synthesis of fatty acids. The NDPH is primarily generated in the cytosol as the mitochondrial membrane is not permeable to nucleotides. The cytosolic enzymes required for NADPH production are glucose-6-phosphate dehydrogenase, 6-phosphogluconate dehydrogenase, NADP-malate dehydrogenase, and NADP-isocitrate dehydrogenase.

Glucose-6-phosphate dehydrogenase and 6-phosphogluconate dehydrogenase play a pivotal role in NADPH generation through pentose phosphate pathway. Glucose-6-phosphate dehydrogenase converts glucose-6-phospate into 6-phosphogluconolactone with the generation of one molecule of NADPH. The enzyme 6-phosphogluconate dehydrogenase converts 6-phosphogluconate into ribulose-5-phaophate and produce one NADPH.

The enzyme NADP-malate dehydrogenase generates NAPDH via a portion of the citrate cleavage pathway. The oxaloacetate is converted to citrate via the TCA cycle in the mitochondria by citrate synthase. The citrate then translocates from mitochondria to cytosol and converted to oxaloacetate again by citrate cleavage enzyme. The oxaloacetate is converted into malate by NAD-malate dehydrogenase. The malate thus produced is transported into the mitochondria and NADP-malate dehydrogenase catalyzes the reversible conversion of malate to oxaloacetate by malate transhydrogenation cycle. This reaction occurs in two steps: first, malate is converted to pyruvate by NADP-malate dehydrogenase that generates NADPH, then pyruvate is converted into oxaloacetate by pyruvate carboxylase.

NADP-isocitrate dehydrogenase generates reducing equivalents for fatty acid synthesis through a cycle that involves diffusion of citrate (or isocitrate) from the mitochondria to cytosol and its conversion into isocitrate by the enzyme aconitase. The isocitrate then converts into a-ketoglutarate by NADP-isocitrate dehydrogenase with the generation of NADPH.

7.2.5.1 Species Differences in the NADPH-Generating Enzymes

The pathways for the generation of reducing equivalents differ between species (Table 7.3). The activities of glucose-6-phosphate dehydrogenase, 6-phosphogluconate dehydrogenase, and NADP-malate dehydrogenase increase during the initiation of lactation in rats, which supports the notion that pentose phosphate pathway and malate transhydrogenation cycle are the main pathways of NADPH generation in this species, whereas NADP-isocitrate plays a minor role in the generation of reducing equivalents in the rat mammary gland. In contrast, the enzyme NADP-malate dehydrogenase is absent in the mammary gland of rabbits and sows. Along with the absence of NADP-malate dehydrogenase, the mammary gland of rabbit also lacks pyruvate carboxylase in the cytosol.

The enzyme NADP-isocitrate dehydrogenase was increased up to eightfold in the mammary gland of rabbit and guinea pigs from late pregnancy to mid-lactation. The enzyme activity NADP-isocitrate dehydrogenase is nearly three times higher in the rabbit mammary gland than the rat mammary tissue.

In ruminant mammary gland, the activity of ATP-citrate lyase and NADP-malate dehydrogenase is very low, which coincides with the lack of glucose incorporation into fatty acids and rules out the malate transhydrogenation cycle to generate NADPH.

The activity of glucose-6-phosphate dehydrogenase is lower in the ruminant mammary gland compared to nonruminant mammary gland, whereas the activity of 6-phosphogluconate dehydrogenase was similar in ruminant and nonruminant.

Table 7.3 Species differences in the NADPH-generating enzymes

Enzyme activities (nmoles/mg cytosol protein/minute)	Species						
	Mouse	Rat	Rabbit	Pig	Sow	Cow	Sheep
Glucose-6-phosphate dehydrogenase	243	468	260	432	343	74	78
6-Phosphogluconate dehydrogenase	–	31	170	96	28	35	169
NADP-malate dehydrogenase	139	218	0	–	1	1	<1
NADP-isocitrate dehydrogenase	–	52	57	368	82	989	1007
References	Bartley et al. (1966)	Bauman et al. (1970)	Gul and Dils (1969)	Bauman et al. (1970)	Bauman et al. (1970)	Bauman et al. (1970)	Bauman et al. (1973)

NADP-isocitrate dehydrogenase plays a significant role in the generation of NADPH in the ruminant mammary gland, which is supported by the consistent availability of citrate in the cytosol due to the absence of the citrate cleavage pathway.

7.2.6 Reactions of Fatty Acid Synthase Complex

Fatty acid synthase (FASN) is the main enzyme that performs most of the enzymatic steps during fatty acid synthesis. It adds seven malonyl-CoA molecules with one acetyl-CoA to produce 16-carbon saturated fatty acid (palmitic acid). The other products of FASN are myristic acid and stearic acid.

FASN is a multifunctional polypeptide enzyme composed of seven domains, namely β-ketoacyl synthase (KS), acetyl/malonyl-CoA transferase (MAT), β-hydroxyacyl dehydratase (DH), enoyl reductase (ER), β-ketoacyl reductase (KR), acyl-carrier protein (ACP), and thioesterase I (TE I).

Step 1: Two carbon fragments of acetyl-CoA are transferred to ACP moiety of FASN. Then the acetyl unit is transferred from ACP to the cysteine residue of the enzyme to vacate the site of ACP.

Step 2: This vacant place of ACP is occupied by malonate of malonyl-CoA. Both of these reactions are catalyzed by MAT.

Step 3: The acetyl unit attached to cysteine residue is transferred to malonyl group bound to ACP and the malonyl moiety undergoes decarboxylation to produce β-ketoacyl ACP. The reaction is catalyzed by the enzyme KS.

Step 4: The enzyme KR reduces β-ketoacyl ACP to β-hydroxyacyl-ACP with the help of reducing equivalents supplied by NADPH.

Step 5: The enzyme DH causes dehydration of β-hydroxyacyl ACP. One molecule of water is eliminated with the introduction of a double bond between α and β carbon.

Step 6: In the next step, ER produces acyl-ACP (butyryl-ACP)) through a second NADPH-dependent reduction. The butyryl group is attached to the ACP as four-carbon unit.

The four-carbon unit is then transferred to cysteine residue. Steps 2–6 are repeated for 6 times, and in each step the two carbon units are added to fatty acids. Thus, after seven cycles, a 16-carbon fully saturated fatty acid (palmitate) is produced, which is still attached to the ACP.

Step 7: In this step, the enzyme thioesterase separates palmitic acid from ACP moiety of FASN.

7.2.7 Fatty Acid Desaturation

This process involves the dehydrogenation of saturated fatty acids to form monounsaturated fatty acids by the enzyme stearoyl-CoA desaturase (SCD). The enzyme SCD is present in the membrane of endoplasmic reticulum. In cattle, two forms of SCD are found: SCD1 and SCD5. In the mammary gland and adipose tissue, SCD1 is predominantly expressed, whereas SCD5 is expressed in the brain. SCD1 converts palmitic acid (C16:0) and stearic acid (C18:0) into palmitoleic acid (C16:1) and oleic acid (C18:1), respectively. It was reported that the expression of SCD1 is seen during lactation.

7.2.8 Synthesis of Glycerol and Glycerides

The glycerol-3-phosphate is derived from two sources: triose phosphate generated during glycolysis and phosphorylation of glycerol. The primary precursor for glyceride glycerol in the mammary gland is glucose. It was estimated that as high as 95% glyceride is derived from glucose in rabbits and as low as 40% in the sow and intermediate (70%) in cows.

The remaining glyceride glycerol is produced from the phosphorylation of free glycerol catalyzed by the enzyme glycerokinase. This enzyme is localized in the mammary gland of guinea pig, rat, sow, cow, and goat, and its activity is increased during the onset of lactation.

7.2.9 Triglyceride Synthesis

Milk triglycerides are synthesized through the esterification of fatty acids (received from the blood and de novo in the mammary gland) and glycerol. The exact cellular localization of milk fat triglyceride is yet to be explored. But it was a general agreement that both mitochondria and microsomes could be the probable site. The formation of triglycerides involves two pathways, namely α-glycerol phosphate pathway and monoglyceride pathway.

7.2.9.1 α-Glycerol Phosphate Pathway

It is the predominant pathway of milk triglyceride synthesis. In this pathway, two fatty acids (CoA derivatives) are esterified with α-glycerol phosphate to form phosphatidic acid, which is subsequently converted to 1,2-diglyceride. The detailed pathway is operated as follows:

1. Acylation of glycerol-3-phosphate at N-1 position by the enzyme glycerol-3-phosphate acyltransferases (GPATs).
2. Binding of fatty acyl-CoA to the sn-1 site of glycerol-3-phosphate by the enzyme glycerol-3-phosphate acyltransferase (GPAM) to form lysophosphatidic acid (LPA).

3. The enzyme 1-acylglycerol-3-phosphate O-acyltransferase 6 (AGPAT6) facilitates the binding of another fatty acyl-CoA to glycerol-3-phosphate at the sn-2 site to form phosphatidic acid (PA).
4. Lipin 1 (LPIN1), a phosphatidyl phosphatase and transcriptional co-activator, transfers a phosphate group from PA to form 1,2 diacylglycerol (DAG). The enzyme diacylglycerol acyltransferase (DGAT) transfers acyl groups from the fatty acyl-CoA to N-1, 2 DAG to form triglycerides.

7.2.9.2 Monoglyceride Pathway

In this pathway, the fatty acids are converted into DAG by the enzyme monoacylglycerol acyltransferases (MOGATs). The DAG is converted to triglycerides by DGAT. This pathway mainly operates in the enterocytes. A study reported that monoacylglycerol pathway for triacylglycerol synthesis does not exist in the goat mammary gland (Hansen et al. 1986).

7.2.10 Synthesis of Phospholipid

Phospholipids constitute nearly 1% of milk fat and mostly appear in the milk in the form of milk fat globular membrane. Predominant milk phospholipids are sphingomyelin, phosphatidyl choline, phosphatidyl serine, phosphatidyl ethanolamine, and phosphatidyl inositol. Each of these phospholipids contains each containing 25–30 fatty acids. Though some of the phospholipids are absorbed directly from the blood, major portions of milk phospholipids are synthesized de novo in the mammary gland. The phospholipids absorbed in the mammary gland are metabolized, and the fatty acids are reutilized for triglyceride synthesis. In the mammary gland of goats, circulating phospholipids do not contribute to milk phospholipids; rather, the mammary gland synthesizes phospholipids by using a common phosphate pool for both milk inorganic phosphate and phosphorus required for milk phospholipid synthesis.

7.2.11 Milk Cholesterol Synthesis

Cholesterol and cholesterol esters comprise 0.5% of milk fat. They are synthesized de novo from acetate within the mammary gland and directly taken from the blood.

Synthesis of milk cholesterol is a multistep process and the enzymes for cholesterol biosynthesis are present in the cytosol and microsomal fractions of the cell. Acetate is the main source of carbons of cholesterol. At the beginning, two moles of acetyl-CoA condense to form acetoacetyl-CoA. One molecule of acetyl-CoA is again added to acetoacetyl-CoA to form β-hydroxy β-methylglutaryl CoA (HMG CoA) by the enzyme HMG CoA synthase. HMG CoA is then reduced to mevalonate with the help of enzyme HMG CoA reductase. The reducing equivalents are coming from NADPH. In the next step, mevalonate is converted to 3-phospho 5-pyrophosphomevalonate, which is decarboxylated to form isopentenyl pyrophosphate (IPP) and its isomer dimethylallyl pyrophosphate (DPP). These reactions are catalyzed by different kinases. The IPP and DPP are 5-carbon isoprenoid units and condense to yield 10-carbon geranyl pyrophosphate (GPP). In the next step, GPP again combines with another IPP to form a 15-carbon compound called farnesyl pyrophosphate (FPP). Two units of FPP join together and subsequently form 30-carbon squalene. The squalene is converted to lanosterol through hydroxylation and cyclization with the help of epoxidase hydroxylase cyclase with the utilization of O2 and NADPH. Lansosterol undergoes a series of about 19 enzymatic reactions to yield cholesterol through the production of intermediary compounds like desmethyl lanosterol, zymosterol, cholestadienol, and desmosterol. The immediate intermediate before cholesterol biosynthesis is 7-dehydrocholesterol, which is reduced to give cholesterol.

7.2.12 Secretion of Milk Lipids

Milk lipids are secreted in the form of milk droplets composed of triglycerides (95%) with lesser amounts of sterols, partial glycerides, phospholipids, glycolipids, and hydrocarbons. The droplets are encapsulated by a membrane called milk fat globule membrane (MFGM) composed of polar lipids and proteins. The MFGM is derived from either apical plasma membrane or endoplasmic reticulum. Milk droplets are of two types: cytoplasmic lipid droplets (CLDs) (size 1–5 μm) and microlipid droplets (MLDs) (size 0.5 μm or less).

There are two routes of milk lipid secretion:

Apical vesicle route: In this route, lipid droplets originate in the rough endoplasmic reticulum as MLDs and transport toward the apical membrane alone or in combinations to form CLDs. The MLDs are fused together to form CLDs during their transit.

Secretory vesicle route: In this pathway, CLDs are surrounded by secretory vesicles. Later they form intracytoplasmic vacuoles and transported toward the apical membrane.

In both the cases, the contents of apical and secretory vesicles are released by exocytosis.

A combination of both apical and secretory vesicle routes may also help to release milk fat droplets.

7.2.13 Regulation of Milk Fat Synthesis

The synthesis of milk fat is regulated by two main transcription factors: namely peroxisome proliferator-activated receptor γ (PPARγ) and sterol-regulatory element-binding protein (SREBP) 1 and 2.

Table 7.4 MicroRNAs (miRNAs) regulate fatty acid synthesis

Name	Function	Species	Reference
miR-103	Promotes the expression of fatty acid synthase	Goat	Ji et al. (2012)
miR-143	Induces the expression of Smad3 to induce lipid droplet formation	Bovine	Zhang et al. (2020)
miR-25	Inhibits triglyceride synthesis by regulating Peroxisome proliferator-activated receptor γ coactivator 1 (PGC-1β)	Goat	Ma et al. (2018)
miR-27a	Decreases triglyceride synthesis	Goat	Lin et al. (2013)
miR-183	Inhibits milk fat metabolism by controlling macrophage stimulating 1 (Mst1) gene	Goat	Chen et al. (2018)
miR-106b	Regulating cholesterol metabolism through ATP-binding cassette subfamily A-1 (ABCA1)	Bovine	Chen et al. (2019)

PPARγ forms a heterodimer with retinoid X receptor (RXR) and binds with peroxisome proliferator-activated receptor (PPAR) response elements (PPRE), which induces the expression of genes responsible for fatty acid synthesis (fatty acid synthase, acetyl-CoA carboxylase, and stearoyl-CoA desaturase) and fatty acid transport (CD36). Long-chain fatty acids (LCFA) are the potent agonist of PPARγ. Polyunsaturated fatty acids (PUFAs) are the natural ligands of PPARγ in nonruminants.

SREBP 1 and 2 are present in the endoplasmic reticulum with their activator called SREBP-cleavage activating protein (Scap). Decreased cholesterol stimulates Scap, which facilitates the transport of SREBP to nucleus to the expression acetyl-CoA carboxylase α (ACACA), fatty acid synthase (FASN) genes to promote fatty acid synthesis and HMG-CoA synthase and HMG-CoA reductase for cholesterol biosynthesis.

Another important transcriptional regulator of fatty acid synthesis is mammalian target of rapamycin (mTOR). This mTOR activates SREBP to induce the biosynthesis of fatty acid synthesis genes and CD36.

There are some microRNAs (miRNAs) that is also involved in the post-transcriptional regulation of fatty acid synthesis genes (Table 7.4).

7.3 Protein Metabolism of the Mammary Gland

The mammary gland is the major organ of nitrogen utilization. However, the efficiency to transform dietary nitrogen into milk proteins is low (25–30%). The synthesis of proteins is a highly active process that involves energy expenditure from ATP, GTP, NADH, and NADPH. It was estimated that half of the available ATP is utilized for mammary tissue protein synthesis in goats. The major milk protein precursors are amino acids derived from blood. The proportion of plasma amino acids corresponding to their residues in the milk was estimated to be 84% for arginine, 86% for methionine, 96% for phenylalanine, 85% for threonine, and 96% for valine. Some nonessential amino acids are synthesized in the mammary gland from arginine and ornithine. The glutathione of erythrocytes and plasma oligopeptides also makes a minor contribution to milk protein synthesis. A substantial portion of amino acids is also derived from tissue protein. It was estimated that 90–430 g of amino acids/day is supplied from tissue protein in cows. The value for the same in goats is 2–66 g/day.

7.3.1 Amino Acid Uptake by the Mammary Gland

The main precursors for milk protein synthesis are free amino acids (AAs) and peptide-bound amino acids (PBAAs). It was estimated that 10–30% of the total AAs for milk protein synthesis come from PBAAs in lactating goats. In cows, nearly 25% of AAs are derived from rumen bypass peptides.

7.3.1.1 Uptake of Free Amino Acids

The amino acids are taken up by the mammary secretory cells at their basolateral membrane. There are two different classes of amino acid transporters Na+-dependent transporters and Na + -independent transporters. The Na-dependent transport is energy-dependent process and they facilitate unidirectional transport amino acids utilizing electrochemical gradients of Na+ and other ions. In contrast, Na^+-independent transport in nonenergy-dependent and favors bidirectional transport of amino acids. Based on the amino acid specificity, both Na^+-dependent and independent transporters are different for basic, acidic, and neutron amino acids (Table 7.5).

Na^+-dependent transporters utilize the electrochemical gradients of Na^+ and other ions to actively transport amino acids. These transporters are also energy-dependent

Table 7.5 Na+-dependent transporters in the mammary gland in different species

Na+-dependent transporters	Types	Amino acids involved	Species	References
Transporters for basic and acidic AA	L-type amino acid transporter-2 (LAT-2)	Lys, Arg, His, Leu, Ile, Met, Ala, Ser, Thr, Val	Pig, human, rat	Bröer (2008), Karunakaran et al. (2011)
	L-type amino acid transporter-2 (LAT-2)	Lys, Arg, His, Gln, Leu, Met, Ala, Cys	Pig	Closs (2002), Bionaz and Loor (2011)
Neutral amino acid transporters	Sodium-coupled neutral amino acid transporter (SNAT)	Ala, Ser, Gly, Pro, Cys, Gln	Rat, mouse, cow	Bröer (2008)
	Alanine, serine, cysteine amino acid transport protein (ASCT)	Ala, Ser, Gly, Val, Thr, Cys, Gln	Pig, human, rat, cow	Sharma and Kansal (2001), Bröer (2008)

Table 7.6 Na+-independent transporters in the mammary gland in different species

Na+-independent transporters	Types	Amino acids involved	Species	References
Transporters for basic and acidic AA	Cationic amino acid transport protein (CAT) (y+ system $y^{+}L$ system, $b^{0,+}$ system and $B^{0,+}$ system	Lys, Arg, His, Ornithine	Pig, human, rat, cow	Bröer (2008), Karunakaran et al. (2011)
	Amino acid transporter rB (rBAT)	Lys, Arg, Ornithine, Cystine, Leu	Pig	Closs (2002), Bionaz and Loor (2011)
	Excitatory amino acid transporter (EAAT)	Asp, Glu	Mouse, rat	Bionaz and Loor (2011)
Neutral amino acid transporters	L-type amino acid transporter (LAT)	Ala, Ser, Val, Thr, Leu, Ile, Met, Phe, Tyr, Trp, His	Mouse, rat, cow	Bröer (2008)
	T-type amino acid transporter (TAT)	Phe, Tyr, Trp	Mouse	Sharma and Kansal (2001), Bröer (2008)

and facilitate unidirectional amino transport. Based on the amino acid specificity, Na^{+}-dependent transporters may be of two types (Table 7.6).

7.3.1.2 Uptake of PBAA

The PBAAs undergo hydrolysis by small peptide hydrolase to yield free AAs at the basement membrane of mammary epithelial cells before their transportation through AA transporters. Some of the small peptides are absorbed intact through their specific transports such as peptide transporters 1 (PepT1) and 2 (PepT2). The expression of PepT2 in the mammary gland of cows was reported to increase in response to lactogenic hormones (i.e., prolactin, hydrocortisone, and insulin) and specific substrate.

7.3.2 Utilization of Amino Acids

After entering the mammary secretory cells, the amino acids may have either of the following fates. They may be utilized for milk protein synthesis through RNA-directed polymerization, may form tissue proteins and retained into the cells, undergo metabolic reactions to form urea, polyaminine, and other nonessential amino acids, or may pass unchanged into the blood.

The amino acid uptake by the mammary gland is equal to its output in milk for cows, goats, sows, and ewes. However, it varies considerably between different amino acids (Table 7.7). The amino acids having uptake:output ratios more than

Table 7.7 Mammary amino acid uptake:output ratios in different mammals

Species	Uptake: output ratios	Amino acids	References
Cows	= 1	Methionine, histidine, tryptophan, phenylalanine, and tyrosine	Omphalius et al. (2019), Haque et al. (2015), Raggio et al. (2006)
	> 1	Valine, isoleucine, leucine, lysine, and arginine	
	< 1	Nonessential amino acids	
Goats	= 1	Methionine, histidine, tryptophan, phenylalanine, and tyrosine	Mepham and Linzell (1966)
	> 1	Valine, isoleucine, leucine, lysine, and arginine	
	< 1	Serine, glutamine, proline, and asparagine	
Sows	= 1	Methionine, histidine, and lysine	Trottier et al. (1997)
	> 1	Arginine, leucine, isoleucine, valine, tryptophan, phenylalanine, glutamate, glutamine, alanine, and glycine	
	< 1	Proline, aspartate, and asparagine	
Ewes	= 1	Methionine, phenylalanine, tyrosine, threonine, and histidine	Davis et al. (1978)
	> 1	Valine, isoleucine, leucine, and arginine	
	< 1	Nonessential amino acids (except for serine)	

1 indicate that these amino acids can be metabolized into urea, polyaminine, and other nonessential amino acids.

7.3.3 Milk Protein Synthesis

Hormone-induced transcription factors initiate the expression of milk protein genes. The casein gene locus was identified in chromosome 6 in cattle, sheep, and goats, chromosome 5 in mice and chromosome 4 in human. β-Lactoglobulin-encoding gene locus has been identified in chromosome 3 in sheep and chromosome 11 in cows and goats. The α-lactalbumin-encoding gene is localized in chromosome 12 in man, chromosome 3 in sheep, chromosomes 5 in bovine and goats, and chromosome 5 in pigs.

The transcription of genes requires binding of specific transcription factors to its promoter region.

The synthesis of milk proteins includes several steps.

7.3.3.1 Activation of Transcription Factors

The process of transcription involves the synthesis of RNA from DNA. The functional unit of DNA that is transcribed is called a gene. In this process, one DNA strand acts as a template (noncoding strands) to transcribe into RNA molecules, which are complementary to the template strand; another DNA strand is called the coding strand, which does not participate in transcription, but it regulates the process of transcription. The enzyme RNA polymerase helps in the process of transcription. RNA polymerase binds to a sequence near the beginning of a gene. This binding site is called a promoter. RNA polymerase attaches to the promoter site with the help of transcription factors.

The minimal requirement for the initiation of gene transcription is the binding of an appropriate set of transcription factors to its 5′-upstream region. There are specific DNA sequences for the binding of transcription factors. Major transcription factors associated with milk protein synthesis are signal transducer and activator of transcription 5 (Stat5), musculoaponeurotic fibrosarcoma (MAF), CCAAT/enhancer-binding proteins (C/EBP), nuclear factor 1 (NF1), and glucocorticoid receptor (GR). The transcription factor Stat5 is activated by prolactin and induces the genes for milk protein. After binding with its receptors, prolactin activates tyrosine kinase JAK2, which leads to the initiation of cascades of reactions to phosphorylate cellular proteins including Stat5. The phosphorylated Stat5 translocates into the nucleus to bind with specific DNA sequence motif for the transcription of milk protein genes. Growth hormone and placental lactogen also stimulate the expression of milk protein genes.

The amino acids transported into the mammary gland also facilitate the transcription of milk protein gene through the activation of Janus kinase 2-signal transducer and activator of transcription 5 (JAK2-STAT5). Other than this, they also activate seryl-tRNA synthetase (SARS), AA taste 1 receptor member 1/3 (TAS1R1/TAS1R3), phosphatidylinositol-3-kinase (PI3K-AKT) that ultimately upregulate mammalian target of rapamycin (mTOR) signaling pathway to initiate transcription of milk protein genes.

7.3.3.2 Post-Transcriptional Modifications of RNA

The RNAs produced during the transcription are called primary transcripts. The primary transcript produced by RNA polymerase II in eukaryotic cells is called heterogeneous nuclear RNA (hnRNA), which is processed further to produce mRNA. The primary transcripts or mRNAs produced during transcription undergo post-transcriptional modifications to become active. These modifications include the following:

The 5′ capping: In this process, 5′ end of mRNA undergoes capping with 7-methylguanosine by an unusual 5–5′ triphosphate linkage. S-Adenosylmethionine is the methyl group donor. The capping stabilizes the structure of mRNA.

Poly-A tail: It is an additional chain of adenine nucleotide at the 3′-end of the mRNA that stabilizes the mRNA. The enzyme responsible for adding poly(A) tail is poly (A) polymerase (PAP) and poly(A)-binding protein (PABP) in the cytosol of the epithelial cells binds with the poly(A) in mRNA and protect mRNA from exoribonucleases. The degree of polyadenylation determines the half-life of casein mRNA in the mammary gland.

mRNA splicing: In this mechanism, the noncoding sequence of mRNA (introns) is removed from the newly synthesized mRNA by spliceosome and the coding sequences (exons) are joined together.

7.3.3.3 Amino Acid Activation

The amino acids are activated and attached to the tRNAs by two-step reactions. At the beginning, amino acids are combined with ATP to form amino acid and adenosine monophosphate (AMP) by the enzyme aminoacyl tRNA synthetase. These activated amino acids are transferred to 3′ end of the tRNA to form aminoacyl tRNA.

The acceptance capacity (nmoles AA/mg of tRNA) of bovine tRNAs to different amino acids varied considerably. The highest capacity was reported for phenylalanine followed by glutamic acid, leucine, and glycine in the virgin mammary gland of cows. But in the lactating mammary gland, glutamic acid predominates followed by leucine, phenylalanine, and glycine.

7.3.3.4 Translation

The process of biosynthesis of proteins or polypeptide is called translation. Each tRNA contains the anticodon, three nucleotide base sequence that recognizes their complementary bases at mRNA known as codon.

The translation occurs on the ribosomes, which are in association with the rough endoplasmic reticulum (RER).

The process of translation is divided into three distinct stages, namely initiation, elongation, and termination.

At the initiation stage, ribosomes attach to the mRNA at the start codon. The initiation requires special proteins called eukaryotic initiation factors (eIFs). The initiation process occurs through several steps. At the beginning, dissociation of ribosome occurs. The 80S ribosome is dissociated to form 40S and 60S subunits. The initiation factors, eIF-3 and eIF-1A, bind with 40S subunit to prevent its reassociation with 60S subunit. A ternary complex of aminoacyl tRNA (methionyl tRNA) binds to the 40S ribosomal subunit to form 43S preinitiation complex. This binding is facilitated by the eIF-2 with the help of GTP. The 43S preinitiation complex is stabilized by eIF-3 and eIF-1A. The binding of mRNA with 43S preinitiation complex results in the formation of 48S initiation complex. In the next step, eIF-4F complex is formed win association with eIF-4G, eIF-4A, and eIF-4E. The initiation factor eIF-4E binds with the 5′ cap of mRNA, eIF-4G, which binds to both eIF-4E at the 5′ cap and PABP at the 3′ poly-A tail. The mRNA is transferred to the 43S complex. The initiation complex at the ribosome scans mRNA to identify the initiation codon AUG. The 48S initiation complex then binds with 60S ribosomal subunit to form 80S initiation complex through the hydrolysis of GTP that binds with eIF-2. The initiation factor eIF-5 favors the formation of 80S initiation complex. The 80S ribosome has three tRNA-binding sites, namely P (peptidyl), A (aminoacyl), and E (exit).

In the elongation step, polypeptide chains are formed by the addition of amino acids by the sequence of the codons in the specific mRNA. First, the aminoacyl tRNA (methionyl tRNA) is attached at the P site, leaving the A site empty. The second aminoacyl tRNA is carried to the A site. This is facilitated by the involvement of elongation factor 1a (EF-Ia) with GTP. The methionine present in the P site is transferred to aminoacyl tRNA at the A site and a peptide bond is formed with the help of peptidyltransferase. After the formation of peptide bond, the ribosome proceeds to the next codon of the mRNA and the growing polypeptide chain moves from A-site to P-site. This process is augmented by EF-2 and GTP.

The termination of translation occurs when a stop codon (UAA, UAG, or UGA) comes into the A site. The cells do not have any tRNA having complementary anticodons for these stop codons; hence, no tRNA is able to bind with the A site. An eukaryotic release factor (eRF-1) recognizes these stop codons and binds with A site to release the completed polypeptide chain and facilitates the dissociation of tRNA and mRNA from the ribosome.

7.3.3.5 Intracellular Transport and Processing of Milk Proteins

The newly synthesized protein in the ribosomes is in the form of a long poly peptide chain. Protease cleaves a short peptide of 16–30 amino acids present at the N-terminus called signal sequence. This sequence is identified by the receptors in the endoplasmic reticulum, and the newly synthesized protein is translocated into the endoplasmic reticulum. After the translocation, folding of nascent polypeptides occurs with the formation of disulfide bond between cysteine-rich peptide residues by the enzyme disulfide isomerase (PDI). The formation of disulfide bond favors the transport of proteins into the Golgi complex. Along with the disulfide bond formation, N-glycosylation of α-lactalbumin and oligomerization of caseins also occur as co-translation modifications. The newly synthesized protein is transported from endoplasmic reticulum to Golgi complex through ER–Golgi intermediate compartment (ERGIC), tubule vesicular network between endoplasmic reticulum, and Golgi complex. At the Golgi complex, several post-translational modifications occur.

7.3.4 Post-Translational Modifications of Milk Proteins

The newly synthesized milk proteins undergo post-translational modifications such as phosphorylation and glycosylation for their stability and micelle formation. αs1-, αs2-, and β-caseins undergo phosphorylation, whereas glycosylation occurs in the κ-casein at the Golgi complex.

7.3.4.1 Phosphorylation

The enzyme protein kinase phosphorylates the Ser or Thr residues after the identification of Ser/Thr-X-Glu/SerP/Asp tripeptide motif (X stands for any AA residue and P represents phosphorylation). The casein kinase is a cAMP-dependent kinase that facilitates casein phosphorylation and the ATP acts as ATP as the phosphate donor. Divalent cations such as Ca^{2+} or Mg^{2+} are required for this reaction. The phosphorylation facilitates caseins to form micelle after interacting with calcium phosphate. The degree of phosphorylation varies between different casein isoforms. Bovine αS1 casein has two common phosphorylated isoforms such as αS1-CN-8P and αS1-CN-9P. In αS2-casein, αS2-CN-10P and αS2-CN-13P are the two isoforms. The β-casein appears as β-CN-5P or 4P and κ-casein is found as κ-CN-1P or 2P.

The whey proteins such as β-actoglobulin and α-lactalbumin are generally not phosphorylated.

7.3.4.2 Glycosylation

The glycosylation is one of the important post-translational modifications that occurs in the Golgi complex with the help of enzymes N-acetylgalactosaminyltransferase, galactosyltransferase, and sialyltransferase. The κ-caseins are mostly glycosylated. There are two types of glycosylation: O-glycosylation for serine- or threonine-linked glycans and N-glycosylation for asparagine-linked glycans. But κ-casein undergoes only O-glycosylation. It was estimated that 60% of κ-casein is glycosylated. The major glycans for this glycosylation are tetrasaccharide (56%) composed of galactose (Gal), N-acetylgalactosamine (GalNAc), and sialic or neuraminic acid (NeuAc). However, monosaccharide (0.8%), disaccharide (6.3%) and trisaccharide (36.9%) are also found. After phosphorylation of caseins in the Golgi apparatus, calcium ions are attached to the casein ester phosphate groups in the terminal Golgi to yield calcium caseinate phosphate and form micelles.

7.3.4.3 Formation of Casein Micelle

The predominant milk protein casein appears as casein micelles that constitute 95% casein protein and 5% minerals in the form of micellar calcium phosphate (MCP). Though the primary components of MCP are calcium and phosphate, a trace amount of magnesium, citrate, and other minerals is also present in the casein micelle. The size of casein micelle in bovines ranges from 50 to 500 nm. In the casein micelle, αS1, αS1, β, and κ-casein fraction are present in the proportion of 40%, 10%, 35%, and 15%, respectively. The α-caseins have properties of molecular chaperon that stabilizes its structure and prevents coagulation. The self-assembling properties of casein micelle are exhibited by the amphiphilic structure and intermolecular hydrophobic interactions between different casein fractions. The κ-casein constitutes the hydrophilic layer due to the presence of carbohydrate moiety. The initial aggregation of caseins occurs in the *cis*-Golgi stacks. The final micelle aggregates are formed in the prosecretory granules or trans-Golgi network (TGN).

7.3.5 Secretion of Milk Proteins

The major milk proteins (caseins, α-lactalbumin, and β-lactoglobulin) are secreted by exocytosis. The initial submicelle formation occurs at the cis-Golgi stacks, which undergo further aggregation and formation of casein micelle at pro-secretory granules analogous to trans-Golgi network (TGN). The time taken by the casein protein to reach from ER to Golgi requires 15–25 min. Their concentration in the secretory vesicles was appreciated after 25-45mins and their accumulation in the lumen after 60mins. The secretory vesicles reach the apical membrane and their contents are subsequently released by exocytosis. The fusion of casein-containing secretory vesicles and apical membrane is facilitated by a group of proteins called soluble N-ethylmaleimide–sensitive fusion (NSF) attachment protein receptor (SNARE) proteins. There are two classes of SNARE proteins: R-SNAREs present on the membrane of secretory vesicle and Q-SNAREs on the apical membrane. These two classes of SNARE proteins that fuse with each other to form SNARE complex and exocytosis occurs. The dissociation of SNARE complex is facilitated by NSF adenosine triphosphatase and its adaptor protein synaptosomal-associated protein (SNAP). Studies have shown that SNAP23, VAMP8/endobrevin, and Syntaxins (Stx3, 6, 7,12) are important SNARE proteins involved in casein exocytosis.

The hormone prolactin helps in the exocytosis of secretory vesicle by modulating SNARE proteins in the mammary epithelial cells. Prolactin induces the production of arachidonic acid and phospholipase A2 (PLA2) after binding with its receptors through a calcium-independent mechanism. This arachidonic acid is believed to be interacting with SNARE complex to facilitate exocytosis.

7.3.6 Metabolism of Amino Acids in the Mammary Gland

The mammary gland is an important site for amino acid synthesis and catabolism. Excess uptake of amino acids leads to catabolism and is not considered to be limiting for milk protein synthesis. The catabolism only happens when the acyl-tRNA is fully saturated because the Km value for activation of acyl-tRNA synthetases is about 100 times lower than the Km value for the enzymes required for amino acid catabolism. Table 7.8 shows the uptake of amino acids and their output in the milk proteins in lactating sow.

7.3.6.1 Metabolism of Branched Chain Amino Acids (BCAAs)

BCAA such as leucine, isoleucine, and valine are catabolized in the mammary gland to form glutamate and glutamine. At the beginning, BCAAs undergo transamination by BCAA transaminase (BCAT) with the help of α-ketoglutarate to form branched-chain α-ketoacids (BCKA) (α-ketoisovalerate, α-ketoisocaproate, α-keto β-methyl valerate, respectively, from valine, leucine, and isoleucine), and glutamate. The

Table 7.8 Amino acid uptake and their output in milk protein in the mammary gland of lactating sow

Amino acid	Uptake by the mammary gland (g/day)	Output in milk (g/day)	Difference (g/day)
Arginine	31	6	+25
Proline	26	40	−14
Branched chain amino acids (BCAA)	76	46	+30
Glutamine	16	36	−20

Lei et al. (2012), Li et al. (2009) and Trottier et al. (1997)

BCKA are decarboxylated by the enzyme BCKA dehydrogenase complex (BCKAD) to form their corresponding acyl-CoA derivatives (sobutyryl CoA, isovaleryl CoA, and α-methylbutyryl CoA, respectively, from valine, leucine, and isoleucine). The BCKAD enzyme complex is located in the inner mitochondrial membrane; so, if the transamination of BCAA occurs in the cytosol, the BCKA must enter the mitochondria to form acyl-CoA derivatives or they may release from the cells. However, in cows, the majority of BCKA is released into the extracellular space rather converted to acyl-CoA derivatives.

There are two different isoforms of BCAT in cows and sows. BCAT is present in the cytosol, while $BCAT_m$ is located in the mitochondria. But in rat mammary gland, $BCAT_m$ is only present.

The glutamate derived from BCAA forms either glutamine or transaminated to form alanine (or aspartate). Glutamine synthetase and glutaminase are the two important enzymes for these reactions. The activity of glutaminase is absent in lactating mammary gland; hence, the production of glutamine predominates over its catabolism. It has been estimated that the catabolism of 30 g/d BCAA yields 20 g/d glutamine in the mammary gland of lactating cows.

7.3.6.2 Metabolism of Arginine

The uptake of arginine by the mammary gland of sow is greater than its output. Hence, it is obvious that a substantial portion of arginine is catabolized into the mammary gland. It was estimated that nearly 81% of the arginine is degraded locally into the mammary gland of sows.

There are different pathways of arginine catabolism by the lactating mammary gland. A part of arginine is hydrolyzed into ornithine and urea via the arginase pathway, and another minor portion is catabolized to form polyamine and nitric oxide via the arginase and nitric oxide synthase (NOS) pathways. The ornithine derived from arginine is converted to proline, whereas nitric oxide acts as an endothelium-dependent relaxing factor to control mammary blood flow.

The enzyme arginase catalyzes the conversion of arginine into urea and ornithine. The two different arginase isoforms, namely arginase I and II, are located in the cytosol and mitochondria, respectively, in the cows', sows', and rats' mammary epithelial cells. The ornithine can be utilized for the synthesis of polyamines by enzymes ornithine decarboxylase (ODC) and spermidine synthase. A relatively high concentration of polyamine in the milk of rats, sows, and human milk is due to the activity of these enzymes.

A part of the arginine-derived ornithine can enter mitochondria to form Δ^1-l-pyrroline-5-carboxylate (P5C) by ornithine aminotransferase (OAT). This P5C can lead to the production of glutamic acid by Δ^1-l-pyrroline-5-carboxylate dehydrogenase (P5CD) or proline by Δ^1-l pyrroline-5-carboxylate reductase (P5CR). However, the activity of enzyme P5CR is 56-fold higher than P5CD. Hence, the majority of arginine is converted to proline rather than glutamic acid.

The conversion of arginine into nitric oxide is facilitated by the enzyme nitric oxide synthase (NOS). This nitric oxide acts as a vasodilator and increases mammary blood flow, favoring the supply of precursors of milk synthesis.

7.3.6.3 Metabolism of Lysine

The uptake of lysine by the mammary gland is the highest among all other essential amino acids. Lysine is one of the major limiting amino acid for milk protein synthesis. But a substantial portion of lysine is oxidized in the mammary gland of cows, ewes, and sows. The incorporation of lysine into the milk protein was estimated to be 67% and 23% and undergoes oxidative losses. The exact pathway of lysine catabolism is yet to be explored. But it was assumed that lysine could be utilized for the synthesis of several nonessential amino acids.

7.3.6.4 Metabolism of Methionine and Cysteine

Methionine and cysteine are two essential sulphur-containing amino acids required for protein synthesis. It was estimated that 95% of extracted methionine can be incorporated into milk protein. The uptake of methionine by the mammary gland closely matched its protein output. A minor portion of methionine could be utilized for the synthesis of phospholipids, creatine, polyamine, and carnitine.

7.3.6.5 Metabolism of Phenylalanine and Tyrosine

Mammary uptake of phenylalanine is matched with its secretion in milk proteins. A portion of phenylalanine generates tyrosine via the phenylalanine hydroxylase pathway.

7.3.7 Transcytosis of Milk Proteins

Proteins such as albumin, immunoglobulins, transferrin, hormones, and growth factors are transported across the mammary epithelial cells through the transcytosis pathway. The major advantage of transcytosis is that the bioactive molecules are carried, avoiding the degradation. Hence, the milk contains several intact bioactive molecules for the neonates. The process of transcytosis involves three steps: endocytosis of the materials, followed by endosomal trafficking and, finally, the exocytosis.

The endocytosis is mediated by a clathrin-dependent or a clathrin-independent mechanism through membrane-bounded vesicles. The fluids are taken up by pinocytosis or fluid-phase endocytosis. Clathrin is a protein that interacts with the plasma membrane proteins like a cage in the form of coated pits. The plasma membrane adapter complex termed as AP-2 is required for the transport and packaging of materials into clathrin-coated vesicles.

The clathrin-independent mechanism is also called caveolae-mediated endocytosis (CavME). Myoepithelial cells surrounding the alveolar epithelium contain small vesicles (50–80 nm) called caveoli. Caveolin-1 is the integral membrane protein of caveoli. The phosphorylation of caveolin-1 facilitates the internalization of caveolae with the cargo materials.

After the internalization, the vesicle undergoes fusion with the early endosome for sorting. Then they undergo retrograde trafficking mechanisms through trans-Golgi network (TGN) and finally exocytosis. Some vesicles are transported to the lysosome through the late endosome/multivesicular body (MVB) for degradation or recycled back to plasma membrane by recycling endosomes.

7.3.7.1 Transcytosis of Transferrin

The transferrin (Tf), along with its receptor (TfR), undergoes endocytosis by coated vesicles. After the internalization, Tf-TfR complex is transported into the endosomal compartment. The acidic pH of endosomes facilitates the release of iron (Fe^{+3}) and the complex is recycled to basolateral membrane. The Tf-TfR complex can also be directed to multivesicular bodies (mvb) for degradation.

7.3.8 Transport of Water and Electrolytes Across the Mammary Gland

The plasma and milk are isosmotic in aqueous phage, but their ionic composition varies a lot. This difference in the ionic composition maintains a concentration gradient across transepithelial membrane, which favors the transepithelial ion transport across the apical and basolateral membrane of mammary epithelial cells. The ionic composition of mammary epithelial cells, extracellular fluid, and milk is depicted in Table 7.9.

The distribution of ions across the mammary epithelium generates an electrochemical gradient where the interior of epithelial cells is electrically negative compared to milk (−41 mv vs 3 mv). This electrochemical gradient is chiefly maintained by Na^+-K^+-ATPse pump in the basolateral membrane and passive transport of Na^+ and K^+ at the apical membrane.

7.3.8.1 Water Transport

The water transport in the mammary gland occurs through the transcellular route, and the major driving force of this transportation is the osmotic gradient produced by milk lactose. The transport of water across the mammary epithelial cells is mediated by aquaporins (AQP), water-permeable membrane protein. The AQP creates pores in the membrane to facilitate the transport of water influenced by osmotic gradients. There are different types of AQP identified in the mammary epithelial cells of different species (Table 7.10).

AQP are activated by arginine-vasopressin via V2-R receptors at the basolateral membrane of the mammary epithelial cells. The AQPs exist as intracellular vesicles

Table 7.9 The concentrations of different ions between extracellular fluid and mammary epithelial cells in guinea pig

Ions	Extracellular fluid	Mammary epithelial cell	Milk
Sodium (Na^+)	150 mM	43 mM	8 mM
Potassium (K^+)	4.5 mM	143 mM	24 mM
Chloride (Cl^-)	116 mM	62 mM	12 mM

Linzell and Peaker (1971)

Table 7.10 Aquaporins in the mammary gland of different species

Aquaporin	Species	References
AQP1, AQP2, AQP3, AQP4, AQP5, AQP6, and AQP7	Rat	Matsuzaki et al. (2005)
AQP1 and AQP3	Human	Mobasheri et al. (2005)
AQP1, AQP3, AQP4, and AQP7	Bovines	Mobasheri et al. (2011)

and arginine-vasopressin mediates their translocation into the membrane. The binding of arginine-vasopressin with its receptors initiates intracellular signaling cascade that involves activation of adenylate cyclase (AC) and increased intracellular cAMP. The AQP is phosphorylated at serine-256 by protein kinase A (PKA). The phosphorylated AQP then moves to the plasma membrane and fuses with it. The insertion of AQP in the plasma membrane creates water channels for the movement of water.

7.3.8.2 Transport of Sodium, Potassium, and Chloride

The sodium, potassium, and chloride are responsible for maintaining the osmolality of milk in the species with a low lactose content in the milk. There is an active gradient of Na^+, K^+, and Cl^- between the milk and plasma maintained by Na^+-K^+-ATPase pump and Cl^- transporters at the basolateral surface and Na^+, K^+, and Cl^- channels at the apical surface.

The basolateral Na^+-K^+-ATPase pump maintains higher K^+ and lower Na^+ inside the mammary epithelial cells. At the apical surface, the distribution of Na^+ and K^+ is maintained by ion channels due to the electrical potential difference across the membrane.

The concentration of Cl^- is more inside the cells due to the presence of Na^+-K^+-Cl^- co-transporters at the surface facing the blood. The higher chloride concentration inside the cells favors the secretion of ions and water across the apical membrane.

The transport of Na^+, K^+, and Cl^- depends upon the prolactin concentration. The concentration of Na^+ is decreased and K^+ is increased in response to prolactin. It also upregulates Na^+-$K^{+-}Cl^-$ co-transporters in rat mammary epithelium.

7.3.8.3 Calcium Transport

The milk is rich in calcium, and the mammary gland receives a large amount of calcium from the blood to maintain high calcium concentration in the milk in the form of casein micelles, free ionized calcium, or complexed with phosphate and citrate. But accumulation of large quantities of intracellular calcium may lead to cellular toxicity. Thus, there must be an efficient mechanism to maintain low intracellular calcium in the mammary epithelial cells that pumps the intracellular calcium into the Golgi complex. Calcium enters the mammary gland via the transcellular route as calcium is unable to cross the tight junctions. At the basolateral membrane of mammary epithelial cells, calcium is taken up by stretch-activated calcium channel. Then, calcium is pumped into the Golgi membrane across the Golgi membranes by a Ca^{2+}-ATPase pump identified in cows, rats, and mice mammary gland. These pumps are of two types: Ca-ATPases (SPCA1 and SPCA2) and plasma membrane calcium ATPase isoform 2 (PMCA2). There are calcium-sensing receptors called CaR that regulates the calcium transport across the Golgi membrane. Increased intracellular calcium upregulates PMCA2 through CaR signaling. The release of Ca^{2+} into milk is mediated by the exocytosis of Golgi vesicles, along with lactose, casein, and citrate.

7.3.8.4 Phosphate Transport

The phosphate in the milk exists in three forms: inorganic orthophosphate (Pi) as solution as HPO_4^- and $H_2PO_4^{\ 2-}$, colloidal phosphate in the form calcium casein phosphate and bound to casein micelle. In goat milk, out of a total of 20.5 mM phosphate, 6.7 mM is present as inorganic orthophosphate, 8.9 mM as colloidal suspension, and 4.9 mM bound to casein protein. The primary source of phosphate in the milk is the phosphate derived from the plasma, phosphate produced in the Golgi body by the hydrolysis of UDP during the synthesis of lactose, and the phosphate generated during the process phosphorylation of casein. The mammary gland derives phosphate from the plasma. In lactating rats, the entire plasma phosphate pool is replaced every 10 mins. The uptake of phosphate from the plasma occurs at the basolateral membrane of the mammary epithelial cells via two pathways: Na1-Pi co-transport mechanism and anion-exchange system. The secretion of phosphate in the milk is through exocytosis along with casein.

7.3.8.5 Transport of Citrate

Citrate is present in the milk in the form of calcium citrate, Cit^{2-}, and Cit^{3-}, and the citrate is considered a good milk buffer. The mammary gland is impermeable to citrate. Therefore, it is obvious that citrate is synthesized within the mammary gland. The synthesis of citrate in the mammary gland occurs from glucose and acetate in goats. The secretion of citrate occurs through the Golgi vesicular route at the apical membrane of mammary epithelial cells.

7.3.8.6 Iodide Transport

The concentration of iodide in the milk is 20–30 times more than the plasma, and the mammary gland has a remarkable ability to incorporate iodide in the milk for the thyroid function of the neonates. The iodide enters the mammary gland through sodium/iodide symporter (NIS) on the basolateral membrane of mammary epithelial cells. The NIS is produced in the endoplasmic reticulum and carried to Golgi for post-translational modification. It has been reported that glycosylation of NIS by the enzyme dolichyl-phosphate (UDP-N-acetylglucosamine) acetylglucosaminephosphotransferase 1 (DAPGT1) favors its translocation onto the basolateral membrane. Another protein called valosin-containing protein (VCP) also modulates the function of NIS by altering its folding pattern. The unfolded or misfolded NIS proteins are prone to degradation by the proteasomes, which decreases the iodide uptake. Studies in rats showed that the intake of iodine upregulated DPAGT1 and downregulated VCP to regulate iodide uptake by the mammary epithelial cells and iodine content in milk.

7.3.8.7 Choline Transport

The choline concentration is nearly 10–20-fold higher in the milk compared to plasma. In milk, choline exists in three forms: phosphatidylcholine, sphingomyelin, and unesterified choline. The choline uptake is mediated by two pathways, namely hemicholinium-3-sensitive route and simple diffusion. It has also been reported that mammary is capable of synthesizing choline de novo by the methylation of phosphatidylethanolamine to form phosphatidylcholine by phosphatidylethanolamine N-methyltransferase.

7.3.8.8 Transport of L-Carnitine

The concentration of L-carnitine is higher in milk (320 mM) compared to plasma (35 mM). The mammary gland contains a sodium-dependent L-carnitine carrier that facilitates the influx of L-carnitine in the mammary gland. However, the efflux of L-carnitine is Na independent.

Exercises

Objective Questions

1. The mammary gland is unable to synthesize glucose from other precursors due to the lack of ______________________enzyme.
2. Facilitated diffusion of glucose in the mammary gland occurs through __________________.
3. The substrate for de novo fatty acid synthesis in the ruminants is ____________________.
4. Ruminants are not able to utilize glucose carbon for fatty acid synthesis due to the lack of two key enzymes of citrate cleavage pathway, namely ___________________ and ____________________.
5. The key enzyme for de novo fatty acid synthesis is ____________________.
6. The major site for post-translational modifications of protein is _______________.
7. Proteins such as albumin, immunoglobulins, transferrin, hormones, and growth factors are transported across the mammary epithelial through the ___________________ pathway.
8. Aquaporin water channels are activated by ____________________ hormone.
9. Higher K^+ and lower Na^+ inside the mammary epithelial cells are maintained by ____________________
10. For synthesis of one molecule of lactose ____________________ molecules of glucose are required.

Subjective Questions

1. Briefly describe the molecular mechanism that regulates fatty acid synthesis in the mammary gland.
2. Write a short note on the transcellular pathways of nutrient uptake in the mammary gland.
3. Describe the details of the utilization of glucose by the mammary gland with the help of a flow diagram.
4. Describe in brief the transport of water in the mammary epithelial cells.
5. Write in brief the transcytosis of milk proteins.

Answers to Objective Questions

1. Glucose-6-phosphatase
2. Glucose transporters (GLUT)
3. Acetate
4. ATP-citrate lyase and NADP-malate dehydrogenase
5. Fatty acid synthase
6. Golgi complex
7. Transcytosis
8. Arginine-vasopressin
9. Na^+-K^+-ATPase pump
10. Two

References

Books

Bauman DE, Davis CL (1974) Biosyn thesis of milk fat. In: Larson BL, Smith VR (eds) Lactation: a comprehensive treatise, vol 2. Academic, New York, pp 31–75

Mukherjee J, Das PK, Banerjee D (2023) Lactation physiology. In: Das PK, Sejian V, Mukherjee J, Banerjee D (eds) Textbook of veterinary physiology. Springer, Singapore. https://doi.org/10.1007/978-981-19-9410-4_25

Vernon RG (1988) The partition of nutrients during the lactation cycle. In: Garnsworthy PC (ed) Nutrition and lactation in the dairy cow. Butterworths, London, pp 32–52

Research Articles

Agius L, Robinson AM, Girard JR, Williamson DH (1979) Alterations in the rate of lipogenesis in vivo in maternal liver and adipose tissue on premature weaning of lactating rats: a possible regulatory role of prolactin. Biochemist J. 180:689–692

Bartley JC, Abraham S, Chaikoff IL (1966) Activity patterns of several enzymes of liver, adipose tissue, and mammary gland of virgin, pregnant, and lactating mice. Proc Soc Exp Biol Med 123(3):670. https://doi.org/10.3181/00379727-123-31

Bauman DE, Brown RE, Davis CL (1970) Pathways of fatty acid synthesis and reducing equivalent generation in mammary gland of rat, sow, and cow. Arch Biochem Biophys 140(1):237–244. https://doi.org/10.1016/0003-9861(70)90028-7

Bauman DE, Mellenberger RW, Derrig RG (1973) Fatty acid synthesis in sheep mammary tissue. J Dairy Sci 56:1312–1318

Bionaz M, Loor JJ (2011) Gene networks driving bovine mammary protein synthesis during the lactation cycle. Bioinform Biol Insights 5:83–89

Bröer S (2008) Amino acid transport across mammalian intestinal and renal epithelia. Physiol Rev 88:249–286

Chen Z, Shi H, Sun S, Luo J, Zhang W, Hou Y, Loor JJ (2018) MiR-183 regulates milk fat metabolism via MST1 in goat mammary epithelial cells. Gene 646:12–19. https://doi.org/10.1016/j.gene.2017.12.052

Chen Z, Chu S, Wang X, Fan Y, Zhan T, Arbab AAI, Li M, Zhang H, Mao Y, Loor JJ, Yang Z (2019) MicroRNA- 106b regulates milk fat metabolism via ATP binding cassette subfamily a member 1 (ABCA1) in bovine mammary epithelial cells. J Agric Food Chem 7(14):3981–3990. https://doi.org/10.1021/acs.jafc.9b00622

Closs EI (2002) Expression, regulation and function of carrier proteins for cationic amino acids. Curr Opin Nephrol Hypertens 11:99–10

Davis S, Bickerstaffe R, Hart D (1978) Amino acid uptake by the mammary gland of the lactating ewe. Aust J Biol Sci 31:123–132

Gul B, Dils R (1969) Enzymic changes in rabbit and rat mammary gland during the lactation cycle. Biochem J 112(3):293–301. https://doi.org/10.1042/bj1120293

Hansen HO, Jensen SS, Knudsen J (1986) Absence of monoacylglycerol pathway for triacylglycerol synthesis in goat mammary gland. Biochem J 238:173–176

Haque M, Guinard-Flament J, Lamberton P, Mustière C, Lemosquet S (2015) Changes in mammary metabolism in response to the provision of an ideal amino acid profile at 2 levels of metabolizable protein supply in dairy cows: consequences on efficiency. J Dairy Sci 98:3951–3968

Ji Z, Wang G, Xie Z, Zhang C, Wang J (2012) Identification and characterization of microRNA in the dairy goat (Capra hircus) mammary gland by Solexa deep- sequencing technology. Mol Biol Rep 39:9361–9371

Kanto U, Clawson AJ (1980) Effect of energy intake during pregnancy and lactation on body composition in rats. J Nutr 110:1829–1839

Karunakaran S, Ramachandran S, Coothankandaswamy V, Elangovan S, Babu E, Periyasamy-Thandavan S, Gurav A, Gnanaprakasam JP, Singh N, Schoenlein PV, Prasad PD, Thangaraju M, Ganapathy V (2011) SLC6A14 (ATB0,+) protein, a highly concentrative and broad specific amino acid transporter, is a novel and effective drug target for treatment of estrogen receptor-positive breast cancer. J Biol Chem 286(36):31830–31838

Lei J, Feng D, Zhang Y, Zhao FQ, Wu Z, SanGabriel A, Fujishima Y, Uneyama H, Wu G (2012) Nutritional and regulatory role of branched-chain amino acids in lactation. Front Biosci 17:2725–2739

Li P, Knabe DA, Kim SW, Lynch C, Hutson S, Wu G (2009) Lactating porcine mammary tissue catabolized branched-chain amino acids for glutamine and asparate synthesis. J Nutr 139:1502–1509

Lin XZ, Luo J, Zhang LP, Wang W, Shi HB, Zhu JJ (2013) miR-27a suppresses triglyceride accumulation and affects gene mRNA expression associated with fat metabolism in dairy goat mammary gland epithelial cells. Gene 521(1):15–23. https://doi.org/10.1016/j.gene.2013.03.050

Linzell JL, Peaker M (1971) Mechanism of milk secretion. Physio Reviews 51:564597

Ma L, Qiu H, Chen Z, Li L, Zeng Y, Luo J, Gou D (2018) miR-25 modulates triacylglycerol and lipid accumulation in goat mammary epithelial cells by repressing PGC-1beta. J Anim Sci Biotechnol 9:48. https://doi.org/10.1186/s40104-018-0262-0

Matsuzaki T, Machida N, Tajika Y, Ablimit A, Suzuki T, Aoki T, Hagiwara H, Takata K (2005) Expression and immunolocalization of water-channel aquaporins in the rat and mouse mammary gland. Histochem Cell Biol 123(4–5):501–512

Mepham T, Linzell J (1966) A quantitative assessment of the contribution of individual plasma amino acids to the synthesis of milk proteins by the goat mammary gland. Biochem J 101:76–83

Mobasheri A, Wray S, Marples D (2005) Distribution of AQP2 and AQP3 water channels in human tissue microarrays. J Mol Histol 36(1–2):1–14

Mobasheri A, Kendall BH, Maxwell JE, Sawran AV, German AJ, Marples D, Luck MR, Royal MD (2011) Cellular localization of aquaporins along the secretory pathway of the lactating bovine mammary gland: an immunohistochemical study. Acta Histochem 113(2):137–149

Omphalius C, Lapierre H, Guinard-Flament J, Lamberton P, Bahloul L, Lemosquet S (2019) Amino acid efficiencies of utilization vary by different mechanisms in response to energy and protein supplies in dairy cows: study at mammary-gland and whole-body levels. J Dairy Sci 102:9883–9901

Raggio G, Lemosquet S, Lobley G, Rulquin H, Lapierre H (2006) Effect of casein and propionate supply on mammary protein metabolism in lactating dairy cows. J Dairy Sci 89:4340–4351

Romsos DR, Muiruri KL, Lin PY, Leveille GA (1978) Influence of dietary fat, fasting, and acute premature weaning on in vivo rates of fatty acid synthesis in lactating mice. Proc Soc Exp Biol Med 159:308–312

Sharma R, Kansal VK (2001) Heterogeneity of transport systems for L-glutamine in mouse mammary gland. Indian J Biochem Biophys 38(4):241–248

Trottier N, Shipley C, Easter R (1997) Plasma amino acid uptake by the mammary gland of the lactating sow. J Anim Sci 75:1266–1278

Zhang M, Ma L, Liu Y, He Y, Li G, An X, Cao B (2020) CircRNA-006258 sponge- adsorbs miR-574-5p to regulate cell growth and milk synthesis via EVI5L in goat mammary epithelial cells. Genes 11(7):718. https://doi.org/10.3390/genes11070718

Galactopoiesis

8

Contents

Abstract

Galactopoiesis refers to the physiological maintenance of lactation once milk secretion has been established. In dairy cows, milk yield follows a characteristic bell-shaped lactation curve, rising steadily to a peak at 4–6 weeks postpartum and then declining gradually until drying off before the next calving. The lactation period is commonly categorized into early (14–100 days), mid (100–200 days), and late (200–305 days) stages, with peak yield typically occurring during

J. Mukherjee et al., *Veterinary Lactation Physiology*,
https://doi.org/10.1007/978-3-032-21123-1_8

5–6 weeks of lactation. During early lactation, cows experience a marked negative energy balance because nutrients are preferentially directed toward milk synthesis, but this imbalance generally resolves by 5–7 weeks postpartum. The shape and persistency of the lactation curve are primarily determined by the number and activity of mammary secretory cells. Maintenance of milk production is governed by several endocrine and metabolic regulators, including prolactin, somatotropin, glucocorticoids, and thyroid hormones, which support milk component synthesis and effective gland emptying. Milk yield and composition remain highly dynamic traits influenced by genetic factors such as breed and parity, as well as environmental and managerial conditions, including nutrition, milking frequency, and climate.

Graphical Abstract

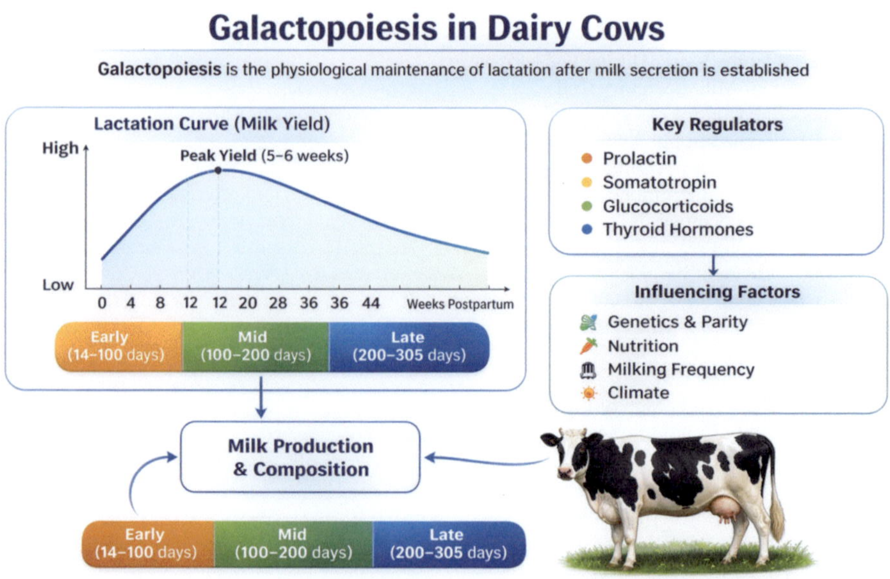

Description of the graphic: Galactopoiesis is the process that maintains lactation after milk secretion begins. Dairy cows show a typical bell-shaped lactation curve, with milk yield peaking at 4–6 weeks and gradually declining thereafter. The lactation cycle is divided into early (14–100 days), mid (100–200 days), and late (200–305 days) stages. Early lactation is marked by negative energy balance, which usually resolves by 5–7 weeks postpartum. Lactation persistency depends on the number and activity of mammary secretory cells and is regulated by hormones such as prolactin, somatotropin, glucocorticoids, and thyroid hormones. Milk yield and composition are highly influenced by genetics, nutrition, management, and environmental conditions

Keywords

Galactopoiesis · Lactation curve · Persistency of lactation · Endocrine factors · Milk yield · Milk composition

Inside the Chapter

- *Energy Homeostasis During Galactopoiesis*
- *Activity of Milk Secretory Cells*
- *Endocrine Control of Galactopoiesis*
  - Somatotropic Axis
  - Prolactin
  - Thyroid Hormones
  - Glucocorticoids
  - Insulin
  - Ovarian Steroids
  - Leptin
- *Factors Affecting Milk Yield and Composition*
  - Breed
  - Genetics
  - Parity and Stage of Lactation
  - Body Condition Score (BCS)
  - Environment
  - Nutrition
  - Milking Management
  - Photoperiod
  - Pregnancy and Dry Period

Learning Objectives

- Lactation curve and persistency of lactation.
- Energy homeostasis during galactopoiesis.
- Endocrine regulation of galactopoiesis.
- Factors affecting milk yield and composition.

Galactopoiesis refers to the process responsible for maintaining milk secretion once lactation is established. In dairy cows, milk production follows a characteristic lactation curve that illustrates changes in yield throughout the lactation period. This curve reflects the combined effects of genetic and environmental factors within a herd. Typically, the curve shows a steady increase in milk output from calving until it reaches a maximum at peak lactation, after which production gradually declines until the end of the cycle. Most cows reach their peak yield around 5–6 weeks after calving, although this can vary widely depending on breed and physiological factors (Table 8.1). Following this peak, milk yield steadily decreases. The lactation cycle of dairy cows has been divided into three stages: early lactation (14–100 days), mid lactation (100–200 days), and late lactation (200–305 days) (Mukherjee et al. 2023).

Table 8.1 Peak yield and day to attain peak yield in different breeds of cows

Breed	Peak yield (kg/d)	Day of peak	References
Friesian	20.1 ± 0.4 (milked once) 26.2 ± 0.4 (milked twice)	31 ± 2 (milked once) 37 ± 2 (milked twice)	Hickson et al. (2006)
Jersey	14.8 ± 0.4 (milked once) 17.8 ± 0.4 (milked twice)	28 ± 2 (milked once) 36 ± 2 (milked twice)	
Brown Swiss	15 kg	30 days	Bytyqi et al. (2007)
Sahiwal	10.64 ± 0.14	51.68 ± 1.13	Ratwan et al. (2020)
Gir cow	9.53 ± 0.14	61.25 ± 2.50	Singh and Shukla (1986)

Unlike cows, species such as pigs and rodents attain their highest milk production at weaning, approximately three weeks after lactation begins. Guinea pigs, rabbits, and humans, on the other hand, reach peak milk yield roughly midway through their lactation period. In dairy cows, the early and peak stages of lactation are often marked by a negative energy balance due to the high energy demands of milk synthesis, which can adversely affect the animal's health and body condition.

Persistency of lactation refers to a cow's ability to sustain its peak milk yield throughout the lactation period. It can also be described as the rate at which milk production declines following the peak. A more persistent lactation is reflected by a flatter lactation curve. Farm profitability is closely linked to this trait, as cows with high persistency experience only a gradual decrease in milk yield, whereas low persistency is associated with a faster drop after peak production. On average, milk output decreases by about 7% per month once peak yield has been reached. Generally, first-lactation (primiparous) cows exhibit greater lactation persistency than cows in later lactations (multiparous).

Knowledge Corner...
Elephants have longest lactation periods among mammals (up to 4–6 years). Milk composition changes drastically over time, with increasing fat as the calf ages. Lactation overlaps with long gestation period (22 months).

There are several methods to estimate persistency of lactation, such as the ratio method, the variation of yields method, and mathematical lactation. But, the ratio method proposed by Rao and Sundaresan has been proven to be the most effective method of evaluating lactation persistency. It uses the following formula to calculate lactation persistency.

$$\text{Persistency (P)} = \text{Lactation milk yield}/\text{Peak yield}$$

Pregnancy decreases the persistency of lactation. This effect is mainly mediated by estrogen secreted from the fetal–placental unit. The negative effect of pregnancy on lactation can be seen from 100 days of gestation.

8.1 Energy Homeostasis During Galactopoiesis

Energy demand reaches its maximum during peak lactation, and dietary intake alone is insufficient to meet this requirement. As a result, the cow draws on its body reserves—primarily fat and muscle—to supply the additional energy needed for milk synthesis. It is estimated that roughly one-third of the energy normally used for maintenance is redirected toward milk production. During this period of negative energy balance, glucose becomes the primary metabolic fuel allocated to the mammary gland. This preferential glucose supply is facilitated by peripheral insulin resistance and glucose-sparing mechanisms, as previously explained in the lactogenesis chapter.

Alterations in blood metabolites during different stages of the lactation cycle are presented in Table 8.2.

As milk production declines, the severity of energy imbalance decreases; however, the exact point at which cows return to a positive energy balance varies widely. Most studies report that cows typically regain positive energy balance between 5 and 7 weeks postpartum. Interestingly, milk yield itself shows no significant association with energy balance, whereas dry matter intake is strongly and positively correlated with it. Parity has little influence on the time required to achieve positive energy balance. Estimates indicate that about 92% of primiparous cows and 73% of multiparous cows reach positive energy balance by the seventh week after calving, though this difference is not statistically significant.

Assessing energy balance on farms is challenging because accurate measurement requires direct or indirect calorimetry. Although energy balance can be estimated indirectly by calculating net energy intake (NEI) and comparing it with energy requirements, these values are based on predictions and may not represent true physiological conditions. Changes in body weight are also unreliable indicators, as they are influenced by variations in tissue mass and gastrointestinal fill. Instead, body condition score (BCS) has been shown to be a useful tool for estimating a cow's energy balance. However, it too has limitations, since noticeable changes in BCS typically take at least three weeks after a cow returns to a positive energy balance.

8.2 Activity of Milk Secretory Cells

The form of the lactation curve is largely determined by the number and functional activity of mammary secretory cells. Higher milk production is associated with a greater population of active mammary epithelial cells and minimal tissue remodeling. In cows, early lactation is marked by heightened activity of the secretory epithelium without an increase in cell numbers, as evidenced by unchanged levels of Ki-67, a marker of cell proliferation, throughout this period (Table 8.3). As lactation progresses, milk yield gradually declines due to a reduction in cell numbers. At calving, approximately 83% of mammary cells are epithelial, but this proportion

Table 8.2 Alterations in blood metabolites during different stages of the lactation cycle

Blood metabolites	Days in lactation				
	0–60 days	61–120 days	121–180 days	180–240 days	>240 days
Glucose (mg/dl)	59.14 ± 6.47	57.33 ± 6.02	51.11 ± 5.13	49.44 ± 8.50	50.25 ± 3.20
Triglycerides (mg/dl)	18.29 + 2.50	17.44 ± 2.13	18.11 ± 3.10	18.56 ± 3.94	19.75 ± 2.36
Total cholesterol (mg/dl)	130.14 ± 56.51	153.00 ± 36.18	141.78 ± 45.05	150.78 ± 37.35	154.50 ± 68.38

Fauci et al. (2023)

Table 8.3 Mammary cell turnover, enzyme activity, and gene expression in dairy cows during the lactation cycle

Parameters	Days relative to calving			
	14	42	88	172
Ki-67 positive cells (%)	0.75	0.57	0.38	0.60
Apoptotic cells (TUNEL positive) (%)	0.76	0.13	0.25	0.08
DNA (μg/g)	1406	1243	1225	1198
RNA (μg/g)	6909	7147	8046	7129
RNA:DNA ratio	4.9	5.7	6.4	5.9
ACC (nmol/min per mg)	109	127	115	144
FAS (pmol/min per mg)	806	1172	1051	1079
GT (nmol/min per mg)	36	41	44	43
Caspase-3 (fold mRNA expression)	2.0	1.0	0.5	1.3
IGFBP-5 (fold mRNA expression)	3.5	1.9	1.7	1.8

Sorensen et al. (2006)

falls to about 74% in late lactation. Between 90 and 240 days of lactation, the epithelial cell population decreases from roughly 79% to 73%.

During peak lactation, about 0.3% of mammary cells undergo proliferation each day. Apoptotic (TUNEL-positive) cells decrease from early to peak lactation and then rise again afterward (Table 8.3). The increase in apoptosis later in lactation is likely linked to the elimination of senescent or undifferentiated cells. This peak in cell death aligns with elevated expression of apoptotic mediators such as caspase-3 and IGFBP-5. Caspase-3 aids in breaking down essential cellular components, causing chromatin condensation, DNA fragmentation, and formation of apoptotic bodies. IGFBP-5 promotes apoptosis by blocking IGF signaling and activating pro-apoptotic pathways.

The RNA:DNA ratio was also consistent during different days of lactation (Table 8.3). Enzymes such as acetyl CoA carboxylase (ACC), fatty acid synthetase (FAS), and galactosyl transferase (GT) were reported to be consistent throughout the lactation cycle in dairy cows (Table 8.3).

In contrast to cows, the early lactation period in goats is characterized by an increased number of mammary epithelial cells followed by an increase in secretory activity per cell. After the peak lactation, the decrease in milk production is due to reduced secretory cell number.

8.3 Endocrine Control of Galactopoiesis

Galactopoiesis is regulated by various hormones and growth factors that either promote the synthesis of milk components or facilitate frequent drainage of the mammary gland. Key lactation-supporting hormones include prolactin (PRL), somatotropin (ST), glucocorticoids, and thyroid hormones. In addition, oxytocin released during milking is essential for effective milk ejection. Once lactation is established, the somatotropic axis—comprising growth hormone (GH), insulin-like growth factor-1 (IGF-1), IGF-binding proteins, and the receptors for GH and IGF-1—plays a central role. Thyroid hormones such as thyroxine (T4) and triiodothyronine (T3) contribute to mammary gland metabolism. Although PRL supports the differentiation and maintenance of mammary epithelial cells, its role in sustaining milk production in ruminants remains debated.

8.3.1 Somatotropic Axis

It comprising growth hormone (GH), the GH receptor (GHR), IGF-I, and IGF-binding proteins (IGFBP) plays pivotal role in nutrient partitioning during lactation. The GH secretion is increased in response to the primary negative feedback loop through IGF-I. During parturition, circulating IGF-1 concentration decreased rapidly along with lowered expression of GHR mRNA, which triggers the release of GH.

8.3.1.1 Growth Hormone

Earlier, it was believed that growth hormone (GH) did not exert direct effects on mammary tissue because mammary glands were thought to lack GH receptors, and adding GH to mammary cell cultures in vitro failed to enhance casein or fat synthesis. Consequently, the galactopoietic action of GH was considered to be primarily indirect. Proposed mechanisms included nutrient partitioning toward milk production during early lactation, improved feed intake, and enhanced efficiency of converting feed to milk after about five weeks of lactation, as well as increased nutrient delivery through elevated mammary blood flow.

GH supports energy supply during negative energy balance by stimulating lipolysis in adipose tissue and promoting gluconeogenesis in the liver. In dairy cows, exogenous GH administration for a 10–12-week period has been shown to increase milk yield by approximately 40%. It also raises the proportion of cardiac output directed to the udder—from about 14.4% to 18.7%. A summary of GH's effects on peripheral tissues in lactating cows is presented in Table 8.4.

Subsequently, immunoreactive GH receptors (GHR) were detected in mammary epithelial cells (Sinowatz et al. 2000), indicating that the galactopoietic effects of GH may also involve direct action within the mammary gland. During early lactation, GHR mRNA was found in the cytoplasm of glandular epithelial cells. By peak lactation (around the tenth week), GHR became visible in the secretory alveoli, and in late lactation, both alveolar and ductal epithelial cells showed GHR expression. These observations provide strong evidence supporting a direct role of GH in mammary function.

Further research demonstrated that GH helps maintain secretory epithelial cell populations and supports milk synthesis rates. Prolonged GH administration prevented the typical decline in mammary epithelial cell numbers observed as lactation progresses. Additionally, GH treatment in cows and goats increased the activity of key enzymes associated with lactogenesis—such as acetyl-CoA

Table 8.4 Effects of GH on the peripheral tissues of lactating cows

Tissue	Role in lactation
Mammary gland	Increases the milk synthesis with normal composition Increases the nutrient uptake Increases the number and activity of secretory cells Increases blood flow consistent with an increase in milk yield
Liver	Increases gluconeogenesis Decreases the ability of insulin to suppress gluconeogenesis
Adipose tissue	Increases lipogenesis during positive energy balance and lipolysis during negative energy balance Decreases the ability of insulin to stimulate lipogenesis Decreases the ability of adenosine to inhibit lipolysis Increases the ability of catecholamines to stimulate lipolysis
Muscle	Decreases glucose uptake
Kidney and intestine	Increases the production of 1,25-vitamin D3 Increases the absorption of ca, P, and other minerals required for milk Increases the ability of 1,25-vitamin D3 to stimulate the ca-binding protein
Whole body	Decreases glucose oxidation Increases oxidation of non-esterified fatty acids in a negative energy balance Increases cardiac output consistently Increases productive efficiency (milk per unit of energy intake)

Bauman (1999)

carboxylase, acetyl-CoA synthetase, and fatty acid synthase. GH also enhances protein synthesis, as shown by increased RNA content per mammary gland following somatotropin treatment.

The concentration of GH decreased as the lactation advanced (Table 8.5) in cows and buffaloes, and a decline in the milk yield with the advancement of lactation was positively correlated with GH concentration.

However, the relatively low abundance of GHR in mammary tissue compared with the liver led researchers to explore additional mediators of GH action in the mammary gland, bringing attention to the role of somatomedins. Several key observations support the coordinated involvement of GH and IGFs: the mammary gland contains abundant receptors for both IGF-I and IGF-II; bovine somatotropin (bST) administration increases IGF-I secretion; and close-arterial infusion of IGF-I or IGF-II enhances milk yield, whereas direct close-arterial infusion of GH does not. These findings highlight the importance of IGFs in mediating GH's galactopoietic effects.

The use of exogenous somatotropin is associated with certain adverse outcomes. Research indicates that recombinant bovine somatotropin can reduce fertility by about 40% and elevate the incidence of clinical mastitis by 25% and lameness by 50%.

8.3.1.2 Insulin-like Growth Factors (IGF) System

The IGF system includes two somatomedin ligands—IGF-I and IGF-II—their receptors, six high-affinity binding proteins (IGFBP-1 to IGFBP-6), and the

Table 8.5 Concentration of GH (ng/mL) during different stages of the lactation cycle in cows and buffaloes

Species	Days in lactation					
	65 days	80 days	95 days	110 days	125 days	150 days
Cattle	3.77 ± 0.27	4.27 ± 0.57	2.76 ± 0.28	2.60 ± 0.42	2.56 ± 0.34	1.75 ± 0.15
Buffalo	3.30 ± 0.25	3.16 ± 0.25	2.52 ± 0.37	2.79 ± 0.45	1.90 ± 0.27	1.20 ± 0.08

Jindal and Ludri (1990)

Table 8.6 Concentration of IGF-I and IGF-II in plasma and milk of different species

Species	IGF-I (ng/ml)		IGF-II (ng/ml)		References
	Day 1	Day 5	Day 1	Day 5	
Plasma					
Cow	31 ± 4	76 ± 11	182 ± 7	182 ± 7	Vega et al. (1991) and Skaar et al. (1991)
Horse	297 ± 23	171 ± 13	No report	No report	Hess-Dudan et al. (1994)
Sow	57 ± 20	15 ± 7	231 ± 58	492 ± 17	Donovan et al. (1994)
Rat	743 ± 187	501 ± 71	9.3 ± 6.7	7 ± 0.1	Donovan et al. (1991)
Milk					
Cow	176 ± 16	5 ± 2	199 ± 40	1 ± 0.1	Vega et al. (1991) and Skaar et al. (1991)
Horse	259 ± 10	11 ± 1	No report	No report	Hess-Dudan et al. (1994)
Sow	71 ± 11	11 ± 1	165 ± 18	16 ± 1	Donovan et al. (1994)
Rat	30 ± 10	17 ± 8	1.3 ± 0.5	<1	Donovan et al. (1991)

acid-labile subunit (ALS). IGFs function primarily through autocrine and paracrine pathways to regulate mammary activity. IGF-I is mainly produced in the liver in response to GH, while IGF-II is synthesized during pregnancy and plays a key role in fetal development, earning it the name "fetal growth factor." Circulating IGF-II levels are minimally influenced by GH.

The liver is the primary site of IGF production. When somatotropin binds to its receptors in hepatic tissue, it stimulates the synthesis of IGF-I. The presence of somatotropin receptors in the mammary parenchyma also suggests that IGF-I may be produced locally within the mammary gland to act in a paracrine manner (Table 8.6). This idea is further supported by findings that deleting hepatic IGF-I dramatically lowers circulating IGF-I levels—by about 75%—while IGF-I mRNA expression remains preserved in the mammary gland.

Somatomedin production is strongly influenced by an animal's nutritional status. In undernourished animals, bST administration leads to only a modest rise in circulating IGF-I, whereas well-nourished animals show a marked increase in IGF-I levels following GH treatment. Under conditions of severe nutritional deficiency, GH is unable to elevate IGF-I concentrations at all.

In dairy cows experiencing negative energy balance, circulating IGF-I remains low despite elevated GH levels (Table 8.6). Hepatic IGF-I mRNA expression is also lowest during early lactation, indicating reduced liver synthesis of IGF-I. As lactation progresses, liver IGF-I mRNA expression increases, resulting in higher circulating IGF-I concentrations during mid- and late lactation. In contrast, IGF-II levels do not vary with lactation stage.

IGFs exert their effects through two receptor types. Type 1 IGF receptors share structural features with insulin receptors, while type 2 receptors resemble the cation-independent mannose-6-phosphate receptor. Both receptor types have been identified in the mammary glands of several species, including cows, sheep, and rats. Type 1 receptors are the primary mediators of IGF-I and IGF-II actions. When IGF-I levels are high, it can also activate insulin receptors. The density of IGF receptors in the mammary gland decreases as pregnancy progresses and during lactation. During lactation, type 2 receptors become more abundant than type 1, suggesting a downregulation of IGF receptors due to reduced IGF demand in the mammary gland, or that these receptors play a greater role in mammary development than in milk production.

Insulin-like growth factors (IGFs) play multiple crucial roles during lactation. IGF-I contributes to mammary gland development by promoting the proliferation of mammary stem cells and driving the differentiation of luminal progenitor cells into mature luminal and alveolar epithelial cells. It also enhances mammary blood flow by stimulating nitric oxide production via activation of endothelial nitric oxide synthase. Through its receptor, IGF-1R, IGF-I supports cell survival and boosts the rate of DNA replication. Research further indicates that IGF-I participates in the synthesis of β-casein. Lipid production in the mammary gland is also influenced by IGF-I, as it upregulates the expression of Sterol Regulatory Element-Binding Protein (SREBP). In addition, IGF-I raises plasma glucose levels and promotes glucose delivery to the mammary gland, thereby supporting lactose synthesis.

8.3.1.3 IGF-Binding Proteins (IGFBP)

The IGF-binding proteins (IGFBPs) consist of six structurally similar proteins that bind IGF-I and IGF-II with high affinity. Nearly 99% of circulating IGFs remain associated with these binding proteins. Mammary epithelial cells are the primary source of IGFBP-2, IGFBP-3, IGFBP-4, and IGFBP-5.

The central role of IGFBPs is to regulate the IGF system. They can inhibit IGF-I or IGF-II actions by competing with IGF receptors (IGF-IR or IGF-IIR) or enhance IGF activity by increasing their availability at the cell surface. IGFBPs also facilitate the movement of circulating IGFs into the extracellular compartment. IGFBP-1 and IGFBP-2 usually form binary complexes with IGF-I, whereas IGFBP-3 associates with IGF-I and the acid-labile subunit (ALS) to form a ternary complex, which carries most of the IGF-I in the bloodstream.

During lactation, IGFBP-3 levels remain fairly stable, while IGFBP-2-concentrations rise in early lactation. Notably, lactating ewes exhibit higher IGFBP-2 expression in the liver but reduced expression in the mammary gland.

IGFBP-1 and IGFBP-2 generally lower the amount of IGF-I available to peripheral tissues. Their binding affinity for IGF-I increases during the negative energy balance of early lactation, restricting IGF-I action and thereby limiting glucose uptake by the mammary gland when blood glucose levels are low. As lactation progresses to mid-lactation, the affinity of IGFBP-1 and IGFBP-2 for IGF-I decreases, reflecting a shift in metabolic priorities as nutrient supply to the mammary gland becomes less critical than in early lactation.

8.3.2 Prolactin

The galactopoietic role of prolactin is well documented in rodents, primates, and certain livestock species such as sheep and pigs. However, its function in major dairy animals like cows and goats remains uncertain. In rabbits, treatment with the prolactin inhibitor bromocriptine for three days completely halted lactation, which could be readily reversed by administering prolactin. Similarly, mice treated with bromocriptine showed a roughly 30% decrease in milk production.

However, in cows and goats, bromocriptine treatment markedly reduced circulating prolactin without leading to a decline in milk yield. This led to the early assumption that prolactin has a minimal role in sustaining lactation in ruminants. Supporting this view, studies reported weak correlations between milk yield and prolactin levels, as well as no significant difference in prolactin concentrations between high- and low-producing cows.

Yet, later evidence challenged this hypothesis. Cows treated with quinagolide—a prolactin inhibitor approximately 200 times more potent than bromocriptine—showed a steady decline in milk production beginning in the first week of a 9-week treatment period. Similarly, cabergoline, another prolactin antagonist, caused a 28% reduction in milk yield within a day of a single injection and also decreased milk production in goats. Conversely, administering exogenous prolactin increased milk yield in cows and counteracted the suppressive effects of quinagolide. Domperidone, a dopamine antagonist, was also shown to raise prolactin levels alongside milk production in dairy cows. Together, these findings strongly support a galactopoietic role for prolactin in bovines.

Milking itself triggers roughly a threefold increase in prolactin release, but as lactation progresses, this milking-induced prolactin surge diminishes, contributing to the natural decline in milk yield.

The precise mechanism through which prolactin supports galactopoiesis is still not fully understood. It is proposed that prolactin enhances the secretory activity of mammary epithelial cells. Upon binding to its receptors, prolactin activates multiple signaling cascades that stimulate genes involved in epithelial cell proliferation, differentiation, and lactogenesis. In the mammary gland, prolactin action appears to follow an inverse pattern in which higher PRL concentrations are associated with lower prolactin receptor expression.

Recent research has highlighted the involvement of Suppressors of Cytokine Signaling (SOCS) proteins in regulating prolactin signaling within the mammary gland. SOCS proteins downregulate prolactin activity by inhibiting the JAK/STAT pathway. SOCS1, SOCS2, and SOCS3 have been identified in the bovine mammary gland. Notably, the prolactin surge triggered by milking has been linked to a decrease in SOCS3 expression, thereby enhancing prolactin signaling in dairy cows.

8.3.3 Thyroid Hormones

Thyroid hormones—triiodothyronine (T3) and thyroxine (T4)—help to regulate overall energy metabolism by influencing carbohydrate, protein, and lipid metabolism, as well as by activating enzymes that enhance tissue oxygen consumption. They also support normal sodium–potassium ATPase activity, thereby maintaining the balance between energy intake, use, and storage within tissues. These hormones are crucial for proper mammary gland growth, development, and the continuation of lactation. Their secretion is controlled by thyroid-stimulating hormone (TSH).

Administration of thyroxine has been shown to increase milk yield by about 25%, although it simultaneously reduces milk protein concentration. Beyond its role in energy regulation, thyroxine also elevates cardiac output by roughly 20% and enhances mammary blood flow by about 35%, improving nutrient delivery to the mammary gland.

The thyroid gland primarily secretes T4, a prohormone that is converted into the active hormone T3 through 5′-deiodination, catalyzed by the selenium-dependent enzyme 5′-deiodinase. This enzyme exists in three isoforms—type I (D1), type II (D2), and type III (D3)—with tissue-specific distributions. D1 is largely found in the liver, kidneys, and thyroid gland; D2 is abundant in the skin, central nervous system, and brown adipose tissue. In the bovine mammary gland, D2 predominates, while sow mammary tissue contains both D1 and D2, and rat mammary tissue shows mainly D1 activity. D1 is considered the main source of circulating T3. Under hypothyroid conditions, D1 activity falls, and D2 activity rises, whereas the opposite pattern occurs in hyperthyroidism.

Levels of TSH, T3, and T4 fluctuate noticeably across the lactation cycle (Table 8.7). TSH concentrations remain fairly constant from 0–60 days through 180–240 days of lactation, rising only between 240 and 300 days. T3 levels are highest in early lactation and then decline, reaching their lowest point between 120 and 180 days and again near late lactation. Free T3 (fT3) remains relatively stable throughout lactation, with only a slight rise toward the end.

T4 concentrations drop from early lactation (0–60 days) to 60–120 days. Seasonal effects also influence these hormone patterns. During fall, total T3 is highest in early lactation and lowest in mid-lactation, with moderate levels in late lactation. In winter, T3 shows no significant variation across stages, whereas in spring T3 peaks during mid-lactation. T4 remains unchanged across lactation stages in fall, but in winter and spring, higher T4 levels appear in early lactation.

As lactation advances, liver type I 5′-deiodinase activity increases, while mammary type II 5′-deiodinase activity declines. Dairy cows enter a functionally hypothyroid state in early lactation due to reduced hepatic type I deiodinase activity and elevated mammary type II activity. Consequently, plasma thyroid hormone concentrations are lowest during this period, while colostrum contains the highest levels.

Supplementing the diet with thyroprotein can enhance milk yield for 2–4 months and also raise the butterfat percentage. Prolonged feeding of thyroid hormones or thyroproteins increases milk production during early lactation, but this is followed

Table 8.7 Concentration of TSH and thyroid hormones during different days of the lactation cycle in cows

Hormones	Days in lactation				
	0–60 days	61–120 days	121–180 days	180–240 days	>240 days
TSH (ng/ml)	0.17 ± 0.06	0.12 ± 0.04	0.13 ± 0.07	0.11 ± 0.06	0.09 ± 0.05
T3 (ng/dL)	72.24 ± 9.37	81.34 ± 14.26	68 ± 19.26	62.26 ± 30.77	63.93 ± 17.78
fT3 (pg/ml)	2.08 ± 0.42	2.18 ± 0.35	2.31 ± 0.61	1.69 ± 0.58	2.17 ± 0.91
fT4 (ng/ml)	1.05 ± 0.44	1.27 ± 0.34	1.10 ± 0.29	1.06 ± 0.61	1.57 ± 0.43

Fauci et al. (2023)

by a sharp decline later in the lactation period. Some researchers caution against administering thyroid hormones during negative energy balance, as they further elevate metabolic demands. Thyroid hormones are also known to enhance the galactopoietic effects of hormones like prolactin, particularly in stimulating lactose and casein synthesis.

8.3.4 Glucocorticoids

Glucocorticoids (GCs) are hormones produced through the hypothalamic–pituitary–adrenocortical (HPA) axis. In cattle and goats, the primary GC is cortisol, whereas rodents mainly produce corticosterone. These hormones play key roles in regulating metabolism, energy balance, immune responses, stress adaptation, and behavior. Their effects are mediated by glucocorticoid receptors (GRs), which influence gene expression through direct DNA binding or protein–protein interactions. GCs are essential for proper mammary gland development; however, the impact of cortisol on milk production varies among species (Table 8.8).

Multiple in vitro studies have shown that glucocorticoids stimulate milk protein synthesis in a dose-dependent manner. Moderate levels of cortisol can double the production of α-lactalbumin, while low cortisol concentrations suppress its expression. Dexamethasone has also been found to enhance the intracellular transport and

Table 8.8 Effects of GCs on milk yield in different species

Species	Sources of GCs	Effects on milk yield	Reference
Cow	Dexamethasone (large dose)	Decreased milk production along with a decrease in milk fat protein and lactose content	Ollier et al. (2016) Ponchon et al. (2017)
	Flumethasone (oral)	Increased milk production	van der Kolk (1990)
Goat	Endogenous cortisol	Promote milk synthesis	Bomfim et al. (2022)
	Cortisol (systemic infusion)	Increase milk yield	Thompson (1984)
	Endogenous cortisol	Reduced milk production and milk lactose	Hooper et al. (2021)
Pigs	Lower endogenous cortisol	Improved suckling	Baxter et al. (2023)
Mice	Dexamethasone	Increased β-casein expression and secretion	Kobayashi et al. (2017)
Rat	Cortisol-21-acetate (long term)	Increased milk production	Thatcher & Tucker (1970)

secretion of milk proteins by increasing the expression of soluble N-ethylmaleimide–sensitive factor attachment protein receptor (SNARE) proteins.

In cows, the effects of administering cortisol externally on lactation are inconsistent. High doses of dexamethasone have been shown to cause a sudden drop in milk yield. While cortisol can promote gluconeogenesis during early lactation, giving glucocorticoids exogenously reduces glucose uptake by the mammary gland—as indicated by decreased arteriovenous glucose differences—and leads to lower milk lactose levels without altering milk protein or fat content. Similar findings have been reported in goats, where glucocorticoids decrease milk output and lactose concentration, and also inhibit IGF-1–stimulated milk production.

8.3.5 Insulin

Insulin lowers blood glucose by enhancing glycogenesis while suppressing glycogenolysis and gluconeogenesis. It also inhibits lipolysis and promotes lipogenesis, thereby reducing circulating free fatty acids. In lactating animals, insulin plays an important role in regulating glucose metabolism and energy balance across different physiological stages.

During early lactation, plasma insulin levels are low (Table 8.9), which promotes hepatic gluconeogenesis, reduces peripheral glucose utilization, and increases the mobilization of fatty acids and amino acids from adipose tissue and muscle to support milk synthesis. At peak lactation, plasma glucose levels are reduced, but as milk yield declines after peak production, the demand for glucose decreases. As a result, basal glucose concentration rises between day 50 and days 100–150 of lactation. The increase in blood glucose stimulates greater insulin secretion, leading to elevated insulin levels in mid-lactation. These higher insulin concentrations are generally maintained during late lactation, especially in cows receiving high-energy diets.

According to the glucogenic-insulin theory of milk fat depression, feeding cows high-concentrate and low-roughage diets elevates insulin levels, directing nutrients toward adipose tissue rather than the mammary gland, ultimately reducing milk fat synthesis. Administration of insulin alone lowers milk yield and milk lactose content due to reduced glucose availability for lactose formation. However, when insulin is administered alongside supplemental glucose, milk production increases. Research in mice indicates that insulin is essential for maintaining mammary cells in vitro.

Table 8.9 Concentration of insulin hormone during different days of the lactation cycle in cows

Hormones	Days in lactation				
	0–60 days	61–120 days	121–180 days	180–240 days	>240 days
Insulin (mUI/ml)	0.58 ± 0.17	0.88 ± 0.17	0.73 ± 0.17	0.73 ± 0.28	1.12 ± 0.00

Fauci et al. (2023)

Insulin itself does not influence mammary uptake of acetate, β-hydroxybutyrate, triglycerides, amino acids, or glucose.

8.3.6 Ovarian Steroids

Exogenous administration of 17β-estradiol has been shown to reduce milk yield in dairy cows. Similarly, ovariectomy in nonpregnant cows has been found to enhance lactation persistency, and women using estrogen-containing oral contraceptives also experience reduced milk production. These findings support the idea that estrogen is a key factor contributing to the decline in lactation persistency during pregnancy.

Although the exact mechanism by which estrogen influences milk synthesis is still unclear, research in primates indicates that estrogen can inhibit the lactogenic activity of prolactin in mammary tissue. But, estrogen administration did not alter prolactin signaling in cows. So, there may be some other way to control lactation in cows. Another hypothesis proposed that estrogen interferes with growth hormone (GH) signaling by reducing JAK2 phosphorylation, thereby preventing the galactopoietic effects of growth hormone.

Progesterone negatively affects lactogenesis, but during galactopoiesis—or the established phase of lactation—it does not influence milk yield. This may be because mammary tissue lacks progesterone receptors during active lactation, and progesterone tends to associate more readily with milk fat than with its own intracellular receptor.

8.3.7 Leptin

Leptin is a protein-based hormone primarily produced by white adipose tissue. It plays a central role in regulating feed intake and energy balance, thereby influencing nutrient partitioning during pregnancy and lactation. Besides adipose tissue, leptin is also synthesized in the placenta, fetal tissues, stomach, muscles, and the mammary gland. In sheep, mammary adipocytes have been shown to secrete leptin during lactation, and leptin receptor mRNA has been identified in the mammary epithelial cells of both sheep and cattle.

Leptin levels fluctuate markedly across different lactation stages in cows. Concentrations are lowest in early lactation and increase significantly by the eighth month. The reduced leptin level during early lactation is likely linked to adipose tissue mobilization associated with the negative energy balance at this stage. Leptin influences feed intake by suppressing hunger through receptors in the lateral hypothalamus and enhancing satiety via the medial hypothalamus. Thus, reduced leptin in early lactation promotes higher feed intake to help meet the elevated energy demand.

Prolactin is crucial for leptin's actions. It increases leptin receptor expression in bovine mammary epithelial cells by nearly 25-fold and enhances leptin-mediated fatty acid synthesis. Leptin, in the presence of prolactin, also upregulates the expression of α-casein and β-lactoglobulin. Despite these physiological roles, genetic variations in the leptin gene (LEP) have not been associated with differences in milk yield or milk fat and protein content in several cattle breeds.

8.4 Factors Affecting Milk Yield and Composition

Milk production is a highly flexible trait influenced by both genetic and environmental factors that determine milk yield and its components. Animal-related factors such as breed, parity, and stage of lactation, along with management and environmental factors like feeding practices, milking routines, and climatic conditions, play important roles in shaping milk output and composition. High-yielding breeds typically produce more milk than indigenous breeds, making crossbreeding a useful approach for enhancing milk productivity. However, selecting animals solely for higher yield can adversely affect fertility and increase susceptibility to diseases. Moreover, the metabolic strain associated with high production weakens the immune system, leaving cows more vulnerable to metabolic and infectious disorders, which subsequently diminishes milk yield and alters its composition. Intramammary infections, whether subclinical or clinical mastitis, also lead to substantial reductions in milk production and negatively impact milk quality.

Knowledge Corner. . .
Milk and its constituent synthesis follow a diurnal pattern that is influenced, but not entirely governed, by the timing of feed intake. When feed consumption is more evenly spread throughout the day, the fluctuations in milk yield and in circulating metabolites and hormones become less pronounced, suggesting that milk synthesis is regulated by an intrinsic circadian rhythm that is only partially modulated by feeding-related cues and is also responsive to non-nutritional factors.

8.4.1 Breed

Milk yield shows marked variation across different cattle breeds (Table 8.10). In general, larger breeds tend to produce greater volumes of milk than smaller breeds. Because zebu cattle have comparatively lower body weight, their milk production potential is typically lower than that of exotic dairy breeds. Among zebu breeds, milk composition also differs significantly, with the exception of lactose content, which remains relatively consistent. Fat percentage is notably higher in breeds such as Jersey and Guernsey, whereas Holstein Friesian and Ayrshire cows usually produce milk with comparatively lower fat levels. Within-breed variation is most pronounced for milk fat content, followed by solids-not-fat (SNF), protein, and lactose. This indicates that fat content is the most variable milk constituent across individuals of the same breed. The detailed comparative composition of milk components across

Table 8.10 Milk yield of different cattle and buffalo breeds

Species	Types	Breeds	Milk yield (kg/lactation)	References
Cattle	Zebu	Sahiwal	2000–4000	Department of Animal Husbandry and Dairying. Govt. of India, New Delhi (Department of Animal Husbandry and Dairying n.d.)
		Red Sindhi	2000–4000	
		Tharparkar	1800–3500	
		Gir	2000–6000	
		Haryana	1000–2000	
	Exotic	Holstein	6000–8000	TANU Agritech portal, Tamil Nadu veterinary and Animal Science University, Chennai, India (TANU n.d.)
		Ayrshire	4000–6000	
		Jersey	3000–5000	
		Brown Swiss	4000–6000	
		Guernsey	3000–5000	
	Cressbred	Karan Swiss (Sahiwal and Red Sindhi X Brown Swiss)	5000–6000	Thiagarajan (2014)
		Karan Fries (Tharparkar X Holstein Friesian)	3000–4000	
Buffalo		Murrah	1500–2500	TANU Agritech portal, Tamil Nadu Veterinary and Animal Science University, Chennai, India
		Nili ravi	1500–1850	
		Jaffarabadi	100–1200	
		Surti	900–1300	
		Mehsana	1200–1500	
		Godavari	1200–1500	

various breeds of cattle and buffalo is summarized in Table 8.11, highlighting the diversity in milk quality and nutritional traits among different genetic groups.

8.4.2 Genetics

Milk production is a polygenic trait, and genetic improvement is a major focus for modern livestock producers aiming to increase yield. Marker-assisted selection provides an effective way to identify high-producing animals and disseminate their superior genetics to boost overall milk production. Techniques such as quantitative trait loci (QTL) mapping, genome-wide association studies (GWAS), RNA sequencing, whole-genome sequencing, and candidate gene analyses have been widely used to identify genes or specific mutations linked to milk production traits. To date, numerous candidate genes and gene polymorphisms have been discovered that show strong positive associations with milk yield and related performance traits in dairy cattle.

Table 8.11 Milk composition of different cattle and buffalo breeds

Species	Breeds	Fat (%)	Protein (%)	Lactose (%)	Total solid (%)	References
Zebu cattle	Sahiwal	4.23 ± 0.18	3.60 ± 0.05	5.38 ± 0.07	13.99 ± 0.23	Sarkar et al. (2006)
	Tharparkar	4.37 ± 0.20	3.92 ± 0.05	5.35 ± 0.08	14.22 ± 0.25	Sarkar et al. (2006)
Exotic cattle	Holstein	3.56	3.01	4.61	11.91	
	Ayrshire	3.97	3.28	4.63	12.69	
	Jersey	4.97	3.65	4.78	15.15	
	Brown Swiss	3.8	3.18	4.8	12.69	
	Guernsey	4.58	3.49	4.78	13.69	
	Karan fries	3.91 ± 0.14	3.58 ± 0.04	5.39 ± 0.5	13.69 ±:0.7	Sarkar et al. (2006)
Buffalo	Murrah	7.53 ± 0.19	4.03 ± 0.05	–	16.53 ± 0.20	Misra et al. (2008)
	Bhadawari	7.43 ± 0.26	3.92 ± 0.07	–	17.70 ± 0.28	
	Mehsana	6.46 ± 0.17	3.87 ± 0.05	–	5.59 ± 0.18	
	Surti	6.17 ± 0.20	3.93 ± 0.05	–	4.96 ± 0.21	

Several genes show markedly different expression patterns across tissues in relation to milk production and mastitis. For milk production, genes such as TSC1, FRAP1, GSK3A, EIF4EBP2, MAPK14, and DGAT1 have been identified as key regulators. In contrast, numerous genes have been associated with mastitis, including LOC515333, LOC100335608, APOC2, NFKBIA, CD14, SAA3, STAT3, STAT5A, SPEF2, DHX58, CCND2, KCNH4, KRT32, IMMP2L, NFKB1, FAM151A, BoLA-DRA, B2M, FCER1G, NFKBIA, SDS, CD74, and GLYCAM1. These genes serve as important biomarkers for understanding the genetic basis of milk production efficiency and mastitis resistance.

Genome-wide association studies (GWAS) have identified thousands of genetic variants linked to complex traits in cattle, including production, reproductive performance, body conformation, and disease resistance.

Milk yield shows moderate heritability ($\approx$0.25), while milk fat, protein, and lactose percentage have higher heritability ($\approx$0.5). Traits such as lactation persistence, peak yield, and milking rate are also moderately heritable, whereas mastitis resistance has low heritability (Table 8.12). Milk yield is highly repeatable (0.95), and protein and SNF percentages also show high repeatability (0.85 and 0.90) (Table 8.13). In contrast, fat percentage has lower repeatability (0.60). Traits with moderate to high repeatability are more amenable to genetic improvement. Additionally, fat, protein, SNF, and total solids exhibit negative genetic correlations with milk yield (Table 8.14).

Table 8.12 Heritability of different milk production traits in cows

Traits	Heritability
Milk yield	0.25
Fat %	0.50
Protein %	0.50
Peak yields	0.30
Milking rate	0.40
Persistency	0.40
Mastitis resistance	0.10

Wilcox (1992)

Table 8.13 Repeatability of different milk production traits in cows

Traits	Repeatability
Milk yield	0.95
Fat %	0.60
Protein %	0.85
SNF%	0.90

Wilcox (1992)

Table 8.14 The correlation coefficients between milk yield and various milk constituents

Traits	Correlation coefficient
Fat %	−0.3
Protein %	−0.3
SNF%	−0.2
Total solid %	−0.3

Wilcox (1992)

8.4.3 Parity and Stage of Lactation

The milk-producing capacity of cows increases with successive lactations as the mammary gland enlarges with skeletal growth and increased body size, allowing for a larger udder. Typically, cows reach peak production around the 5th lactation, at about 7–8 years of age, when their skeletal size is roughly 30% greater than during the first lactation. Production then stabilizes and gradually declines after 12 years of age. The greatest improvement occurs between the 1st and 2nd lactations (about 13%), followed by smaller gains from the 2nd to 3rd (9%), 3rd to 4th (5%), and 4th to 5th (3%) lactations.

Milk composition also varies with the lactation stage. Reports indicate that fat and SNF decrease slightly—by approximately 0.05% and 0.1%, respectively—with each subsequent lactation, although some studies suggest parity does not significantly affect these components. As lactation progresses, protein content tends to rise while lactose content declines, particularly up to the eighth month of lactation.

8.4.4 Body Condition Score (BCS)

Body condition scoring (BCS) serves as an indirect indicator of a cow's fat reserves. Changes in these reserves over time, especially those related to tissue mobilization, help assess the animal's energy balance. During periods of negative energy balance, dairy cows may lose 30–40% of their fat stores because nutritional demands exceed energy intake. BCS typically declines early in lactation, followed by a gradual improvement during mid-lactation. The greatest loss in body condition usually occurs within the first 30 days after calving and may continue until about 90 days, after which BCS begins to rise again. Some studies report the lowest BCS occurring between 60 and 80 days of lactation.

Primiparous cows generally have higher BCS than multiparous cows, yet they tend to lose condition more rapidly and reach a lower minimum BCS. However, they also recover body condition faster than older cows. Body reserve mobilization shows a strong positive association with milk production, and cows with lower BCS are often higher milk producers. Cows with a BCS of around 3.5 have been reported to achieve the highest 60-day milk yields.

Overconditioned cows at calving typically have reduced dry matter intake compared with thinner cows. As a result, their dietary energy intake is lower, leading to a greater gap between energy consumption and energy requirements, which pushes them into a more severe negative energy balance. This excessive fat mobilization increases the risk of fatty liver syndrome and negatively impacts both productivity and reproductive performance.

8.4.5 Environment

Meteorological factors such as temperature, humidity, wind speed, and duration of sunshine strongly influence milk production. Climate impacts dairy performance in two ways: directly by affecting the animal's comfort and physiology, and indirectly by determining forage availability and disease occurrence. Cattle have a thermal comfort zone of 5–20 °C, within which they maintain normal productivity. Temperatures outside this range significantly impair milk yield. Lactating cows tolerate cold well and can maintain production even when temperatures drop to −5 °C, owing to their higher metabolic heat output. However, this same metabolic heat makes high-yielding cows highly vulnerable to heat stress as ambient temperature rises, making them more sensitive to heat than cold.

Heat stress also reduces feed intake, further lowering milk yield. Critical Temperature Humidity Index (THI) values associated with production loss are approximately 64 (minimum), 72 (mean), and 76 (maximum), although thresholds vary across agro-climatic regions. In subtropical climates, milk production declines around a THI of 72, while cows in temperate areas show thresholds of 60–68. In tropical regions, each unit increase in THI above 72 has been associated with a 0.2-kg drop in milk yield.

The severity of thermal stress is further influenced by solar radiation, wind speed, and rainfall. Increased precipitation has been linked to reduced milk output because rainfall limits grazing time and increases the energy required for movement under muddy conditions. Wet seasons also elevate disease risks, including vector-borne infections, mastitis, and endometritis.

Solar radiation itself generally does not alter milk yield or composition in cows and ewes. However, hot and humid conditions can affect milk quality by modifying its composition and physicochemical traits. Among milk components, fat and protein show notable changes under thermal stress. High temperatures typically reduce milk fat percentage and total protein content. Casein levels tend to decline in summer compared to spring, whereas concentrations of α-lactalbumin, α-casein, and β-lactoglobulin remain largely unaffected by rising temperatures.

8.4.6 Nutrition

Proper nutritional management is an effective approach not only for enhancing milk yield but also for altering its composition. The secretory epithelial cells of the mammary gland need a continuous supply of nutrient precursors to sustain milk synthesis. In dairy cows, milk output—and therefore energy expenditure—typically reaches its highest level between 4 and 8 weeks after calving, while peak dry matter intake (DMI), representing peak energy intake, does not occur until around 10 weeks postpartum.

To optimize milk yield, cows should be encouraged to increase their feed intake, helping to boost production and reduce the severity of negative energy balance. It is estimated that every extra kilogram of dry matter consumed can support an additional 2–2.4 kilograms of milk.

The dry matter intake can be estimated by the following equation:

$$\begin{aligned}\text{DMI (\%body weight)} = 4.048 - 0.00387 \times \text{body weight (kg)} + 0.0584 \\ \times\ 4\%\text{fat corrected milk (FCM) (kg)}\end{aligned}$$

where

$$4\%\text{FCM} = (0.4 \times \text{actual milk yield in kg/day}) + (15 \times \text{milk fat in kg/day})$$

A general guideline for dry matter intake (kg) for lactating dairy cows is presented in Table 8.15.

On a dry matter basis, the minimum forage to concentrate ratio of 40:60 is required to ensure milk fat percentage above 3.6 with an average forage length of 0.65 cm. Finely ground diets decrease milk fat and protein content due to altered rumen metabolism. Protein supplementation at 17–19% is recommended to compensate for the body protein mobilization that occurs in early lactation. Of the total dietary protein, about 30% should be in the soluble form, and approximately 30–35% should consist of rumen-degradable protein.

Table 8.15 General guidelines for dry matter intake (kg) for lactating dairy cows

Time	1st lactation	2nd lactation
Week 1	14	16 (2.5% BW)
Week 2	15–16	19 (2.9% BW)
Week 3	17	21 (3.4% BW)
Week 4	18	22 (3.6% BW)
Week 5	18–19	24 (4% BW)

(Department of Animal Science, McGill University)

Milk fat is the component most responsive to dietary modification, with its level varying by up to 3 percentage units. In contrast, the major milk fatty acids remain largely unaffected by diet, digestion, or mammary biosynthesis. Lactose content is also generally stable and cannot be altered through normal dietary changes, except under rare or extreme feeding conditions. Milk protein levels can be influenced by diet, but they are less responsive to dietary changes than milk fat.

Dietary strategies can modify milk fat and protein concentrations by roughly 0.3% and 0.6%, respectively, while lactose content generally remains unaffected. Milk fat synthesis relies mainly on acetate and butyrate, so lowering the roughage-to-carbohydrate ratio reduces these precursors and leads to a drop in milk fat. Propionate levels show an inverse relationship with milk fat but support milk protein formation by increasing glutamate availability. Milk fat percentage can also be enhanced by including at least 28% neutral detergent fiber in the diet. Adding saturated fatty acids has been shown to raise milk fat content, whereas unsaturated fatty acids tend to lower it. Starch-rich feeds improve microbial protein production, which in turn boosts milk yield and protein levels. Certain feed additives—such as sodium bicarbonate, magnesium oxide, and methionine hydroxy analog—can further stimulate milk fat synthesis, especially when used with high-energy diets, by aiding the transport of blood lipids to the mammary gland.

8.4.7 Milking Management

Maximum lactation persistency is maintained only when milk is removed regularly; otherwise, milk stasis increases intramammary pressure and triggers feedback inhibition, eventually leading to cessation of lactation and mammary involution. Increasing milking frequency beyond twice daily can raise milk yield by 10–20%, although milking three times a day may reduce milk fat percentage. However, more frequent milking reduces feeding time, so higher milking frequency must be supported with improved nutrition.

Milking interval also influences yield. Cows milked at unequal intervals produce less than those milked at equal intervals. Longer intervals between milking decrease total milk yield but increase fat and SNF percentages. More frequent milking lowers intramammary pressure and stimulates oxytocin release, enhancing milk secretion. Machine milking and automated systems generally yield more milk than traditional hand-milking practices.

8.4.8 Photoperiod

Increasing day length has been shown to enhance milk production in dairy cows and several other species. Extending photoperiods from 12 h to 16–18 h can raise milk yield by nearly 25 kg per cow. Photoreceptors in the retina transmit inhibitory signals to the pineal gland via the retino-hypothalamic tract, suppressing N-acetyltransferase activity and reducing melatonin synthesis. This altered melatonin profile influences various endocrine pathways that regulate growth, reproduction, and lactation. Although long-day photoperiods elevate prolactin secretion, prolactin has only a minor role in ruminant lactation, suggesting that other factors mediate the photoperiod-induced increase in milk yield.

One such factor is IGF-I, and its circulating levels rise under long-day lighting. IGF-I supports mammary gland development, prepares the gland for the next lactation, and inhibits apoptosis of mammary epithelial cells. Longer photoperiods also increase dry-matter intake, helping animals better meet the energy demands associated with negative energy balance.

Research further indicates that exposing cows to a short-day photoperiod during the dry period enhances their response to long-day lighting after calving, resulting in higher milk production in the following lactation. Therefore, regulating photoperiod during the dry period is an important management tool for improving milk yield. Light intensity also affects production: optimal milk yield occurs at around 50 Lux, but declines at 100 and 200 Lux. However, higher fat and total solids have been recorded at 100 Lux compared to 50 Lux, while milk protein levels remain unaffected by light intensity.

8.4.9 Pregnancy and Dry Period

The reduction in milk production observed during pregnancy is primarily attributed to nutrient partitioning toward fetal development. Although decreases in milk yield, fat, and protein have been noted from around 90 days of gestation, these changes were not statistically significant. This is likely because the fetus has minimal energy requirements until approximately 190 days of pregnancy. Overall, pregnancy does not have a significant impact on milk yield or milk composition (Table 8.16).

Table 8.16 Alterations in the milk yield and composition in Holstein cows during pregnancy

Trait	Nonpregnant	Pregnancy stage		
		1–120 d	121–210 d	211–300 d
Milk yield (kg/day)	28.5	28.3	27.4	25.2
Fat %	3.83	3.77	3.88	4.03
Protein %	3.40	3.42	3.43	3.47
Lactose %	4.90	4.89	4.91	4.91

Penasa et al. (2016)

The dry period is an essential stage in a dairy cow's production cycle, occurring between two lactations and allowing the mammary gland to regenerate damaged cells in preparation for the next lactation. The ideal dry period ranges from 42 to 60 days, though it may vary depending on breed, management practices, and individual cow factors. Studies have shown that cows given a 60-day dry period produce more milk than those with only 30 days. However, an extended dry period of around 70 days can negatively affect both milk yield and fertility. Conversely, shortening the dry period to 28–35 days or eliminating it altogether reduces milk production by 4.5% and 19%, respectively. While milk fat content remains unaffected by dry period length, shorter dry periods have been associated with increased milk protein, lactose, and SNF levels.

Exercises

Objective Questions

1. Most cows reach their peak yield around ________________ weeks after calving.
2. ________________ is a useful tool for estimating a cow's energy balance by visual assessment.
3. IGF-I is mainly produced in the ________________ in response to GH.
4. T4 is converted into the active hormone T3 by the enzyme________________.
5. ________________ hormone plays a central role in regulating feed intake and energy balance.
6. Milk yield is high/moderate/low heritable character. Pick up the right answer.
7. Cows reach peak production around the ______________ lactation.
8. Cattle have a thermal comfort zone between ________________°C within which they maintain normal productivity.
9. _____________ component of milk is most susceptible to dietary modification.
10. The ideal dry period in cows ranges from ________________ days.

Subjective Questions

1. Briefly describe the lactation curve of cows. What do you mean by the persistency of lactation?
2. How does the somatotropic axis regulate milk production in cows?
3. Describe the role of dietary manipulation to alter milk yield and composition in dairy cows.
4. How does light exposure cause the regulation of melatonin secretion? Write down the effect of photoperiod in cows.
5. Describe in brief the environmental effects on milk yield and composition.

Answer to Objective Questions

1. 5–6
2. Body condition scoring
3. Liver
4. 5′-deiodinase
5. Leptin
6. Moderate
7. 5th
8. 5–20
9. Fat
10. 42–60

References

Books

Mukherjee J, Das PK, Banerjee D (2023) Lactation physiology. In: Das PK, Sejian V, Mukherjee J, Banerjee D (eds) Textbook of veterinary physiology. Springer, Singapore. https://doi.org/10.1007/978-981-19-9410-4_25

Thiagarajan R (2014) Textbook of animal breeding. Satish Serial Publishing House, New Delhi

Research Articles

Bauman DE (1999) Bovine somatotropin and lactation: from basic science to commercial application. Domest Anim Endocrinol 17:101–116

Baxter EM, Hall SA, Farish M, Donbavand J, Brims M, Jack M, Lawrence AB, Camerlink I (2023) Piglets' behaviour and performance in relation to sow characteristics. Animal Int J Anim Biosci 17(2):100699

Bomfim GF, Merighe GKF, de Oliveira SA, Negrao JA (2022) Acute and chronic effects of cortisol on milk yield, the expression of key receptors, and apoptosis of mammary epithelial cells in Saanen goats. J Dairy Sci 105(1):818–830

Bytyqi H, Ødegård J, Mehmeti H, Vegara M, Klemetsdal G (2007) Environmental sensitivity of Milk production in extensive environments: a comparison of Simmental, Brown Swiss, and Tyrol Grey using random regression models. J Dairy Sci 90(8):3883–3888

Department of Animal Husbandry and Dairying (n.d.). Govt. of India, New Delhi, India

Department of Animal Science, Faculty of Agricultural and Environmental Sciences, Macdonald Camus of McGill University. Feeding the dairy cow during lactation. Dairy Cattle Production 342-450A

Donovan SM, Hintz RL, Wilson DM, Rosenfeld RG (1991) Insulin-like growth factors I and II and their binding proteins in rat milk. Pediat Res 29:50–55

Donovan SM, McNeil LK, Jimtnez-Flores R, Odle J (1994) Insulin-like growth factors and insulin-like growth fac- tor binding proteins in porcine serum and milk throughout lactation. Pediat Res 36:159–168

Fauci DL, Bionda A, Liotta L, Crepaldi P, Chiofalo V, Lopreiato V, FAZIO E. (2023) Effects of pregnancy and lactation on thyroid hormones, insulin, and metabolic blood parameters of modicana dairy cows. Large Anim Rev 29:1–7

Hess-Dudan E, Vacher PY, Bruckmaier RM, Weishaupt MA, Burger D, Blum JW (1994) Immunoreactive insulin-like growth factor I and insulin in blood plasma and milk of mares and in blood plasma of foals. Equine Vet J 26:134–139

Hickson RE, Lopez-Villalobos N, Dalley DE, Clark DA, Holmes CW (2006) Yields and persistency of lactation in Friesian and Jersey cows milked once daily. J Dairy Sci 89:2017–2024

Hooper HB, Dos Santos SP, de Oliveira SA, Merighe GKF, Titto CG, Negrão JA (2021) Long-term heat stress at final gestation: physiological and heat shock responses of Saanen goats. Int J Biometeorol. 65(12):2123–2135

Jindal SK, Ludri RS (1990) Growth hormone concentrations in lactating crossbred cows and buffaloes. Asian J Acad Stud 3(4):319–322

Kobayashi K, Oyama S, Kuki C, Tsugami Y, Matsunaga K, Suzuki T, Nishimura T (2017) Distinct roles of prolactin, epidermal growth factor, and glucocorticoids in beta-casein secretion pathway in lactating mammary epithelial cells. Mol Cell Endocrinol 440:16–24

Misra SS, Sharma A, Bhattacharya TK, Kumar P, Saha RS (2008) Association of breed and polymorphism of α-s1and α-s2casein genes with milk quality and daily milk and constituent yield traits of buffaloes (Bubalus bubalis). Buffalo Bull 27:294–301

Ollier S, Beaudoin F, Vanacker N, Blouin R, Lacasse P (2016) Effect of reducing milk production using a prolactin-release inhibitor or a glucocorticoid on metabolism and immune functions in cows subjected to acute nutritional stress. J Dairy Sci 100(7):5782–5791

Penasa M, De Marchi M, Cassandro M (2016) Effects of pregnancy on milk yield, composition traits, and coagulation properties of Holstein cows. J Dairy Sci 99:4864–4869

Ponchon B, Zhao X, Ollier S, Lacasse P (2017) Relationship between glucocorticoids and prolactin during mammary gland stimulation in dairy cows. J Dairy Sci 100(2):1521–1534

Ratwan P, Chakravarty AK, Kumar M (2020) Lactation wise performance of Sahiwal cattle at an organized herd of northern India. Ind J Anim Sci 90(8):1179–1185

Sarkar U, Gupta AK, Sarkar V, Mohanty TK, Raina VS, Prasad S (2006) Factors affecting test day milk yield and milk composition in dairy animals. J Dairying Foods HS 25(2):129–132

Singh J, Shukla KP (1986) Relationship of lactation persistency with some economic traits in Gir cattle. Ind Vet J 63:494–499

Sinowatz F, Schams D, Kölle S, Plath A, Lincoln D, Waters MJ (2000) Cellular localization of GH receptor in the bovine mammary gland. J Endocrinol 166:503–510

Skaar TC, Vega JR, Pyke SN, Baumrucker CR (1991) Changes in insulin-like growth factor-binding proteins in bovine mammary secretions associated with pregnancy and parturition. J Endocrinol. 131:127–133

Sorensen MT, Nørgaard JV, Theil PK, Vestergaard M, Sejrsen K (2006) Cell turnover and activity in mammary tissue during lactation and the dry period in dairy cows. J Dairy Sci 89:4632–4639

TANU Agritech Portal, Tamil Nadu Veterinary and Animal Science University (n.d.), Chennai, India.

Thatcher WW, Tucker HA (1970) Lactational performance of rats injected with oxytocin, cortisol-21-acetate, prolactin and growth hormone during prolonged lactation. Endocrinol. 86(2): 237–240

van der Kolk JH (1990) The bovine pituitary-adrenocortical axis and milk yield. Vet Quart 12(2): 114–120

Vega JR, Gibson CA, Skaar TC, Hadsel DL, Baumrucker CR (1991) Insulin-like growth factor (IGF)-I and -II and IGF binding proteins in serum and mammary secretions during the dry period and early lactation in dairy cows. J Anim Sci 69:2538–2547

Wilcox CJ (1992) In: Horn V (ed) Genetics: Basic concept, vol 4. Large Dairy Herd Management

Milk Ejection

9

Contents

J. Mukherjee et al., *Veterinary Lactation Physiology*,
https://doi.org/10.1007/978-3-032-21123-1_9

Abstract

Milk ejection, also known as the "milk let-down" reflex, represents one of the most important examples of neuroendocrine integration in mammalian physiology. It is a rapid, highly coordinated process through which milk, which is stored in the alveoli of the mammary gland, is expelled into the larger ducts and cisterns in response to the suckling stimulus. This phenomenon primarily depends on the secretion of oxytocin from the posterior pituitary gland, which then acts on myoepithelial cells surrounding the alveoli and results in contraction of alveoli and milk expulsion. Although the reflex has been extensively studied in dairy science due to its direct relation to milk yield, its physiological, evolutionary, and neurobiological implications extend far beyond dairy importance. The milk ejection reflex (MER) provides a window into neuroendocrine control of behavior, maternal bonding, and the plasticity of the hypothalamo–hypophyseal system. Understanding the comparative aspects of this reflex across species offers insights into adaptive lactation strategies, the evolution of maternal behavior, and the regulation of oxytocin release in health and disease.

Graphical Abstract

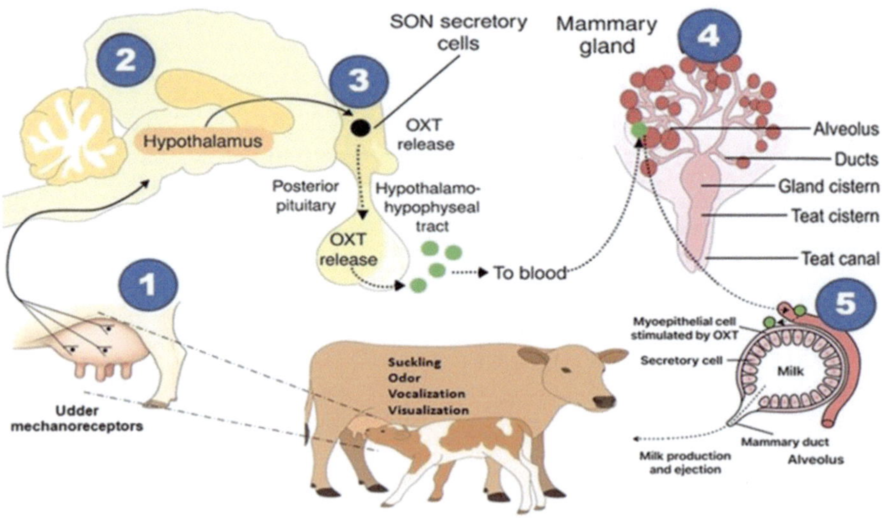

Description of the graphic: Milk ejection or let-down is the physiological process by which milk stored in alveoli and ducts of the mammary gland is propelled toward the teat cistern and delivered to the external duct orifice. The steps of milk let-down are as follows: (1) a stimulus, such as suckling by the calf, activates teat mechanoreceptors; (2) the sensory signal is conveyed to the hypothalamus by neural pathways; (3) stimulation of neurosecretory neurons in the supraoptic nucleus (SON) results in the secretion of oxytocin (OXT); (4) upon reaching the circulation, oxytocin reaches the udder and binds to receptors on alveolar myoepithelial cells; and (5) the oxytocin triggers the contraction of myoepithelial cells and subsequent milk ejection. This physiological pathway, together with sensory stimulation provided by the offspring, explains the importance of manual or mechanical udder stimulation for milk removal

Keywords

Oxytocin · Myoepithelial cells · Neuroendocrine reflex · Paraventricular and supraoptic nuclei (PVN & SON) · Afferent and efferent pathways · Calcium signaling · Stress inhibition · Conditioned reflex · Species variations · Dairy management

Inside the Chapter

- *Introduction*
- *Milk Ejection Reflex*
  - Definition and Overview
  - Components of the Reflex Arc
  - Efferent Pathways and Neurosecretory Response
  - Temporal Dynamics and Phasic Oxytocin Release
  - Milk Flow Patterns During Let-Down

- *Role of Oxytocin in Milk Ejection*
  - Oxytocin Synthesis and Processing
  - Mechanisms of Oxytocin Release
  - Oxytocin Receptors
  - Oxytocin Kinetics, Clearance, and Pharmacology
  - Hormonal Interactions with Oxytocin
- *Factors Affecting the Milk Ejection Reflex*
  - Stage of Lactation and Parity
  - Teat and Udder Stimulation Protocols
  - Ambient Environmental Conditions
  - Stress and Emotional State
  - Offspring Presence and Sensory Cues
  - Milking Interval and Frequency
  - Physiological and Pathological Conditions
  - Nutrition and Metabolic Health
  - Genetic and Individual Variations
- *Disorders of Milk Ejection*
  - Inhibited Milk Ejection
  - Defective Oxytocin Secretion
  - Mammary Gland-Level Disorders
  - Teat Lesions and Injuries

Learning Objectives
After reading this chapter, the reader will be able to:

- Explain the historical and conceptual development of the study of milk ejection and its physiological importance.
- Describe the evolutionary significance of the milk ejection mechanism in mammals.
- Understand the anatomical organization of the mammary gland relevant to milk ejection.
- Discuss the neuroendocrine nature of the reflex and the dual role of oxytocin as hormone and neuromodulator.
- Compare species variations in the mechanism, latency, and behavioral modulation of milk ejection.
- Appreciate the relevance of milk ejection in dairy practice, animal welfare, and clinical veterinary physiology.

9.1 Introduction

Milk ejection (also known as "let-down") is the physiological process by which milk stored in alveoli and ducts of the mammary gland is propelled toward the teat cistern and delivered to the external duct orifice. It is distinct from milk synthesis (i.e., secretion of milk constituents into alveolar lumina) and is essentially a mechanical/

contractile event mediated by myoepithelial cell contraction under neuroendocrine control. Efficient milk ejection is critical in lactating animals to ensure complete removal of milk, maintain high milking flow rates, and avoid residual milk that can compromise mammary health and achieve optimal yield.

In many farm species (cattle, sheep, goats, buffalo, pigs, etc.), a substantial fraction of milk resides in alveolar regions rather than static cisternal reservoirs; successful ejection is thus necessary to harvest most of the milk. The dynamics of ejection, the sensitivity of the reflex, and external influences vary with species, stage of lactation, and husbandry conditions.

9.2 Historical Background

The history of exploration of the milk ejection process dates back to the early nineteenth century, when physiologists first observed rhythmic contractions of the mammary gland following suckling by the offspring. However, the conceptual understanding of milk ejection as a "neuroendocrine reflex" was not established until the mid-twentieth century. Early studies by Starling and others in the 1900s suggested that a "circulating factor" released during suckling might stimulate the mammary gland. This led to the identification of oxytocin, a peptide hormone isolated and characterized by du Vigneaud and colleagues in 1953, as the key mediator of milk let-down.

In pioneering experiments on lactating animals, demonstrated that milk ejection could be prevented by severing the neural connection between the mammary gland and the central nervous system, emphasizing the reflex nature of the response. Subsequent studies by Lincoln and Wakerley (1975) established the concept of phasic release of oxytocin. They also showed that the hormone is secreted in discrete bursts coinciding with the rhythmic contractions of myoepithelial cells. These findings provided direct evidence that the mammary gland acts as an end-organ in a complex neuroendocrine reflex arc.

By the 1970s, electrophysiological studies on the hypothalamic magnocellular neurons in the paraventricular (PVN) and supraoptic (SON) nuclei of lactating rats provided a mechanistic basis for the reflex.

The neuronal synchronization of these nuclei was shown to coincide precisely with the oxytocin pulse, linking central neural activity to peripheral milk ejection. This integration of sensory, neural, and endocrine components established the milk ejection reflex as a classic model for studying hypothalamo-pituitary coordination.

Historically, the term "let-down reflex" was used interchangeably with milk ejection, but the physiological distinction became clearer over time. "Let-down" refers to the expulsion of milk from the alveolar lumen into the cisterns and teats, whereas "milk ejection reflex" (MER) encompasses the entire neural and hormonal sequence that facilitates this process.

Milk ejection studies have contributed immensely to the broader understanding of neurosecretion, which described the transport of hormones from hypothalamic neurons to the posterior pituitary for systemic release. The oxytocin system became the prototype for neurosecretion research and continues to serve as a paradigm for neuroendocrine integration.

From a veterinary perspective, recognition of the MER has guided the development of milking routines, machine design, and animal handling techniques aimed at optimizing oxytocin release and minimizing stress-induced inhibition. Moreover, it has deepened our understanding of maternal behavior, bonding, and welfare, linking physiological reflexes with emotional states.

Knowledge Corner...

The Nobel Prize in Chemistry (1955) was awarded to Vincent du Vigneaud for the synthesis of oxytocin, which is the first peptide hormone ever chemically synthesized. This breakthrough not only confirmed its structure but also laid the foundation for experimental and clinical use of oxytocin in both human and veterinary obstetrics.

9.3 Evolutionary Significance of Milk Ejection

Milk ejection represents a critical evolutionary innovation that ensures efficient transfer of nutrients and immune factors to offspring. The earliest mammals were likely small, nocturnal creatures whose young required frequent feeding. The evolution of a neuroendocrine milk ejection mechanism allowed mothers to synchronize milk delivery with offspring demand, which thereby helps in offspring survival and maternal energy efficiency.

Studies revealed that while milk production is a relatively slow and continuous process, milk ejection is a rapid and episodic event that evolved to match the intermittent suckling behavior of neonates. The development of specialized myoepithelial cells surrounding the alveoli was pivotal in this adaptation, transforming the mammary gland from a passive secreting organ into an active contractile system.

In primitive monotremes such as the platypus and echidna, milk is secreted onto special patches of the skin and licked by the young, suggesting a relatively diffuse let-down mechanism. In contrast, marsupials and eutherian mammals have more advanced mammary structures, with milk stored within alveoli and released through ducts under the control of oxytocin. This indicates a clear evolutionary change from local, passive milk flow to centralized, oxytocin-mediated milk ejection.

The evolution of oxytocin and its receptor also provides evidence of strong selective pressure for efficient maternal–infant transfer. The oxytocin gene is highly conserved among mammals, with only minor variations in sequence and receptor binding affinity, which reflects its ancient and essential role. Furthermore, comparative genomic studies reveal that oxytocin signaling is closely linked to maternal behavior, pair bonding, and stress modulation, indicating that milk ejection and emotional bonding share a common evolutionary origin.

Behaviorally, species differences in nursing patterns correspond to differences in milk ejection dynamics. For example, sows exhibit brief, synchronous bursts of milk flow lasting 20–30 s, synchronized across all glands, whereas rodents display multiple discrete ejection pulses during a nursing bout. In contrast, primates and ruminants show more sustained milk ejection, often modulated by emotional and environmental cues.

The evolutionary refinement of milk ejection thus reflects both neural complexity and behavioral adaptation, which allows mammals to balance the energetic costs of lactation with the survival needs of their offspring.

Knowledge Corner…
Among marine mammals, such as seals and whales, milk ejection has evolved under extreme ecological constraints. High-fat milk is ejected rapidly during brief nursing intervals to conserve heat and energy. The reflex is so efficient that pups can double their body weight within days, reflecting the evolutionary optimization of the oxytocin system for survival in harsh environments.

9.4 Anatomy of the Mammary Gland Relevant to Milk Ejection

Understanding the anatomical basis of milk ejection requires an appreciation of the structural organization of the mammary gland and its relationship with the neuroendocrine system. The mammary gland is composed of lobules, each containing clusters of alveoli lined by secretory epithelial cells. Surrounding each alveolus is a network of myoepithelial cells, the primary effector elements in the milk ejection process. These contractile cells are spindle-shaped, rich in actin and myosin filaments, and oriented longitudinally around the alveolar lumen.

The alveolar epithelium synthesizes milk constituents, i.e., proteins, lipids, and lactose, which are secreted into the lumen by apocrine and merocrine mechanisms. Milk accumulates within these alveoli until the onset of ejection. In species such as cattle and buffalo, a significant portion of milk is stored in the alveolar fraction, which requires oxytocin-induced contraction for release, while the cisternal milk is readily available without stimulation.

The ductal system forms the conduit through which milk travels from the alveoli to the teat. The small intralobular ducts merge into larger ducts and finally into the gland cistern, from which milk flows into the teat cistern. The teat sphincter maintains closure of the teat canal, preventing milk leakage and bacterial entry.

The myoepithelial cell layer is continuous with that of the small ducts, and its contraction exerts radial pressure, propelling milk through the ductal network. These contractions are triggered by oxytocin binding to specific G-protein-coupled receptors on myoepithelial cells, initiating intracellular Ca^{2+} release and activation of the actin–myosin contractile system.

An extensive vascular supply ensures rapid delivery of oxytocin and other hormones to the mammary tissue. The capillary network surrounding the alveoli is richly innervated and highly responsive to hormonal and autonomic regulation. During active milk ejection, increased local blood flow facilitates efficient oxytocin transport and rapid clearance.

The innervation of the mammary gland plays a vital role in initiating the reflex. Afferent fibers from mechanoreceptors located in the teat and skin convey impulses through the spinal cord to the hypothalamus, triggering oxytocin release. These fibers are primarily myelinated Aβ and unmyelinated C fibers, transmitting both tactile and thermal stimuli associated with suckling or milking.

The structural arrangement of the mammary gland varies from species to species, influencing the pattern and efficiency of milk ejection. In ruminants, milk storage is divided between alveolar and cisternal compartments, leading to a relatively rapid ejection phase once oxytocin is released. In rodents, most milk is stored in the alveoli; repeated oxytocin pulses are required for complete emptying. Primates, in contrast, have a predominantly alveolar storage system, and psychological stimuli such as infant cry or visual cues can trigger milk ejection.

The coordination of anatomical, neural, and endocrine elements ensures that milk ejection remains a tightly regulated and adaptive physiological process, essential for both offspring nourishment and mammary health.

Knowledge Corner...

The myoepithelial cells of the mammary gland are embryologically derived from the basal layer of the mammary epithelium and share properties with smooth muscle cells. They not only contract during milk ejection but also play roles in tissue remodeling and protection of the alveolar epithelium against over distension during lactation.

9.5 Biological Purpose and Mammalian Adaptations

Milk ejection is an indispensable physiological event ensuring the transfer of nutrients, energy, and bioactive substances from the mother to the offspring. Its biological purpose extends beyond milk removal; it synchronizes maternal physiology with neonatal demand, preserves mammary gland function, and contributes to the survival and development of the young.

From a functional viewpoint, milk ejection acts as a bridge between milk synthesis and neonatal nourishment. While milk secretion is a relatively slow and continuous process, the ejection mechanism allows for rapid delivery during suckling. This coordination optimizes maternal energy use and minimizes the time the offspring remain exposed to predators, a crucial factor in evolutionary fitness.

In ruminants, milk ejection ensures efficient emptying of the alveolar compartment, which constitutes 80–90% of total milk volume. Without complete milk ejection, alveolar pressure rises, impairing further milk synthesis and predisposing the gland to stasis-related disorders such as mastitis. Therefore, effective ejection is vital not only for nutrient transfer but also for mammary health and production efficiency.

In rodents and rabbits, milk is stored predominantly in the alveoli and is released in short bursts during suckling. The pups typically nurse only once or twice daily, and the entire milk reserve is delivered within a few minutes, demonstrating the critical dependence of lactation on the efficiency of the oxytocin-mediated contraction.

In primates, particularly humans, the biological role of milk ejection extends into the behavioral domain, where it is tightly linked with emotional and social cues such as the infant's cry, touch, or even visual contact. These stimuli evoke oxytocin release, reinforcing mother–infant bonding and caregiving behaviors.

The mammalian adaptations associated with milk ejection include the following:

(i) Structural adaptations: evolution of alveolar organization and myoepithelial cell layers for contractile efficiency.
(ii) Neural adaptations: development of specialized sensory receptors and central neural circuits for reflex initiation and regulation.
(iii) Endocrine adaptations: evolution of oxytocin synthesis, storage, and pulsatile release to match suckling patterns.
(iv) Behavioral adaptations: synchronization of nursing behavior and oxytocin secretion with circadian and reproductive rhythms.

These adaptations ensure that the milk ejection reflex remains one of the most finely tuned examples of maternal physiological integration in mammals.

Knowledge Corner...

In elephants, milk ejection can be stimulated not only by calf suckling but also by the tactile contact of the trunk. This unique sensory adaptation illustrates how diverse mammalian species have evolved specialized mechanisms to ensure successful lactation under varying ecological and behavioral circumstances.

9.6 Neuroendocrine Nature of Milk Ejection

Milk ejection epitomizes a neuroendocrine reflex, in which sensory input from the periphery (the teat) triggers hormonal release from the posterior pituitary. This integration of neural and endocrine responses ensures rapid communication between the suckling stimulus and mammary gland contraction.

9.6.1 Afferent Pathway and Central Processing

The reflex begins when the neonate suckles the teat, stimulating mechanoreceptors located in the dermis and subepithelial tissue of the teat and gland cistern. These tactile impulses are transmitted via the genitofemoral and intercostal nerves to the spinal cord, ascending through the spinothalamic and reticulospinal tracts to reach the paraventricular (PVN) and supraoptic (SON) nuclei of the hypothalamus.

Within these nuclei reside the magnocellular neurosecretory neurons, whose axons project directly to the posterior pituitary (neurohypophysis). Upon activation, these neurons generate synchronized burst discharges, leading to the exocytotic release of oxytocin into the systemic circulation.

The temporal coordination of these discharges was first demonstrated in lactating rats by Lincoln and Wakerley (1975), who observed simultaneous firing of PVN and SON neurons coinciding with pulsatile oxytocin release. Each burst corresponds to a wave of myoepithelial contraction, resulting in a phasic pattern of milk ejection.

9.6.2 Efferent Pathway and Peripheral Response

Once released into the bloodstream, oxytocin reaches the mammary gland within seconds due to the gland's rich vascularization. The binding of oxytocin to its G-protein-coupled receptors (OXTR) on myoepithelial cells triggers activation of the phospholipase C-inositol triphosphate (IP_3)-Ca^{2+} pathway, leading to a rise in intracellular calcium and contraction of the myoepithelial layer. This contraction compresses the alveoli, forcing milk into the ductal system and toward the teat cistern. The reflex is self-limiting; as the alveoli empty and mechanoreceptor stimulation ceases, oxytocin secretion diminishes. The refractory period between successive reflexes ensures that ejection occurs only in response to appropriate stimuli, preventing unnecessary energy expenditure.

9.6.3 Integration and Modulation

The MER demonstrates the functional unity of the hypothalamo–hypophyseal axis, where electrical activity in the brain translates into endocrine secretion. This unique design allows fine-tuned regulation by higher brain centers, including the limbic system, amygdala, and preoptic area, which integrate emotional, sensory, and environmental inputs.

Factors such as stress, pain, and fear can inhibit this reflex by activating the sympathetic nervous system and catecholamine release, which in turn constrict mammary arterioles and suppress oxytocin secretion. Conversely, positive emotional stimuli like the sight or sound of the offspring can trigger anticipatory oxytocin release even before suckling begins, demonstrating the cognitive modulation of the reflex.

In this manner, milk ejection serves as a classic example of how neural, hormonal, and behavioral components converge to maintain physiological homeostasis and maternal responsiveness.

Knowledge Corner...
During hand milking or machine milking, gentle tactile stimulation of the udder and teats serves as the physiological equivalent of calf suckling. This pre-stimulation initiates the afferent limb of the milk ejection reflex, which causes timely oxytocin release and improving milk yield and flow rate in dairy animals.

9.7 Oxytocin: Dual Role as Hormone and Neuromodulator

Oxytocin, the central mediator of milk ejection, occupies a unique position among hormones due to its dual mode of action as a peripheral hormone and as a central neuromodulator.

9.7.1 Peripheral (Hormonal) Role

In the periphery, oxytocin is synthesized by magnocellular neurons in the PVN and SON, and then transported along axons bound to neurophysin I and stored in the posterior pituitary. Upon stimulation, oxytocin is released into the bloodstream and acts on distant target organs, primarily the mammary gland and uterus. Its peripheral effects include:

(i) Milk ejection: Induction of myoepithelial contraction for milk ejection.
(ii) Uterine contraction: Causes uterine myometrial contraction and helps in parturition and postpartum uterine involution.
(iii) Hemostasis: Reduction of postpartum hemorrhage through vascular constriction.

The half-life of oxytocin in circulation is short (1–6 min in cows), allowing precise temporal control of the reflex and preventing prolonged or uncoordinated contractions.

9.7.2 Central (Neuromodulatory) Role

Beyond its classical endocrine function, oxytocin acts as a neuromodulator within the brain. It influences behavior, stress responses, and emotional states. Dendritic release of oxytocin within the hypothalamus and other brain regions allows local autocrine and paracrine signaling, modulating neuronal excitability and synchrony.

Central oxytocin release promotes maternal behaviors, including grooming, nursing posture, and pup retrieval in rodents. It also reduces stress and anxiety by dampening hypothalamic–pituitary–adrenal (HPA) axis activity, thereby supporting calm and attentive maternal care. This duality ensures that physiological and behavioral aspects of lactation occur in harmony.

9.7.3 Oxytocin and Emotional Bonding

Recent neuroimaging and behavioral studies have demonstrated oxytocin's critical role in establishing social and emotional bonds. In mammals, including humans, oxytocin facilitates recognition of offspring, trust formation, and social memory. The repeated activation of oxytocin pathways during lactation fosters long-term neuroplastic changes in the maternal brain, enhancing caregiving motivation and reducing stress reactivity.

9.8 Phasic and Dendritic Release Mechanisms

Oxytocin release occurs through two distinct mechanisms:

1. *Phasic systemic release*: It is triggered by action potentials traveling along axons to the posterior pituitary, leading to hormone exocytosis into the circulation.
2. *Dendritic release*: It is a locally regulated process in which oxytocin is secreted from neuronal dendrites into the extracellular space, modulating neuronal networks independently of peripheral secretion.

These mechanisms may act synergistically, i.e., dendritic release primes the neural circuitry for synchronous burst firing, while systemic release coordinates peripheral organ responses.

9.8.1 Pharmacological and Clinical Implications

Exogenous oxytocin administration has been widely used in veterinary and human medicine for inducing parturition, managing retained placenta, and facilitating milk let-down. However, excessive or inappropriate use may lead to receptor desensitization, uterine hypertonicity, and disruption of natural reflex timing. Therefore, a physiological understanding of oxytocin kinetics and receptor regulation is essential for its responsible clinical application.

Knowledge Corner...
Oxytocin and vasopressin differ by only two amino acids, yet their physiological roles are distinct. While vasopressin primarily regulates water balance and blood pressure, oxytocin governs reproductive and social behaviors. Their close structural relationship underscores their evolutionary origin from a common ancestral peptide.

9.9 Behavioral and Emotional Influences on Milk Ejection

Although the milk-ejection reflex (MER) is fundamentally neuroendocrine, its sensitivity to behavioral and emotional states exemplifies the intimate interaction between physiology and psychology in mammalian lactation.

9.9.1 Stress and Inhibition of Milk Ejection

Emotional stress, pain, or fear activates the sympathetic nervous system, causing the release of catecholamines (epinephrine and norepinephrine) that antagonize oxytocin action in two principal ways.

1. Peripheral inhibition: Catecholamines constrict mammary arterioles, reducing blood flow and consequently the delivery of oxytocin to the gland.
2. Central inhibition: Activation of hypothalamic CRH and noradrenergic pathways suppresses the firing of oxytocin neurons in the PVN and SON.

This dual inhibitory mechanism explains why nervous, frightened, and uncomfortable animals often fail to eject milk despite full alveolar storage. In dairy practice, this manifests as the "inhibited let-down syndrome."

Classical studies demonstrated that even brief stress like loud noise, restraint, or rough handling can stop the MER within seconds, yet calm conditions restore it quickly once stress ceases.

9.9.2 Facilitation by Positive Behavioral Cues

Pleasant sensory cues enhance oxytocin release. The sight, sound, or smell of offspring, rhythmic tactile stimulation, and the habitual routine of milking can all condition the reflex. In cows, conditioned oxytocin release has been recorded merely at the sound of the milking machine, even before udder contact. In primates and humans, the cry of the infant or thoughts of feeding can elicit pre-emptive milk let-down, which is an example of psychogenic oxytocin release.

Gentle animal handling, consistent milking routines, and calm environments promote optimal neuroendocrine function. Many dairy operations now integrate low-stress stockmanship to maintain stable oxytocin secretion patterns. It ultimately increases productivity and reduces the costs of milk production.

9.10 Maternal Behavior and Oxytocin Feedback

Behavioral expression of maternal care further augments milk ejection. Grooming, nuzzling, and licking stimulate tactile afferents in both mother and offspring, generating reciprocal oxytocin release. This mutual feedback loop strengthens maternal-offspring bonding while synchronizing feeding bouts. In rodents, blocking oxytocin receptors in the brain disrupts both milk ejection and core maternal behaviors essential for lactation success.

Knowledge Corner...

In buffaloes, calm temperament and gentle pre-milking massage have been shown to increase milk yield by 8–12%, largely due to enhanced oxytocin release. Conversely, the presence of unfamiliar handlers or abrupt noises can delay milk let-down by up to 2 minutes which is enough to reduce total yield significantly.

9.11 Species Variations in Milk Storage and Let-Down

The dynamics of milk ejection vary markedly among different species, which reflects differences in mammary anatomy, milk-storage distribution, and behavioral nursing patterns.

9.11.1 Ruminants (Cows, Buffaloes, Goats, Sheep)

In ruminants, 70–90% of milk is stored in the mammary alveoli and requires oxytocin-mediated ejection, whereas 10–30% resides in the cisternal compartment and is available immediately. Oxytocin pulses trigger complete milk evacuation within 30–60 s after stimulation. The reflex latency averages 40 s in cows and 60 s in buffaloes.

Environmental stressors prolong latency and diminish milk flow. Goats and sheep possessing smaller udders and less cisternal storage display faster but shorter ejection episodes.

9.11.2 Rodents

Rodents store nearly all milk alveolarly. Nursing occurs once or twice daily, and milk is expelled in multiple discrete pulses lasting a few seconds each. Each oxytocin pulse corresponds to synchronized burst firing of hypothalamic neurons. The entire litter coordinates suckling to maximize the reflex, making the mouse MER a preferred experimental model for studying pulsatile hormone secretion.

9.11.3 Primates

Primates exhibit a predominantly alveolar storage pattern with strong emotional modulation. In humans, psychogenic factors can elicit anticipatory ejection, whereas anxiety or pain can completely inhibit it. The latency of let-down varies widely from 30 s to several minutes, depending on maternal mood, infant cues, and tactile stimulation.

9.11.4 Sows

In pigs, milk ejection is uniquely synchronized across all glands and lasts only 20–25 s. Sows nurse every 50–60 min, and piglets must be fed simultaneously because the brief oxytocin pulse delivers all available milk at once. This short, synchronous burst pattern represents an extreme adaptation of MER to litter-nursing behavior.

9.11.5 Marsupials and Monotremes

In marsupials, milk composition and ejection mechanisms evolve through lactation stages, paralleling pouch young development. In monotremes (e.g., platypus), milk is secreted onto the skin rather than through teats, suggesting diffuse myoepithelial contractions instead of a centralized let-down mechanism.

These inter-species differences highlight the evolutionary flexibility of the oxytocin system in meeting diverse ecological and developmental demands.

Knowledge Corner...

The "milk let-down curve" in dairy cows typically shows a rapid rise in flow rate after oxytocin release, a brief plateau, and a sharp decline as alveolar milk empties. Recording these curves during machine milking is an effective diagnostic tool for assessing udder health and reflex efficiency.

9.12 Importance of Milk Ejection in Dairy Science

Efficient milk ejection is central to milk yield, milking efficiency, and udder health in dairy animals. Understanding the physiology of this reflex allows optimization of milking management and equipment design.

9.13 Milking Routine and Pre-Stimulation

Consistent pre-stimulation, such as udder washing, wiping, or brief hand-stripping, activates tactile receptors and initiates the oxytocin reflex before machine attachment. The recommended pre-stimulation period is 45–60 s, ensuring maximal oxytocin concentration at the start of milking. Premature attachment without stimulation often results in delayed milk flow, incomplete udder emptying, and residual milk accumulation.

9.13.1 Machine Milking and Flow Curves

Milking machines must be synchronized with the physiological timing of milk ejection. Pulsation frequency, vacuum level, and liner design should maintain teat massage while facilitating milk removal during the oxytocin peak. Continuous monitoring of milk-flow curves helps identify inhibited let-down or equipment malfunction.

9.13.2 Stress Reduction and Animal Handling

Low-stress environments enhance MER efficiency. Factors such as gentle human contact, stable social grouping, comfortable ambient temperature, and minimal noise contribute to sustained oxytocin release. Even minor stress immediately before or during milking can halve plasma oxytocin concentrations.

9.13.3 Residual Milk and Udder Health

Incomplete milk removal due to inhibited MER increases residual milk, which elevates intramammary pressure, reduces subsequent milk yield, and predisposes cows to mastitis. Proper stimulation and, when necessary, controlled exogenous oxytocin can prevent these complications. However, chronic or excessive oxytocin use may desensitize mammary receptors and should be minimized.

9.13.4 Training and Welfare Considerations

From a welfare standpoint, the MER reflects the animal's emotional state. Positive human–animal interactions not only improve milk yield but also enhance trust and calmness, reducing cortisol levels and facilitating natural oxytocin release. Modern dairy practice increasingly views efficient milk ejection as an indicator of both productive efficiency and psychological well-being.

Knowledge Corner...
Studies in Holstein cows show that calm, consistent handling can increase plasma oxytocin by 30–40% and shorten milk-flow latency by 20 s compared with stressed animals. Thus, improving the behavioral environment is as crucial as genetic or nutritional interventions for maximizing production.

9.14 Clinical Relevance in Veterinary Practice

Understanding the physiology of milk ejection has direct and extensive clinical implications in veterinary medicine. Disorders of milk let-down, oxytocin release, and myoepithelial responsiveness can significantly affect milk yield, udder health, and reproductive efficiency in domestic animals.

9.15 Inhibited Milk Ejection

Inhibited milk ejection is one of the most frequent functional disturbances encountered in dairy practice. It is usually caused by stress, pain, and environmental change that interferes with the oxytocin reflex. Animals that are frightened, separated from their offspring, or milked in unfamiliar surroundings often fail to eject milk despite full udder distension.

Catecholamines released during stress cause constriction of mammary blood vessels and reduce oxytocin delivery to the gland. In addition, central inhibition of oxytocin neuron firing by noradrenergic inputs further suppresses hormone release. Clinically, inhibited let-down is characterized by low milk flow, prolonged milking time, and incomplete udder emptying.

Management involves calming the animal, restoring familiar environmental cues, and, if necessary, administering exogenous oxytocin (2–5 IU i.m.) shortly before milking to restore ejection temporarily. However, routine dependence on oxytocin injections can lead to receptor desensitization and reduced endogenous reflex efficiency, so behavioral correction remains the preferred approach.

9.15.1 Pain-Induced Inhibition

Pain from teat lesions, mastitis, and udder edema can suppress milk ejection via nociceptive inhibition of hypothalamic oxytocin neurons. Adequate analgesia and mastitis control are therefore essential components of milking management. In such cases, relief of pain restores normal reflex activity more effectively than pharmacological oxytocin administration.

9.15.2 Oxytocin Deficiency and Receptor Dysfunction

Its occurrence is rare. True oxytocin deficiency may occur due to hypothalamic or pituitary lesions. In cows and buffaloes, receptor downregulation or desensitization from chronic oxytocin exposure can also blunt the milk-ejection response. These cases require differential diagnosis to distinguish between neuroendocrine failure and peripheral gland insensitivity.

9.15.3 Diagnostic and Therapeutic Applications

Measurement of plasma or milk oxytocin concentrations can serve as a diagnostic indicator of let-down efficiency. In addition, oxytocin assays are used in research to evaluate stress, welfare, and maternal bonding. Therapeutically, oxytocin is used for inducing milk let-down in animals with inhibited reflexes, facilitating uterine contraction post-partum and in cases of retained placenta and assisting parturition under controlled conditions. In all cases, careful dosing and timing are crucial to avoid side effects such as uterine tetany, milk leakage, and receptor tolerance.

Knowledge Corner...
In dairy buffaloes, the presence of the calf during milking can increase milk yield by up to 20%. This effect is mediated entirely through oxytocin release triggered by the calf's tactile and vocal stimuli, demonstrating the powerful behavioral modulation of the reflex.

9.15.4 Milk Ejection as a Model of Maternal Brain Plasticity

Beyond its reproductive importance, the milk ejection reflex provides a unique experimental and conceptual model for understanding neural plasticity in the maternal brain. During lactation, the hypothalamo–hypophyseal system undergoes profound morphological and functional remodeling that enhances the efficiency and synchronization of oxytocin release.

9.15.5 Structural Plasticity of Oxytocin Neurons

Magnocellular neurons in the paraventricular (PVN) and supraoptic (SON) nuclei exhibit dynamic structural changes during lactation. Dendritic remodeling, synaptic reorganization, and increased glial cell withdrawal create closer neuron–neuron contacts, facilitating electrical coupling and synchronized burst firing. This plasticity ensures that oxytocin neurons discharge in unison, generating the phasic pulses characteristic of the milk ejection reflex.

9.15.6 Functional Plasticity and Burst Firing

Neuronal synchronization during milk ejection depends on excitatory (glutamatergic) and inhibitory (GABAergic) inputs modulated by hormonal and sensory feedback. Each suckling event triggers a cascade of neurotransmitter release that fine-tunes the timing and amplitude of oxytocin pulses. Repeated activation strengthens these circuits through activity-dependent changes, a phenomenon analogous to learning and memory processes.

9.15.7 Behavioral and Emotional Correlates

The neuroplastic adaptations underlying milk ejection also influence maternal behavior. Oxytocin release promotes emotional bonding, reduces anxiety, and enhances social recognition. These behavioral effects stem from oxytocin's action on limbic structures such as the amygdala, nucleus accumbens, and prefrontal cortex. Thus, the milk ejection reflex represents a physiological basis for maternal empathy and nurturing.

9.15.8 Comparative and Translational Significance

Comparative studies across species from rodents to humans demonstrate that the principles of oxytocin-induced plasticity are evolutionarily conserved. Understanding these mechanisms has broader implications for neuropsychiatric research, including conditions such as postpartum depression, social anxiety, and attachment disorders. The MER, therefore, serves as both a veterinary and biomedical model for studying neuroendocrine adaptation and emotional regulation.

Knowledge Corner...

Electron microscopy of lactating rats has shown that astrocytic processes retract from oxytocin neuron membranes during milk ejection, allowing direct neuron–neuron contact. This transient glial withdrawal is a striking example of reversible neuroplasticity driven by physiological demand.

9.16 Milk Ejection Reflex

9.16.1 Definition and Overview

The milk ejection reflex (MER), also termed "let-down reflex," is a neuroendocrine reflex in which sensory stimulation of the mammary gland due to suckling or milking results in the release of oxytocin from the posterior pituitary. This oxytocin acts on the myoepithelial cells surrounding the alveoli and small ducts of the mammary gland, resulting in their contraction and expulsion of milk into the ductal and cisternal systems.

Milk ejection is distinct from milk secretion. Milk secretion involves the synthesis and accumulation of milk within the alveolar lumen, while ejection refers to the active discharge of stored milk in response to a neural stimulus. The reflex occurs within seconds and is critical for effective lactation and milk removal.

The MER is one of the well-characterized examples of neuroendocrine integration in mammals, demonstrating the communication between the nervous and endocrine systems. It can be triggered not only by tactile stimulation of the teat but also by conditioned sensory cues such as sight, sound, and smell of the offspring, highlighting the role of higher brain centers in reflex modulation.

The reflex can be divided into three sequential phases:

1. *Sensory activation:* stimulation of mechanoreceptors in the teat skin during suckling or milking.
2. *Neuroendocrine transmission:* afferent impulses travel to the hypothalamus, leading to synchronized firing of oxytocin neurons and hormone release from the neurohypophysis.
3. *Effector response:* circulating oxytocin acts on mammary myoepithelial cells to induce contraction and milk expulsion.

The entire process typically occurs within 30–60 s after stimulation in most domestic species. Its efficiency depends on emotional calmness, proper sensory stimulation, and intact hypothalamo–hypophyseal function.

Knowledge Corner...

The term neuroendocrine reflex was first coined by Ernst and Berta Scharrer in the 1940s, describing hormonal secretion controlled directly by neuronal activity. The milk ejection reflex remains the classic example of this concept.

9.17 Components of the Reflex Arc

The milk ejection reflex follows the classical organization of a reflex arc, comprising:

1. Afferent limb—sensory input from the mammary gland.
2. Central integration—processing and synchronization within the hypothalamus.
3. Efferent limb—hormonal output via oxytocin secretion and peripheral action.

Each component operates with remarkable temporal precision to achieve coordinated milk expulsion.

9.18 Afferent Pathways and Mechanoreceptor Activation

The reflex begins when the neonate suckles the teat or when mechanical milking stimulates the teat skin and sinus epithelium. Specialized mechanoreceptors and pressure-sensitive nerve endings are present within the dermis of the teat and gland cistern that respond to stretch and tactile sensation.

These receptors include both low-threshold Aβ fibers (rapidly conducting, myelinated fibers responsible for touch and pressure detection) and slow-conducting C fibers (respond to sustained stimulation). The impulses travel through the genitofemoral, iliohypogastric, and pudendal nerves, entering the spinal cord via the lumbar and sacral dorsal roots.

From the spinal cord, impulses ascend through multisynaptic pathways involving the spinoreticular and spinothalamic tracts, ultimately projecting to the brainstem reticular formation and then to the hypothalamus. The transmission involves neurotransmitters such as glutamate and neuropeptides that activate oxytocinergic neurons in the paraventricular (PVN) and supraoptic (SON) nuclei.

These sensory inputs constitute the afferent arm of the reflex and are essential for initiating synchronized neuronal discharge in the hypothalamus. The latency between teat stimulation and oxytocin release is species-dependent, averaging 20–30 s in goats, 40 s in cows, and up to 60 s in buffaloes.

Emotional stress or pain can interrupt afferent transmission through activation of inhibitory descending pathways or sympathetic overactivity and that suppress the oxytocin neuron activation.

9.18.1 Spinal and Supraspinal Transmission

Once activated, sensory signals from the teat ascend through the spinal cord to the brainstem and hypothalamus where they undergo integration and modulation.

At the spinal level, impulses are transmitted via interneurons within the dorsal horn to ascending tracts of the reticular formation. The reticulospinal system acts as a relay to hypothalamic nuclei, and it causes rapid signal transfer.

Electrophysiological recordings in lactating rats and goats have shown that stimulation of the teat produces multi-unit activity in the PVN and SON within a fraction of a second. This demonstrates the remarkable speed of neural transmission involved in the reflex.

The supraspinal centers, particularly the hypothalamic nuclei, serve as the command center. Within these centers, sensory information converges with modulatory inputs from other brain regions such as the amygdala, preoptic area, and brainstem catecholaminergic nuclei. These higher centers can either facilitate or inhibit the reflex depending on the animal's emotional state. Activation of the amygdala during fear or stress inhibits oxytocin neuron activity, whereas stimulation of the preoptic area enhances reflex responsiveness.

9.18.2 Hypothalamic Integration: SON and PVN

The paraventricular nucleus (PVN) and supraoptic nucleus (SON) of the hypothalamus form the central integration site of the milk ejection reflex. Each contains magnocellular neurosecretory neurons that synthesize oxytocin and project their axons to the posterior pituitary (neurohypophysis).

Upon receiving afferent input from the mammary mechanoreceptors, these neurons exhibit synchronized burst firing, which leads to the pulsatile release of oxytocin into the bloodstream. The synchronization is mediated by both electrical coupling and chemical communication through dendro-dendritic release of oxytocin and excitatory neurotransmitters.

This coordinated activity ensures that the entire population of oxytocin neurons discharges simultaneously, generating a systemic pulse of oxytocin sufficient to elicit a contraction of the mammary myoepithelial network. Studies using electrophysiological and calcium imaging techniques have confirmed that oxytocin neurons display burst-pause rhythmicity during milk ejection, corresponding precisely to each wave of milk flow. Furthermore, glial remodeling around oxytocin neurons during lactation facilitates enhanced synaptic contact and neuronal synchronization.

Knowledge Corner...

During lactation, astrocytes in the PVN and SON retract their processes from oxytocin neurons, allowing dendro-dendritic communication and synchronized burst firing a form of functional neuroplasticity unique to the maternal brain.

9.19 Efferent Pathways and Neurosecretory Response

The efferent limb of the milk ejection reflex begins with the discharge of oxytocin neurons in the hypothalamus and ends with the contraction of myoepithelial cells in the mammary gland. This pathway transforms neural excitation into a hormonal and then a mechanical response.

9.19.1 Oxytocin Secretion from the Posterior Pituitary

The action potentials generated in the magnocellular neurons propagate along their axons through the hypothalamo–hypophyseal tract to the posterior pituitary. In the posterior pituitary oxytocin is stored in Herring bodies. The electrical depolarization triggers Ca^2-dependent exocytosis of oxytocin into the capillary plexus of the neurohypophysis. Within 1–2 s, oxytocin enters the systemic circulation and reaches the mammary gland through the blood. Its plasma half-life is short (1–3 min), allowing precise temporal control of the reflex. Each burst of oxytocin secretion produces a transient rise in plasma concentration (up to 10–30 pg/mL in cows), corresponding to a single phase of milk ejection. The temporal relationship between oxytocin release and milk flow has been confirmed by simultaneous hormone assays and milk flow measurements.

9.19.2 Action on the Mammary Gland

In the mammary gland, oxytocin binds to G-protein-coupled oxytocin receptors (OXTR) on myoepithelial cells lining the alveoli and small ducts. This activates the phospholipase C-IP_3-Ca^{2+} signaling cascade, releasing intracellular calcium stores and initiating actin–myosin interaction for contraction. The contraction of the myoepithelial layer exerts radial pressure on the alveolar lumen, forcing milk into the ductal system and eventually into the cisterns and teat canal. In ruminants, this process empties approximately 80–90% of the alveolar milk within 30–60 s.

9.19.3 Termination of the Reflex

The reflex terminates naturally when alveolar pressure decreases, and mechanoreceptor stimulation ceases. Negative feedback through reduced sensory input and declining oxytocin levels prevents prolonged contraction and allows the mammary gland to refill for the next ejection cycle. Refractory periods between oxytocin pulses vary among species; in rats, multiple brief pulses occur per nursing bout, while in cows, a single oxytocin surge suffices for complete milk removal.

9.19.4 Neurovascular Dynamics

The mammary gland's rich vascular network ensures rapid hormone delivery and clearance. During active milk ejection, mammary blood flow increases transiently, enhancing oxytocin uptake. Vasomotor tone in these vessels is modulated by autonomic inputs, providing a link between stress, circulation, and reflex efficiency.

Knowledge Corner...
In ewes, intravenous oxytocin administration produces visible milk flow within 20 s, confirming the speed of hormonal transport and the responsiveness of mammary myoepithelial cells. This property has been utilized experimentally to assess mammary contractility and oxytocin receptor sensitivity.

9.20 Temporal Dynamics and Phasic Oxytocin Release

Milk ejection is a rapid yet precisely timed sequence of neural and hormonal events. The defining feature of this process is the phasic, pulsatile release of oxytocin, which coordinates myoepithelial contraction and milk flow.

9.20.1 Latency and Timing of Oxytocin Surges

Following teat stimulation, there is a short latency period, i.e., the interval between initial sensory input and measurable milk flow. In cows, the latency averages 40–60 s, whereas in goats the latency period is approximately 20–30 s. In buffaloes, it may extend up to 60–90 s because of larger alveolar storage and thicker gland tissue. During this period, afferent impulses reach the hypothalamus, oxytocin neurons synchronize, and the hormone is secreted into circulation. During this time, plasma oxytocin levels rise sharply, reach the peak within 30–45 s after stimulation, and then decline exponentially as milk flow ceases.

9.20.2 Phasic Pattern of Oxytocin Secretion

Electrophysiological studies by Lincoln & Wakerley (1975) revealed that oxytocin neurons discharge in synchronous bursts rather than tonic firing. Each burst results in a discrete pulse of oxytocin release into the bloodstream. In lactating rats, bursts recur every 3–5 min during a nursing bout, producing multiple brief surges. In contrast, cows and humans usually display a single pronounced pulse per milking or feeding event. This phasic pattern ensures that the mammary gland contracts rhythmically, preventing vascular constriction or tissue fatigue. It also conserves oxytocin by releasing only as much as required for effective ejection.

9.20.3 Feedback Control and Self-Limitation

Oxytocin secretion is self-limiting. As alveoli empty and mechanoreceptor stimulation wanes, afferent input decreases, leading to cessation of hypothalamic activity. Additionally, oxytocin has a short plasma half-life (1–3 min) and is rapidly degraded by hepatic and renal oxytocinases. Negative feedback through central inhibitory neurotransmitters (e.g., GABA, opioids) also terminates burst firing, preventing continuous secretion. This tight temporal control maintains the efficiency and reproducibility of the reflex over many lactation cycles.

9.20.4 Central Coordination and Synchronization

Synchronized discharge of oxytocin neurons depends on both electrical coupling and dendritic release of oxytocin within the hypothalamus. This autocrine positive feedback momentarily enhances neuronal excitability, generating a coherent burst that translates into a systemic hormone pulse. The remarkable synchronization across PVN and SON neurons explains the rapid systemic response and is a key model for studying rhythmic neuroendocrine activity.

Knowledge Corner…
Using microdialysis in lactating rats, demonstrated that oxytocin release within the SON precedes peripheral hormone surges by several seconds, evidence that central dendritic release helps initiate neuronal synchrony before blood-borne secretion.

9.21 Milk Flow Patterns During Let-Down

The milk-flow curve recorded during milking or nursing provides a functional signature of the milk ejection reflex (Table 9.1).

9.21.1 Phases of Milk Flow

A typical curve shows three main phases:

1. Lag phase: brief period (20–60 s) of minimal flow while oxytocin levels rise.
2. Rapid rise phase: sudden increase in flow as alveolar milk is expelled.
3. Decline phase: gradual fall as alveoli empty and residual milk diminishes.

Table 9.1 Comparative characteristics of the milk ejection reflex across species

Species	Reflex latency	No. of oxytocin pulses per event	Duration of milk flow	Remarks
Cow	40–60 s	1–2	2–3 min	Single dominant surge
Buffalo	60–90 s	1	3–4 min	Slower onset, prolonged flow
Goat	20–30 s	1–2	1–2 min	Rapid reflex
Sheep	25–35 s	1	1–2 min	Similar to goats
Sow	15–20 s	1	20–25 s	Synchronous across glands
Rat	3–5 min intervals	Multiple	Several sec each	Pulsatile pattern
Human	30 s–3 min	2–4	Variable	Emotionally modulated

In well-stimulated dairy cows, the peak flow occurs within 1 min of oxytocin release and lasts for 2–3 min. Residual milk constitutes about 10–15% of total yield and can be expelled only with sustained oxytocin activity or manual stripping.

9.21.2 Multiple Ejections in Small Species

In rodents and rabbits, milk flow occurs in multiple small bursts, each corresponding to a discrete oxytocin pulse. The total duration of milk ejection is thus spread over several minutes. This episodic flow pattern aligns with the offspring's synchronized suckling behavior.

9.21.3 Influence of Stress and Handling

Emotional disturbance causes delayed or irregular flow curves characterized by a flattened peak and an extended lag phase. Measurement of such deviations is a valuable tool for assessing reflex inhibition and animal welfare in dairy herds.

9.21.4 Practical Implications

Modern milking systems employ flow-rate sensors to monitor let-down efficiency. Optimal machine attachment timing, approximately 45–60 s after udder stimulation, which coincides with the oxytocin peak, ensures maximal flow and minimal residual milk.

Knowledge Corner...
Recording of milk-flow curves originated in the 1950s when German physiologist Hans Tiegs devised electronic lactometers to visualize milk ejection dynamics in cows. These recordings later became indispensable for diagnosing inhibited let-down and evaluating machine milking efficiency.

Knowledge Corner...
In sows, oxytocin release occurs in one of the most synchronized patterns known in mammalian physiology. All mammary glands empty within 25 s and if piglets are prevented from suckling at that exact moment, the milk is reabsorbed. This phenomenon is an example of an evolutionary safeguard against wastage.

9.22 Role of Oxytocin in Milk Ejection

9.22.1 Oxytocin Synthesis and Processing

9.22.1.1 Prepro-Oxytocin, Pro-Oxytocin, and Neurophysin I

Oxytocin is a nonapeptide hormone ($C_{43}H_{66}N_{12}O_{12}S_2$), consisting of nine amino acids: Cys–Tyr–Ile–Gln–Asn–Cys–Pro–Leu–Gly. It differs from its closely related peptide, vasopressin, by only two amino acids, yet the two hormones serve distinct physiological functions, i.e., oxytocin in lactation and reproduction, vasopressin in water balance and vascular regulation. The hormone is synthesized as part of a larger precursor molecule, prepro-oxytocin-neurophysin I, within the magnocellular neurons of the paraventricular (PVN) and supraoptic (SON) nuclei of the hypothalamus.

The biosynthetic process involves the following:

1. Gene transcription of the oxytocin–neurophysin I gene located on chromosome 20 in most mammals.
2. Translation of prepro-oxytocin (comprising oxytocin, neurophysin I, and a signal peptide).
3. Cleavage of the signal peptide in the endoplasmic reticulum to form pro-oxytocin–neurophysin I.
4. Processing in the Golgi apparatus where enzymatic cleavage yields mature oxytocin and its carrier protein neurophysin I.

Neurophysin I binds oxytocin non-covalently, stabilizing it during axonal transport and facilitating its storage within neurosecretory vesicles.

Oxytocin synthesis is upregulated during late pregnancy and lactation, driven by elevated estrogen levels and repeated suckling-induced neuronal activation. This ensures an abundant supply of hormones for the frequent reflexes required in nursing.

Knowledge Corner...
The human oxytocin gene contains a highly conserved promoter region responsive to estrogen. This explains why oxytocin synthesis and receptor expression both increase toward parturition, preparing the mammary gland for effective milk ejection.

9.22.1.2 Transport and Storage in the Posterior Pituitary

Once synthesized in the hypothalamic neurons, oxytocin and neurophysin I are packaged into membrane-bound secretory granules. These granules are transported down the axons via microtubule-dependent fast axonal transport, assisted by kinesin motor proteins. The journey from the hypothalamic soma to the posterior pituitary (neurohypophysis) spans several millimeters, and the transport rate is approximately 1–3 mm per hour. During transport, vesicles accumulate in Herring bodies swellings along the axon terminals that serve as storage reservoirs. Within the neurohypophysis, oxytocin is released by Ca^{2+}-dependent exocytosis in response to electrical impulses propagated from the hypothalamic cell bodies. Each pulse of neuronal activity triggers synchronized vesicular fusion and hormone discharge into the perivascular space, from where oxytocin rapidly enters the systemic circulation. Histologically, the neurohypophysis contains a dense capillary plexus of fenestrated capillaries, ensuring minimal diffusion distance between secretory endings and bloodstream.

Knowledge Corner...
Electron microscopy of the posterior pituitary reveals dense core vesicles approximately 100–200 nm in diameter, containing both oxytocin and neurophysin I. These vesicles represent the final storage form of oxytocin before release.

9.23 Mechanisms of Oxytocin Release

9.23.1 Burst Firing of Magnocellular Neurons

The defining electrophysiological characteristic of oxytocin neurons during lactation is their phasic burst firing pattern. Each milk ejection episode corresponds to a synchronized burst of action potentials across the population of magnocellular neurons in the PVN and SON. The firing pattern typically includes rising phase (where individual neurons begin to discharge irregularly), synchronized burst (during which all neurons fire rapidly), and a silent phase of several minutes (representing neuronal recovery and refilling of vesicular stores). The burst firing is triggered by afferent sensory input from the mammary mechanoreceptors and is coordinated by local dendritic release of oxytocin, which acts back on oxytocin neurons via autocrine positive feedback. This mechanism ensures simultaneous activation of thousands of neurons, resulting in a sharp, systemic oxytocin pulse. Electrophysiological studies have demonstrated that the firing frequency and duration of bursts correlate directly with plasma oxytocin concentration and milk ejection magnitude.

9.23.2 Dendritic Release and Central Effects

In addition to axonal secretion into the bloodstream, oxytocin is also released from dendrites within the hypothalamus. This phenomenon was first demonstrated by Theodosis & Poulain (1993) using immunocytochemistry and in vivo microdialysis. Dendritic release allows oxytocin to act locally on neighboring neurons and glial cells, promoting neuronal synchronization and modulating excitability. This central release is regulated independently of action potentials and often influenced by intracellular calcium waves and neuromodulators. Functionally, dendritic oxytocin acts as a neuromodulator, facilitating maternal behaviors, reducing stress, and reinforcing the emotional bond between mother and offspring. These central effects ensure that physiological milk ejection is accompanied by appropriate behavioral and emotional states, enhancing maternal responsiveness and care.

9.24 Oxytocin Receptors

Oxytocin exerts its physiological effects by binding to specific G-protein-coupled receptors (GPCRs) located on target cells. These receptors belong to the Class I (rhodopsin-like) family of GPCRs and are encoded by the OXTR gene, highly conserved among mammals. The distribution, activation, and intracellular signaling of these receptors determine the magnitude and pattern of the milk ejection response.

9.24.1 Distribution in Mammary Tissue

In the mammary gland, oxytocin receptors are predominantly located on the myoepithelial cells surrounding the alveoli and small ducts. Lesser concentrations are found on vascular endothelial cells and smooth muscle fibers within the gland's microvasculature, contributing to local hemodynamic regulation during ejection. Receptor density increases markedly toward the end of pregnancy and during lactation, under the influence of estrogen and prolactin. Estrogen enhances OXTR gene transcription, while prolactin maintains receptor expression and sensitivity. Receptor distribution varies in different species. In cows and goats, receptor concentration is higher in alveolar and ductal myoepithelia. In humans and primates, additional receptors are present in the mammary stroma and vasculature. In rodents, receptors are uniformly distributed across alveolar walls, which support rapid synchronized contraction.

9.24.2 Receptor Activation and Signal Transduction

Upon oxytocin binding, the receptor undergoes a conformational change that activates Gq/11-type G-proteins (Fig. 9.1). This leads to stimulation of

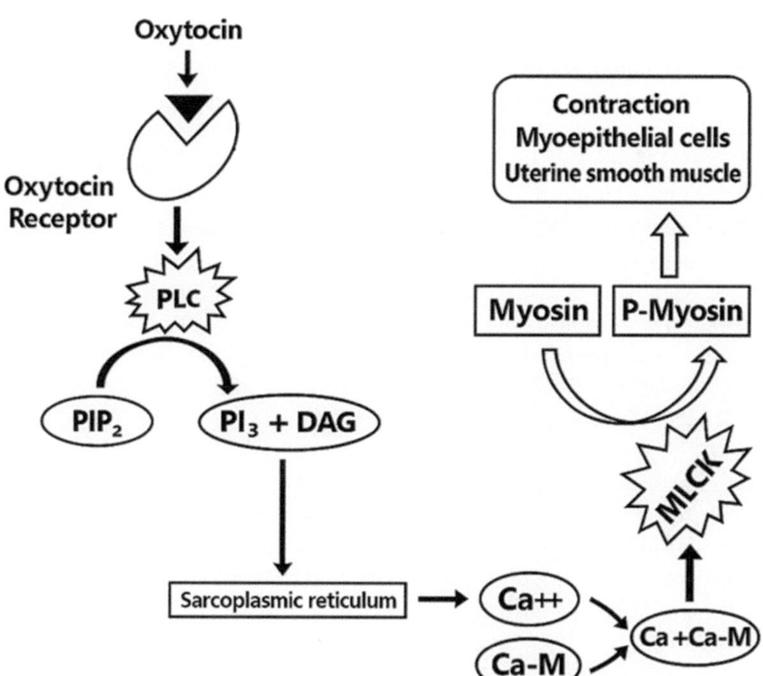

Fig. 9.1 The mechanism of action of oxytocin on mammary myoepithelial cells

phospholipase C-β (PLC-β), which hydrolyzes membrane phosphatidylinositol 4,5-bisphosphate (PIP_2) into two key second messengers, i.e., inositol 1,4,5-triphosphate (IP_3) (mobilizes intracellular Ca^{2+} from endoplasmic reticulum stores) and diacylglycerol (DAG) (activates protein kinase C (PKC), modulating contractile proteins and membrane excitability). The rise in intracellular Ca^{2+} binds to calmodulin, initiating activation of myosin light-chain kinase (MLCK). MLCK phosphorylates myosin light chains, enabling actin–myosin cross-bridge formation and contraction of the myoepithelial cells. This biochemical cascade results in synchronous contraction of the alveolar network, generating pressure for milk expulsion through the ducts.

Oxytocin receptors are members of the rhodopsin-type (Class I) G-protein-coupled receptor superfamily. The binding of oxytocin to its receptor activates phospholipase C (PLC), which catalyzes the hydrolysis of phosphatidylinositol-4,5-bisphosphate (PIP_2) into diacylglycerol (DAG) and phosphatidylinositol-1,4,5-trisphosphate (IP_3). IP_3 induces the release of calcium ions from the sarcoplasmic reticulum into the cytosol. The increased intracellular calcium binds to calmodulin (CaM), forming a Ca^{2+}–CaM complex that activates myosin light-chain kinase (MLCK). MLCK phosphorylates myosin, and this phosphorylation initiates contraction of the mammary myoepithelial cells, resulting in milk ejection.

9.24.3 IP_3-Ca^{2+} Pathway and Contractile Machinery

The IP_3-Ca^{2+} signaling pathway is the final common mechanism translating oxytocin receptor activation into mechanical milk ejection. The steps are as follows:

1. IP_3 binds to its receptors on the endoplasmic reticulum, causing a rapid Ca^{2+} efflux into the cytoplasm.
2. The rise in cytosolic Ca^{2+} triggers actin–myosin filament sliding, mediated by the MLCK pathway.
3. PKC activation modulates ion channels, sustaining contraction and fine-tuning the duration of response.
4. Ca^{2+} is then pumped back to the sarcoplasmic reticulum (SR) by Sarcoendoplasmic Reticulum Calcium ATPase (SERCA) pumps, restoring basal levels and allowing relaxation.

The contraction spreads as a wave across the alveolar network, ensuring uniform milk expulsion. Repeated stimulation or exogenous oxytocin exposure can lead to receptor desensitization, characterized by receptor internalization and reduced coupling efficiency, which is a clinically relevant consideration in veterinary and dairy practice.

9.25 Oxytocin Kinetics, Clearance, and Pharmacology

9.25.1 Kinetics and Half-Life

Oxytocin displays a rapid onset and short duration of action, features essential for its precise physiological control. Following release into the circulation, oxytocin reaches the mammary gland within 10–20 s in most species and is cleared within 1–3 min. The plasma half-life varies slightly among different species. Because of this rapid clearance, continuous sensory stimulation is required to sustain the reflex during prolonged milking or nursing. The short half-life is attributed to enzymatic degradation by oxytocinases, particularly cystine aminopeptidase present in plasma, liver, and kidney. This enzyme cleaves the disulfide bond linking cysteine residues, inactivating the peptide. The placenta also produces oxytocinase during pregnancy, regulating systemic oxytocin exposure and preventing premature uterine contractions.

9.25.2 Distribution and Metabolism

Oxytocin is a small hydrophilic peptide that distributes primarily in the extracellular fluid compartment. It binds weakly to plasma proteins, allowing rapid diffusion to target tissues. The hormone does not cross the blood–brain barrier easily, so peripheral oxytocin acts mainly on peripheral organs, while central oxytocin must be released locally within the brain. Metabolic inactivation occurs chiefly in the liver and kidney, with a smaller fraction degraded in mammary tissue itself. The mammary glands' high perfusion rate ensures both efficient delivery and prompt removal of the hormone after action.

9.26 Hormonal Interactions with Oxytocin

The efficiency of milk ejection is influenced by interactions between oxytocin and other endocrine factors that regulate lactation, stress, and reproductive physiology. These interactions can be synergistic or antagonistic depending on the physiological context.

9.26.1 Prolactin

Prolactin is secreted by the anterior pituitary. It is primarily responsible for milk synthesis. It also modulates oxytocin action. Prolactin enhances oxytocin receptor expression in mammary tissue and sustains receptor sensitivity during lactation. During suckling, prolactin and oxytocin are released concurrently. Prolactin stimulates milk synthesis and oxytocin regulates milk ejection. Their coordinated secretion ensures balance in milk production and release. In rats, chronic blockade of prolactin results in reduced oxytocin receptor density and diminished milk ejection response, which emphasizes the synergistic relationship between the two hormones.

9.26.2 Catecholamines

Catecholamines such as epinephrine and norepinephrine exert a potent inhibitory influence on the milk ejection reflex. Emotional stress, fear, or pain activates the sympathoadrenal system, leading to catecholamine release from the adrenal medulla and sympathetic nerve terminals. These catecholamines cause the following:

(i) Vasoconstriction of mammary arterioles results in a reduction in oxytocin delivery.
(ii) Inhibition of oxytocin neuron firing via α_2-adrenergic receptors in the hypothalamus.
(iii) Direct inhibition of myoepithelial responsiveness through β-adrenergic receptor activation on the mammary gland.

Thus, catecholamines provide a rapid mechanism for stress-induced inhibition of milk ejection.

9.26.3 Estrogen and Progesterone

These ovarian steroids modulate both oxytocin synthesis and receptor expression in a complementary, stage-dependent manner. Estrogen upregulates oxytocin gene transcription in the hypothalamus and increases receptor density in mammary and uterine tissues. Progesterone, on the other hand, antagonizes these effects by downregulating receptor expression and stabilizing the uterus during pregnancy. Toward the end of gestation, progesterone levels fall while estrogen rises, creating an endocrine environment favorable for oxytocin responsiveness. This shift prepares both the uterus for parturition and the mammary gland for lactation and efficient milk ejection. In ruminants, plasma estrogen concentrations peak around calving, coinciding with increased oxytocin receptor mRNA in mammary tissue. These hormonal changes ensure that the first postpartum milking triggers a strong and complete let-down.

9.26.4 Glucocorticoids

Glucocorticoids, particularly cortisol, play a dual role. At physiological levels, they support mammary epithelial differentiation and enhance oxytocin receptor expression. However, under stress, elevated cortisol acts via central pathways to inhibit oxytocin secretion. Cortisol suppresses oxytocin neuron firing by enhancing GABAergic inhibitory tone and modulating CRH (corticotropin-releasing hormone) neurons in the hypothalamus. Consequently, chronic stress or disease can blunt the milk ejection reflex, leading to reduced milk yield and incomplete alveolar emptying. Clinically, managing stress and ensuring metabolic health are crucial for maintaining a normal glucocorticoid–oxytocin balance.

9.26.5 Endogenous Opioids

Endogenous opioid peptides, such as β-endorphin and enkephalins, are important neuromodulators of oxytocin release. These peptides act primarily through μ- and κ-opioid receptors in the hypothalamus, exerting inhibitory effects on magnocellular neuron activity. During stress or pain, elevated β-endorphin levels suppress oxytocin secretion, thereby inhibiting milk ejection. This provides a neuroendocrine link between stress-induced analgesia and reproductive suppression. Experimental studies in lactating rats show that opioid receptor antagonists (e.g., naloxone) can restore oxytocin pulses inhibited by stress, confirming the opioid-mediated inhibition mechanism. Endogenous opioids serve to protect the organism from excessive stress responses. They can also transiently impair milk ejection when activated excessively.

Knowledge Corner...
The interaction of oxytocin with prolactin and estrogen represents one of the most elegant examples of hormonal synergy in mammalian physiology, where synthesis, secretion, and delivery of milk are coordinated through tightly regulated neuroendocrine feedback loops.

9.27 Factors Affecting the Milk Ejection Reflex

9.27.1 Stage of Lactation and Parity

9.27.1.1 Early Lactation

At the onset of lactation, oxytocin secretion and receptor density are maximal. Estrogen priming before parturition upregulates oxytocin receptor expression in mammary tissue, while prolactin and cortisol establish epithelial secretory capacity. The alveolar compartment is highly distended, and myoepithelial cells respond vigorously to oxytocin, producing a rapid, complete let-down of milk.

9.27.1.2 Mid to Late Lactation

As lactation progresses, receptor density and mammary vascular responsiveness gradually decline. Milk yield stabilizes, and oxytocin secretion remains pulsatile but of lower amplitude. In late lactation, partial involution processes may slightly delay the reflex because of increased connective tissue and reduced myoepithelial elasticity.

9.27.1.3 Parity Effects

Multiparous animals generally exhibit shorter reflex latency and higher peak flow rates than primiparous animals. Experience reduces emotional reactivity to handling and enhances conditioned oxytocin release. In contrast, heifers may show inhibited let-down during the first few milkings due to unfamiliar stimuli and incomplete neural conditioning.

9.27.1.4 Physiological Implications

Repeated lactation strengthens neuroendocrine coordination by improving hypothalamic sensitivity to afferent input and maintaining receptor expression. However, over-milking and chronic exogenous oxytocin exposure can reduce responsiveness over successive parities.

Knowledge Corner...

Studies in multiparous buffaloes demonstrate a 25–30% shorter milk-flow latency compared with heifers, directly correlating with higher basal oxytocin receptor expression in mammary tissue.

9.27.2 Teat and Udder Stimulation Protocols

Proper stimulation of the mammary sensory apparatus is critical for initiating the afferent limb of the MER.

9.27.2.1 Manual and Mechanical Stimulation

Gentle washing, wiping, and fore-stripping of the teats provides tactile input that triggers mechanoreceptor activation. Optimal pre-stimulation duration is about 45–60 s, coinciding with peak oxytocin secretion. Mechanical stimulation by milking machines must mimic natural suckling pressure and rhythm to maintain continuous afferent input.

9.27.2.2 Importance of Consistency

Animals quickly associate routine stimuli with milk ejection. Consistent timing, sequence, and handling reduce stress and facilitate conditioned oxytocin release. Abrupt changes in milking procedure or operator behavior can delay or inhibit the reflex.

9.27.2.3 Intensity and Type of Stimulation

Light tactile stimuli elicit optimal responses, whereas excessive stimulation and painful stimulation activate nociceptors that inhibit hypothalamic activity. Overly strong vacuum pressure or faulty liner design may induce stress-related inhibition.

9.27.2.4 Neural Mechanism

Activation of low-threshold Aβ mechanoreceptors in the teat sends impulses via the genitofemoral and pudendal nerves to the spinal cord and hypothalamus and initiates synchronized firing of oxytocin neurons within 30–60 s.

Knowledge Corner...

The classical "let-down" massage practiced by Indian dairy farmersgentle circular rubbing of the udder base has been shown to elevate plasma oxytocin levels by 25–40% within one minute of stimulation, validating indigenous techniques through modern physiology.

9.27.3 Ambient Environmental Conditions

9.27.3.1 Temperature and Thermal Stress

Thermal extremes influence both the animal's comfort and hormonal balance. High ambient temperature induces heat stress, leading to hyperventilation, dehydration, and elevated Cortisol. All of these conditions suppress oxytocin release. In cows, plasma oxytocin during hot, humid conditions can fall by 30–40% relative to thermoneutral periods. Cold stress, conversely, enhances sympathetic tone and peripheral vasoconstriction, delaying oxytocin delivery to the mammary gland. Maintaining optimal barn temperature is therefore vital for reflex efficiency.

9.27.3.2 Lighting and Photoperiod

Adequate light exposure (14–16 h per day) supports the normal circadian rhythm of oxytocin and prolactin secretion. Disrupted lighting schedules or dark, gloomy parlors can lengthen reflex latency. Melatonin secretion in darkness may indirectly dampen oxytocin release.

9.27.3.3 Noise and Handling Environment

Sudden loud sounds trigger startle responses that activate the sympathetic nervous system, instantly suppressing milk flow. Well-designed parlors with low noise (<70 dB) and calm handling areas minimize stress-related inhibition.

9.27.3.4 Olfactory and Visual Stimuli

Familiar odors and sights (e.g., presence of calf, routine environment) enhance anticipatory oxytocin release. Novel or aversive odors activate limbic circuits linked to stress inhibition.

9.28 Stress and Emotional State

9.28.1 Mechanisms of Stress Inhibition

Stress activates the hypothalamo–pituitary–adrenal (HPA) axis and the sympathoadrenal system, releasing cortisol and catecholamines that inhibit both oxytocin neuron firing and mammary vasodilation. This results in a functional block of milk ejection despite adequate secretion.

9.28.1.1 Sources of Stressors

The common sources of stress or stressors are

(i) Rough handling or painful milking techniques.
(ii) Separation from calf or social isolation.
(iii) Loud noise or unfamiliar environment.
(iv) Physical discomfort from mastitis or udder edema.

Each of these stimulates the amygdaloid–hypothalamic pathways that suppress oxytocin release.

9.28.1.2 Physiological Consequences

Under stress, plasma oxytocin concentration may drop below the threshold required for myoepithelial contraction. Milk remains trapped in alveoli, prolonging milking time and predisposing to mastitis. Residual milk also provides substrate for bacterial growth.

9.28.1.3 Mitigation Strategies

Calm, predictable handling, gentle voice contact, and brief tactile pre-stimulation, all these processes counteract stress responses. Some studies report that soft instrumental music during milking lowers cortisol and improves milk yield, which reflects reduced autonomic inhibition of oxytocin neurons.

9.28.2 Offspring Presence and Sensory Cues

The presence of the offspring is one of the most potent natural stimuli for milk ejection. The presence of offspring integrates tactile, auditory, olfactory, and visual inputs into the maternal neuroendocrine network.

9.28.2.1 Multisensory Integration

Tactile cues: suckling stimulates mechanoreceptors that directly initiate the reflex.

Auditory cues: vocalizations of the young evoke anticipatory oxytocin release even before contact.

Olfactory cues: maternal recognition of calf odor triggers hypothalamic activation through the limbic system.

Visual cues: sight of the offspring reinforces conditioned neural pathways associated with previous nursing.

Together, these cues generate both reflexive and emotional activation of oxytocin neurons.

9.28.2.2 Conditioned Responses

Repeated presence of offspring with mother cues with nursing leads to classical conditioning of oxytocin release. Cows often exhibit spontaneous milk leakage upon hearing their calf's call, a reflection of learned neural facilitation.

9.28.2.3 Practical Applications

Allowing the calf to nuzzle or suckle briefly before milking markedly enhances milk yield and reduces inhibited let-down. Some dairy systems use this by permitting "calf-in-sight" or partial suckling during the initial phase of milking, especially in buffaloes.

9.28.2.4 Neurobiological Basis

Offspring cues activate limbic and hypothalamic circuits involving the amygdala, preoptic area, and PVN, converging on oxytocin neurons. Concurrent activation of dopaminergic and opioid pathways contributes to the emotional satisfaction associated with nursing, further reinforcing reflex efficiency.

> **Knowledge Corner...**
> In cross-fostering experiments with ewes, olfactory recognition of the lamb develops within two hours postpartum. Blocking olfactory input prevents milk let-down, proving that sensory bonding is essential for initiating the reflex in this species.

9.28.3 Milking Interval and Frequency

9.28.3.1 Influence on Oxytocin Dynamics

The frequency and regularity of milking play a central role in regulating the sensitivity and efficiency of the milk ejection reflex (MER). Oxytocin release is tightly coupled to the pattern of afferent stimulation. Therefore, long intervals between two milking can disrupt the reflex timing and responsiveness. When milk accumulates in the alveoli for extended periods, intramammary pressure increases, which results in feedback inhibition of secretion and reduces both milk synthesis and myoepithelial responsiveness. This may lengthen reflex latency and diminish the amplitude of oxytocin pulses.

9.28.3.2 Optimum Milking Frequency

Most dairy cows are milked twice daily (12 h interval), which balances production efficiency and mammary health. Increasing frequency to three times daily elevates total milk yield by 10–15%, largely due to more frequent activation of oxytocin release and improved alveolar emptying. However, excessively frequent milking (more than three times a day) can induce stress and fatigue, counteracting hormonal benefits. In buffaloes, longer intervals (14–16 h) are often tolerated due to slower milk secretion rates, but consistency remains crucial. Irregular milking intervals disrupt conditioned oxytocin release and can cause residual milk accumulation.

9.28.3.3 Reflex Conditioning

The hypothalamic oxytocin neurons adapt to consistent timing, displaying anticipatory activation before expected milking times. This conditioning is lost if the schedule varies greatly, resulting in delayed milk flow. Hence, regularity in the milking schedule is as physiologically important as frequency.

9.28.4 Physiological and Pathological Conditions

9.28.4.1 Udder Health and Mastitis

Mastitis alters both local and systemic conditions of the mammary gland, impairing the MER. Inflammatory cytokines (IL-1β, TNF-α) and endotoxins interfere with oxytocin receptor signaling and increase vascular permeability, reducing the contractile response of myoepithelial cells. Pain from infection also activates stress pathways that suppress hypothalamic oxytocin release. Chronic subclinical mastitis often manifests as a prolonged lag phase, reduced peak milk flow, and high residual milk volume, even when secretion remains adequate.

9.28.4.2 Udder Edema

Periparturient udder edema causes mechanical compression of ducts and capillaries, impeding milk flow despite normal oxytocin levels. The condition may delay reflex onset by restricting venous return and hormone delivery to the gland.

9.28.4.3 Systemic Illness and Metabolic Disorders

Diseases causing fever, hypocalcemia, and ketosis compromise smooth muscle and neuronal function. Hypocalcemia, for example, directly reduces the contractile capacity of myoepithelial cells, while systemic acidosis depresses neuronal excitability, both leading to weak milk ejection.

9.28.4.4 Reproductive and Endocrine Status

Pregnancy, pseudopregnancy, and hormonal treatments that elevate progesterone inhibit oxytocin receptor expression. Conversely, postpartum estrogen dominance enhances responsiveness. Endocrine imbalance must therefore be considered when diagnosing reflex failure.

Knowledge Corner...
In cows with experimentally induced mastitis, local infusion of oxytocin fails to restore normal milk flow, demonstrating that inflammation reduces receptor sensitivity, not merely systemic hormone availability.

9.28.5 Nutrition and Metabolic Health

9.28.5.1 Energy and Protein Balance

Adequate nutrition supports both milk synthesis and the neuroendocrine machinery underlying ejection. Negative energy balance (NEB) during early lactation elevates circulating non-esterified fatty acids (NEFA) and ketone bodies, which interfere with hypothalamic neurotransmission and oxytocin release. Protein deficiency affects the synthesis of oxytocin and its carrier protein neurophysin I, as both require peptide precursors. Chronic undernutrition results in blunted reflex responses and prolonged latency.

9.28.5.2 Mineral and Vitamin Status

Calcium: essential for contraction of myoepithelial cells; hypocalcemia directly weakens myoepithelial activity.

Magnesium: required for ATP-dependent calcium transport.

Vitamin E and selenium: protect mammary tissue from oxidative stress, indirectly supporting reflex efficiency.

9.28.5.3 Feeding and Behavioral Conditioning

Feeding during milking enhances calmness and anticipatory oxytocin release through positive behavioral conditioning. Many dairies supply concentrate feed in the parlor to maintain relaxation and consistent reflex activation.

9.28.5.4 Metabolic Diseases

Ketosis, fatty liver, and subclinical hypocalcemia reduce MER efficiency by altering both neuronal activity and mammary contractility. Restoring metabolic balance rapidly normalizes reflex function.

9.28.6 Genetic and Individual Variations

9.28.6.1 Heritable Differences

Genetic selection for milk yield inadvertently affects neuroendocrine traits. High-yielding breeds like Holstein-Friesians often exhibit shorter reflex latency and greater oxytocin release capacity compared to dual-purpose breeds. Polymorphisms in the OXTR gene promoter and neurophysin I gene have been associated with variable oxytocin responsiveness.

9.28.6.2 Breed-Specific Patterns

Buffaloes: inherently slower reflex but higher oxytocin amplitude; require calf presence for maximal ejection.
Zebu cattle: more stress-sensitive; let-down is easily inhibited by environmental change.
Goats and sheep: shorter latency; efficient, rapid milk removal.

These differences likely reflect evolutionary adaptations in mammary storage and behavioral ecology.

9.28.6.3 Individual Temperament

Within the same breed, temperament profoundly influences milk ejection. Calm animals have higher baseline oxytocin and more consistent milk flow. Genetic correlations between docility and milkability have been identified in several dairy breeds.

9.28.6.4 Selective Breeding Potential

Emerging genomic tools enable selection for traits linked to MER efficiency, such as shorter let-down time, smooth milk-flow curves, and low stress reactivity. Understanding genetic determinants of oxytocin pathways could revolutionize breeding for "neuroendocrine robustness" in dairy animals.

Knowledge Corner...
A single nucleotide polymorphism (SNP) in the promoter region of the bovine OXTR gene has been correlated with faster milk let-down and reduced residual milk in Holstein cows, providing molecular evidence for heritable variation in oxytocin sensitivity.

9.29 Disorders of Milk Ejection

9.29.1 Inhibited Milk Ejection

The most frequent and economically significant disorder of lactation in domestic animals is inhibited milk ejection, a transient failure of milk let-down despite normal milk synthesis. This condition results from suppression of oxytocin release or impaired delivery of the hormone to the mammary gland.

9.29.1.1 Pathophysiology

The reflex may be interrupted at three levels:

1. Central inhibition—suppression of hypothalamic oxytocin neuron activity.
2. Peripheral inhibition—reduced mammary blood flow preventing hormone delivery.
3. Local mechanical obstruction—ductal constriction or edema impairing milk flow.

Inhibited ejection is therefore not a deficiency of milk but a failure of the neuroendocrine reflex.

9.29.2 Stress-Induced Inhibition

Emotional stress activates the sympathoadrenal system, releasing catecholamines (epinephrine, norepinephrine) that constrict mammary arterioles and inhibit oxytocin release from the posterior pituitary. Elevated β-endorphins and CRH further suppress hypothalamic neurons. In dairy cows, loud noises, shouting, and rough handling can reduce plasma oxytocin by 50–70%, delaying milk flow by several minutes. In buffaloes, stress sensitivity is even higher, and total inhibition may persist for an entire milking.

9.29.2.1 Clinical Signs

(i) Prolonged lag phase in milk flow curve.
(ii) Firm, distended udder with minimal flow.
(iii) Decreased milk yield despite full alveoli.
(iv) Increased residual milk and mastitis predisposition.

9.29.2.2 Diagnosis

Flow-curve monitoring, behavioral observation, and cortisol assays confirm stress-induced inhibition.

9.29.2.3 Management

(i) Calm handling, quiet environment, and consistent routine.
(ii) Allowing calf presence or visual contact before milking.
(iii) Soft background music and reduced waiting times.
(iv) Administration of mild oxytocin (2–5 IU i.m.) as a temporary corrective.

9.29.3 Pain-Induced Inhibition

Pain from mastitis, udder injury, and rough milking also triggers sympathetic dominance, preventing reflex activation. Activation of nociceptors increases spinal and hypothalamic GABAergic inhibition, suppressing oxytocin neuron firing. Even mild discomfort from cracked teats or cold stimulation can cause partial inhibition. Analgesia, proper liner pressure, and avoiding over-milking are key preventive measures.

9.29.3.1 Environmental or Behavioral Factors

Inhibition can also arise from environmental novelty (new milking parlor, new operator, sudden lighting changes) and separation anxiety in maternal species like buffaloes and goats. Animals conditioned to specific cues (e.g., particular sounds or persons) may temporarily lose reflex synchronization when those cues change. Consistency and retraining restore conditioned oxytocin release within days.

Knowledge Corner...

Epinephrine injection (0.01 mg/kg) can suppress milk ejection in lactating cows for up to 20 min, even if exogenous oxytocin is subsequently administered, demonstrating that vascular blockade can prevent the hormone's access to mammary tissue despite normal plasma levels.

9.30 Defective Oxytocin Secretion

Defective secretion may occur when oxytocin neurons or neurosecretory pathways fail to respond appropriately to afferent stimulation.

9.30.1 Central Causes

Hypothalamic lesions or inflammation: Damage to the PVN or SON reduces oxytocin synthesis.

Pituitary dysfunction: Injury or ischemia in the posterior pituitary impairs hormone release.

Endocrine suppression: High progesterone or glucocorticoid levels inhibit oxytocin gene expression.

9.30.2 Peripheral or Functional Causes

Chronic stress or malnutrition blunts oxytocin responsiveness and synthesis. Long-term exogenous oxytocin use causes negative feedback and depletion of hypothalamic stores. Postpartum fatigue or systemic illness (e.g., hypocalcemia, ketosis) may transiently suppress hypothalamic excitability.

9.30.3 Diagnostic Clues

Defective secretion is distinguished from stress inhibition by the lack of oxytocin rise even under calm conditions. Laboratory assay of plasma oxytocin is done after tactile stimulation (30–60 s post-stimulation). If plasma oxytocin fails to exceed 5–10 pg/mL, secretion is considered impaired.

9.30.4 Treatment

(i) Eliminate underlying disease or stress.
(ii) Support neuroendocrine function with adequate nutrition (Ca, Mg, energy).
(iii) Short-term low-dose oxytocin injections to recondition reflex pathways.
(iv) Avoid chronic use to prevent dependence.

Knowledge Corner...
Repeated oxytocin injections (5 IU daily for 30 days) in buffaloes led to depletion of neurohypophyseal granules and decreased neuronal immunoreactivity—clear evidence that overuse causes secretory exhaustion of oxytocin neurons.

9.31 Mammary Gland-Level Disorders

Local mammary pathology can impair milk ejection even when systemic oxytocin secretion is normal. The most common causes are mastitis, edema, and teat lesions.

9.31.1 Mastitis

Mastitis is the inflammation of the mammary gland. It induces structural and biochemical changes that hinder milk flow. The inflammatory mediators (IL-1β, TNF-α, prostaglandins) interfere with oxytocin receptor signaling. Vasoconstriction and edema reduce perfusion, delaying hormone delivery. Pain and discomfort activate central inhibitory pathways.

9.31.1.1 Clinical Effects

(i) Reduced or irregular milk flow.
(ii) Increased somatic cell count.
(iii) Thickened or clotted milk.
(iv) Elevated residual milk fraction.

9.31.1.2 Management

(i) Immediate anti-inflammatory and antimicrobial therapy.
(ii) Gentle milking to minimize pain.
(iii) Use of warm compresses to promote vasodilation.
(iv) Ensure a hygienic environment to prevent recurrence.

9.31.2 Udder Edema

Edema around parturition is common, particularly in heifers. It mechanically compresses ducts and blood vessels, restricting milk flow despite normal oxytocin levels.

Steps can be taken for prevention.

(i) Controlled salt intake before calving.
(ii) Diuretics (furosemide) if severe.
(iii) Regular milking to relieve pressure.
(iv) Adequate exercise to enhance lymphatic drainage.

9.31.3 Teat Lesions and Injuries

Cracked teats, warts, and trauma from faulty liners cause pain-induced inhibition and direct blockage of ducts. Chronic lesions can lead to scar formation that narrows the teat canals. The following steps can be taken for the prevention of the above conditions:

(i) Regular inspection and maintenance of liners.
(ii) Teat dipping and emollient use.
(iii) Avoiding over-milking and improper pulsation ratios.

Knowledge Corner...
Histological examination of mastitic udders reveals downregulation of oxytocin receptors in myoepithelial cells, confirming that local inflammation can desensitize the gland itself, independent of central oxytocin levels.

The physiology of milk ejection transcends its mechanical role; it represents a window into the adaptive intelligence of the maternal organism, where neural coordination, hormonal signaling, emotion, and behavior converge.

From the first tactile impulse at the teat to synchronized hypothalamic firing and the rhythmic contraction of myoepithelial cells, the process encapsulates the harmony of body and brain that defines mammalian life. As new technologies, molecular tools, and welfare paradigms evolve, understanding the milk ejection reflex will remain central not only to dairy science and veterinary physiology but also to the study of neuroendocrine integration and maternal biology itself.

Exercises

Objective Questions

1. The milk ejection reflex is a ____________ reflex involving both neural and hormonal components.
2. Oxytocin is synthesized in the ____________ and released from the posterior pituitary.
3. Myoepithelial contraction is mediated by the increase of intracellular ____________ ions.
4. The receptor for oxytocin is a ____________ receptor.
5. Emotional stress inhibits milk ejection via the release of ____________.
6. The typical reflex latency in buffaloes is about ____________ seconds.
7. Dendritic oxytocin release contributes to neuronal ____________.
8. The alveolar pressure during milk ejection rises to about ____________ mm Hg.
9. Conditioned reflexes depend on repeated activation of the ____________ system.
10. The principal effector hormone for milk synthesis is ____________, not oxytocin.

Subjective Questions

1. Discuss in detail the "neuroendocrine mechanism of the milk ejection reflex" with an annotated diagram.
2. Explain the "molecular events" linking oxytocin receptor activation to myoepithelial contraction.
3. Describe the evolutionary and comparative aspects of milk ejection among mammals.
4. Elaborate on the factors affecting milk ejection under farm conditions and their management.
5. Write an essay on the role of oxytocin in behavior, emotion, and maternal bonding.
6. Discuss clinical disorders of milk ejection and their veterinary significance.
7. Explain the neurobiological plasticity of oxytocin neurons during successive lactations.
8. Describe how AI and machine-learning technologies assist in predicting milk ejection efficiency.
9. Outline the immune–endocrine interactions in the mammary gland during lactation.
10. Provide a critical summary of future research directions in milk ejection physiology.

Answer to Objective Questions

1. Neuroendocrine
2. Hypothalamus
3. Calcium
4. G-protein-coupled
5. Adrenaline
6. 60–90
7. Synchronization
8. 10–12
9. Limbic
10. Prolactin

References

Lincoln DW, Wakerley JB (1975) Electrophysiological evidence for the milk ejection reflex. J Endocrinol 64:285–297

Theodosis DT, Poulain DA (1993) Activity-dependent neuronal–glial and synaptic plasticity in hypothalamic oxytocin neurons. Neuroscience 57:745–755

Additional Resources for Further Reading

Bruckmaier RM, Blum JW (1998) Oxytocin release and milk removal in ruminants. J Dairy Sci 81: 939–949

Bruckmaier RM, Wellnitz O (2011) Pathophysiology of milk ejection failure in dairy cows. J Dairy Sci 94:530–540

Carter CS (2014) Oxytocin pathways and the evolution of human behavior. Annu Rev Psychol 65: 17–39

Crowley WR, Armstrong WE (1992) Neurochemical regulation of oxytocin secretion in lactation: a review. Endocr Rev 13:33–65

Fuchs AR, Romero R, Keefe D, Parra M, Oyarzun E, Behnke E (1991) Oxytocin and the timing of birth: lessons from laboratory animals. Adv Exp Med Biol 248:319–330

Gimpl G, Fahrenholz F (2001) The oxytocin receptor system: structure, function, and regulation. Physiol Rev 81:629–683

Helminen HJ, Ericsson JLE (1968) Studies on mammary gland involution. II. Ultrastructural evidence for auto- and heterophagocytosis. J Ultrastruct Res 25:214–233

Janssens CJ, Helmond FA, Wiegant VM (1995) The effect of chronic stress on plasma cortisol and oxytocin in pigs. Physiol Behav 57:999–1002

Kendrick KM (2018) Oxytocin, motherhood and bonding in domestic animals. J Neuroendocrinol 30:e12596

Leng G, Sokolov EN (2004) Neuronal population dynamics during milk ejection. Prog Biophys Mol Biol 84:117–145

Neumann ID, Russell JA, Landgraf R (2000) Oxytocin and vasopressin release in the hypothalamus and blood during parturition and suckling: regulation and function. Prog Brain Res 133:101–121

Oftedal OT (2012) The evolution of milk secretion and its ancient origins. Animal 6:355–368

Poulain DA, Wakerley JB, Dyball REJ (1977) Electrophysiological correlates of milk ejection in the rat. J Endocrinol 73:455–463

Singh K, Dobson H, Singh M (2013) Oxytocin receptor regulation and desensitization in buffaloes under exogenous hormone administration. Vet J 197:662–668

Wellnitz O, Kerr DE, Bruckmaier RM (2009) The role of the blood–milk barrier in the immune defense of the mammary gland. J Dairy Sci 92:1–9

Wotjak CT, Kubota M, Liebsch G, Montkowski A, Holsboer F, Neumann ID (1996) Release of oxytocin and vasopressin in the paraventricular nucleus during stress. J Neuroendocrinol 8:327–333

Physicochemical Properties and Composition of Milk

10

Contents

Abstract

Milk is a natural secretion of the mammary gland of healthy lactating animals, characterized by fat dispersed as an emulsion, proteins and certain minerals present in colloidal form, and lactose along with soluble minerals and proteins existing in true solution. The physicochemical properties of milk are fundamental

J. Mukherjee et al., *Veterinary Lactation Physiology*,
https://doi.org/10.1007/978-3-032-21123-1_10

in determining its nutritional quality, stability during storage, and behavior during processing. The first secretion following parturition, known as colostrum, differs markedly from normal milk in composition and is particularly enriched with immunoglobulins that provide passive immunity to the newborn during the early postnatal period when the immune system is not fully developed. Milk composition varies widely among species, reflecting the specific nutritional needs of their offspring. On average, milk contains about 87% water, 4.9% lactose, 3.5% protein, 3.9% fat, and approximately 0.7% minerals along with vitamins and other minor constituents. It comprises a complex array of nearly 200 proteins exhibiting diverse structural and physicochemical properties. In addition to its basic nutritional role, milk serves as an important source of bioactive peptides that confer multiple health benefits, including antihypertensive, antidiabetic, antioxidant, and antimicrobial activities.

Graphical Abstract

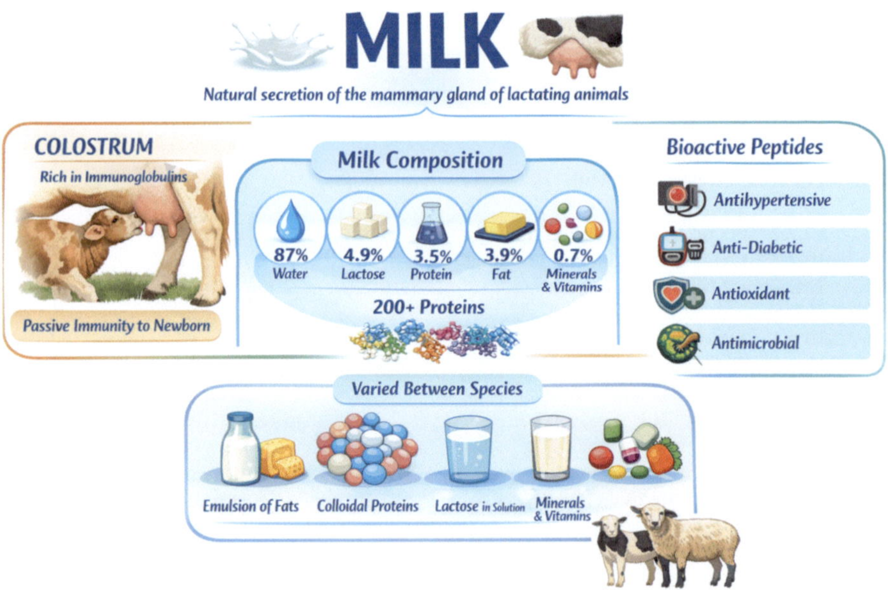

Description of the graphic: Milk is the natural secretion of the mammary glands of healthy lactating animals. The initial post-parturition secretion, colostrum, is compositionally distinct from mature milk and is especially rich in immunoglobulins. On average, milk consists of approximately 87% water, 4.9% lactose, 3.5% protein, 3.9% fat, and 0.7% minerals, vitamins, and other minor components. It contains nearly 200 structurally diverse proteins and is an important source of bioactive peptides exhibiting antihypertensive, antidiabetic, antioxidant, and antimicrobial activities

Keywords

Physicochemical properties · Milk composition · Bioactive compounds · colostrum

Inside the Chapter

- *Physical Properties of Milk*
  - Density and Specific Gravity
  - Viscosity
  - Surface Tension
  - Refractive Index
  - Freezing Point and Boiling Point
  - Electrical Conductivity
- *Chemical Properties of Milk*
  - Titratable Acidity
  - pH or Acid–Base Equilibrium
  - Oxidation–Reduction Potential (Eh)
- *Transition Milk*
- *Colostrum*
  - Interspecies Variability in Colostrum Composition
  - Colostrogenesis
  - Transition of Colostrum into Milk
- *Composition of Milk*
  - Milk Fat
  - Milk Sugar (Lactose)
  - Milk Proteins
    - Casein
    - Whey Proteins
    - Nonprotein Nitrogenous (NPN) Substances
    - Bioactive Peptides in Milk
  - Minerals
  - Vitamins
  - Enzymes

Learning Objectives

- Physicochemical properties of milk.
- Colostrum and its transition into milk.
- Milk composition in different animal species.
- Bioactive peptides present in milk.

Milk can be defined in several ways. According to the Food and Agriculture Organization (FAO) through the Codex Alimentarius, milk is the natural secretion of the mammary gland from healthy milking animals, obtained without any addition or removal of components. It must be produced under hygienic conditions and may be consumed directly or used for processing. FAO also places milk within a core food group and provides standards for safety, quality, and fair trade practices for different types of milk. The International Congress of Food described milk as the product of complete, uninterrupted milking from a healthy, well-nourished dairy female that is not overworked. It must be properly collected and must not contain colostrum (Leseur and Melik 1990). Under the Prevention of Food Adulteration Act (1954), the Government of India defines milk as the whole, fresh, clean lacteal secretion obtained by fully milking one or more healthy milch animals, excluding milk collected 15 days before or 5 days after calving, or for any period needed to ensure it is free from colostrum. It must also meet legally prescribed minimum standards for fat and solids-not-fat (SNF). In general, milk is an opaque white fluid produced by the mammary glands of mammals, where fat exists as an emulsion, proteins and some minerals are present in colloidal form, and lactose along with other minerals and soluble proteins remains in true solution. The secretion produced during the initial days following parturition is called colostrum. For cattle and buffalo, milk is typically considered normal when collected at least 72 h after calving or once it is free of colostrum. The physicochemical characteristics of milk determine its quality, functionality, and suitability for processing. Therefore, understanding these properties is crucial for improving the production, handling, and industrial utilization of cow milk. Milk contains several key components, such as water, proteins, lipids, lactose, vitamins, and minerals. Its important physical properties include viscosity, density, freezing point, and surface tension, while significant chemical properties include pH, dielectric property, oxidation–reduction potential, and titratable acidity.

Milk can also be described as a complex colloidal system in which fat globules, casein, and whey proteins are dispersed in an aqueous phase containing lactose, minerals, and vitamins. It functions as an emulsion or colloid of butterfat droplets suspended in a water-based fluid that holds dissolved carbohydrates, minerals, and aggregated proteins. The gas phase contains some dissolved gases. Milk exists as four physical phases.

Gas phase: When milk is collected without exposure to air, its gas content is about 7–8% by volume, but this increases immediately after milking once the milk comes into contact with air. These gases are present in three forms: dissolved in the liquid, trapped as tiny bubbles (often surrounding fat globules), and as headspace gas. Their levels vary depending on temperature, pressure, and handling conditions. The primary gases in raw milk are nitrogen, oxygen, and carbon dioxide. Typically, raw milk contains about 15 mg/L of nitrogen and 6 mg/L of oxygen.

Fatty phase: The fatty phase in milk is the milk fat, existing as tiny, membrane-covered globules dispersed within the water phase, making milk an oil-in-water emulsion; this fat (butterfat) is primarily triglycerides, providing energy and richness, and its composition (fatty acids) varies with diet, breed, and lactation, influencing flavor, texture, and melting point.

Colloidal phase: Milk is a colloidal emulsion, a heterogeneous mixture where tiny liquid fat globules (dispersed phase) are suspended in a watery solution (dispersion medium), stabilized by proteins like casein, which keeps them from settling out, giving milk its opaque, white appearance and light-scattering properties.

Aqueous phase: The aqueous phase in milk is its water-based continuous liquid, essentially the milk serum or whey, containing dissolved water-soluble components like lactose, whey proteins (casein micelles are also in this phase), vitamins, and minerals, acting as the solvent for the dispersed fat globules, making milk a stable "oil-in-water" emulsion crucial for its fluidity and nutritional profile.

10.1 Physical Properties of Milk

The physical properties of milk are influenced by the solutes present in its continuous phase—such as proteins, fat, lactose, and salts—and by the extent to which these components are dispersed. These constituents play an important role in assessing milk quality. Several of them, particularly properties like thermal conductivity and viscosity, are also critical factors in the design and operation of dairy processing equipment.

10.1.1 Density and Specific Gravity

The density of milk ranges from 1.027 to 1.033 g/m^3 at 20 °C. The density of different milk components at 20 °C is presented in Table 10.1. The determinants of density are composition, storage temperature, stage of lactation, and nutritional status of the cow. Specific gravity is a type of relative density, defined as the ratio between a material's actual density and the density of a chosen reference substance. In most of the cases, the reference substances are water. Specific gravity is useful because its value does not change with the units used to express density, and it varies far less with temperature compared to density itself.

The specific gravity of milk in different species is depicted in Table 10.2.

Table 10.1 Density of different milk components at 20 °C

Components	Density (kg/m^3)
Water	998.2
Fat	918
Protein	1400
Lactose	1780
Other components	1850

Walstra and Jenness (1984)

Table 10.2 Physical properties of milk in different species

Species	Specific gravity	Viscosity (cPas)	Surface tension (dyne/cm)	Refractive index
Cow	1.0258	1.7	51.77 ± 0.184	1.3459 ± 0.000
Buffalo	1.0288	2.2	50.78 ± 0.259	1.3464 ± 0.000
Sheep	1.0318	2.48	–	–
Goat	1.0256	2.12	–	–
Camel	1.0297	2.8	58.39 ± 0.421	1.3423 ± 0.001

Zahoor and Riaz (1991), Park (2007), Yoganandi et al. (2014)

10.1.2 Viscosity

Viscosity refers to a fluid's resistance to flow. In milk, viscosity represents how strongly it resists flowing and is usually expressed in centipoise (cPs). The viscosity of milk varies with its composition and temperature. Milk fat and casein notably influence viscosity, while lactose and whey proteins have only a minor effect. The viscosity of milk varies between species (Table 10.2).

10.1.3 Surface Tension

Surface tension is the force responsible for minimizing a liquid's surface or interfacial area. In milk, it is a key physical property that influences the stability of foams, emulsions, and films, and it plays an important role in processes such as concentration, fractionation, and drying. Surface-active components in milk—such as casein micelles, whey proteins, phospholipids, and fatty acids—lower its surface tension, whereas lactose has no effect. Differences in milk composition among species also lead to variations in surface tension (Table 10.2).

10.1.4 Refractive Index

It is defined as the ratio of the speed of light in air to its speed in a given medium (in this case, milk). The refractive index of milk is influenced by its dissolved components, including whey, casein micelles, proteins, lactose, and minerals. The refractive index of milk fat ranges from 1.4537 to 1.4552 at 40 °C, and these values are often used to quickly assess the purity of milk fat. Refractive index values for milk from different species are provided in Table 10.2.

Knowledge Corner...

Fat globules in buffalo milk are larger and lack carotene, making the milk appear snow white, whereas cow milk is slightly yellow due to carotenoids.

10.1.5 Freezing Point and Boiling Point

The freezing point of cow's milk generally ranges from −0.512 to −0.550 °C and is largely determined by its lactose content. Buffalo milk has an even lower freezing point (around −0.528 °C). Lactose by itself accounts for an estimated freezing point depression of about 0.296 °C. Variations in the freezing point of milk can arise due to factors such as season, feeding regimen, lactation stage, water intake, breed, heat stress, and time of day.

The boiling point of milk is slightly higher than that of water and ranges from 100.2 to 101.0 °C. The boiling point of milk depends on dissolved solids. The addition of salts, acids, sugars, and solids alters the boiling point of milk. The boiling point also depends on pressure.

10.1.6 Electrical Conductivity

The electrical conductivity of milk is determined by the levels of its dissolved anions and cations. It serves as a useful indicator for detecting mastitis, as the concentrations of Na^+ and Cl^- rise during infection, leading to higher conductivity. In healthy cows, milk conductivity typically ranges from 4.0 to 5.5 mS/cm, but it can increase to about 6–8.5 mS/cm in mastitis. The electrical conductivity of cow, buffalo, and goat milk is 4.54 ± 0.52, 4.21 ± 0.55, and 5.97 ± 0.20 mS/cm, respectively (Hariyani et al. 2024).

10.2 Chemical Properties of Milk

The chemical characteristics of milk play a crucial role in determining how milk behaves during storage and processing, as well as its overall nutritional value. These properties are largely influenced by the composition of milk, including its water, fat, protein, lactose, and mineral content. Key chemical attributes that define milk's functional and technological qualities include titratable acidity, pH or acid-base equilibrium, and oxidation–reduction potential.

10.2.1 Titratable Acidity

The titratable acidity of milk reflects its ability to resist changes in pH within the range of 6.6 to 8.3. This buffering action arises from various milk constituents, primarily proteins, phosphate ions, and dissolved carbon dioxide. Titratable acidity serves as an important indicator of the freshness of milk and is particularly valuable in monitoring milk used for fermented dairy products. It is determined by titrating milk with sodium hydroxide (NaOH) until the phenolphthalein endpoint is reached at pH 8.3, and the result is expressed as a percentage of lactic acid. As lactose undergoes bacterial fermentation, it is converted into lactic acid, causing an increase in titratable acidity. The titratable acidity (%) of milk of cow, goat, and buffalo are 0.135–0.139, 0.138–0.139, and 0.137–0.141, respectively.

10.2.2 pH or Acid–Base Equilibrium

The pH of milk serves as a key indicator of its acidity. In cow's milk, the pH typically falls between 6.5 and 6.7 at 25 °C. Colostrum is naturally more acidic, with a pH of about 6.0. Milk obtained from a mastitic or infected quarter shows a distinctly higher pH, often around 7.5. Toward the end of lactation, milk also tends to exhibit an increased pH. Goat milk has a relatively lower pH (around 6.4), which is attributed to its higher content of short- and medium-chain fatty acids, such as capric and caprylic acids. In contrast, sheep and camel milk generally show a higher pH (about 6.7) compared to goat milk.

10.2.3 Oxidation–Reduction Potential (Eh)

It measures milk's tendency to either gain or lose electrons in chemical reactions. The oxidation–reduction potential (Eh) of fresh milk is typically positive, usually falling between +200 and + 400 mV, owing to the presence of dissolved oxygen and other oxidizing substances. During fermentation, however, this value decreases sharply—often reaching negative levels (around −200 mV or lower)—as microorganisms utilize oxygen and create a more reduced environment. This transition from an oxidized to a reduced state plays an important role in cheese ripening, influencing both microbial activity and flavor development. Additionally, methods such as electroreduction can be used to temporarily lower the redox potential.

10.3 Transition Milk

The first mammary secretion produced after parturition is known as colostrum, and its composition differs markedly from that of normal milk. Colostrum is especially rich in immunoglobulins, which are essential for the transfer of passive immunity from the dam to the newborn calf, protecting it during the early life when its own immune system is immature. In addition to antibodies, colostrum contains higher concentrations of proteins, fat, vitamins, minerals, enzymes, hormones, and growth factors compared with milk, supporting early nutrition, metabolism, and gastrointestinal development of the calf.

As lactation progresses, mammary secretions gradually change in composition from colostrum to normal milk. The secretions produced during this intermediate period are referred to as transition milk. Transition milk contains decreasing levels of immunoglobulins and bioactive components and increasing amounts of lactose and milk-specific proteins, reflecting the shift from immune protection to sustained nutritional support until mature milk secretion is fully established.

10.4 Colostrum

It may be described as the initial, energy-dense mammary secretion produced by the dam immediately after parturition, which is rich in immunoglobulins, antimicrobial peptides, and growth factors. Colostrum is often regarded as the "starter kit" for mammals because it supplies essential bioactive components necessary for neonatal survival (Table 10.3). In cattle, mammary secretion produced during the first three days after calving is classified as colostrum. Compared with normal milk, it contains lower lactose but higher concentrations of fat, protein, and minerals. A distinctive characteristic of colostrum is its very high immunoglobulin content, especially IgG.

Ruminant neonates must ingest colostrum as soon as possible after birth to acquire immunoglobulins, since placental transfer of antibodies does not occur and calves are born in a state of hypogammaglobulinemia. The neonatal gut is temporarily permeable to intact immunoglobulins, enabling their absorption and the establishment of passive immunity from the dam. In addition, ruminant colostrum supplies energy and vital nutrients such as proteins, lipids, carbohydrates, minerals, and vitamins, helping the newborn adapt to postnatal challenges, including hypoglycemia, hypoxia, hypercapnia, and hypothermia.

Colostrum is an energy-dense first feed whose primary role is the transfer of passive immunity through antibodies. IgG1 is the dominant immunoglobulin, followed by IgM, IgA, and IgG2, and colostrum feeding markedly reduces calf mortality. Its cellular components, including polymorphonuclear leukocytes and macrophages, secrete protective factors such as lysozyme, complement, and

Table 10.3 Composition of bovine colostrum

Factors	Constituents	Amount	References
Nutritional factor	Energy (kcal/100 ml)	130	Guthrie (1989)
	Protein (g/100 ml)	14.9	
	Lactose (g/100 ml)	2.6	
	Fat (g/ 100 ml)	6.7	
Immune factors	Lactoferrin (mg/ml)	100	Stelwagen et al. (2009)
	IgA (mg/ml)	3.9	
	IgG (mg/ml)	47.6	
	IgG2 (mg/ml)	2.9	
	IgM (mg/ml)	4.2	
Growth factors	Epidermal growth factor (EGF) (mcg/L)	30–50	Stelwagen et al. (2009)
	Transforming growth factor (TGF α) (mcg/L)	2.2–7.2	
	TGF β (mg/L)	1–2	
	Insulin-like growth factor (IGF) (mg/L)	10	
	Vascular endothelial growth factor (VEGF)	NA	
	Growth hormone (GH) (ng/L)	<0.03	
Cellular components	Somatic cells (leucocytes and epithelial cells) (cells/mL)	1,479,000	Ontsouka et al. (2003)

interferon, helping to prevent enterocolitis in the newborn. Colostrum also contains lactoferrin, an iron-binding protein with antibacterial and antiviral activity. Beyond immunity, colostrum influences metabolic and endocrine functions, supports gastro-intestinal development, and promotes cell growth and tissue repair through its growth factors. Additionally, it has a mild laxative effect, facilitating meconium passage and bilirubin excretion.

10.4.1 Interspecies Variability in Colostrum Composition

Neonatal survival strategies vary among species, and these differences influence both the timing of onset and cessation of the colostrum period as well as its composition (Table 10.4). Such variations are closely aligned with species-specific mechanisms of immunoglobulin transfer. In ungulates, the placenta is composed of multiple tissue layers, which restrict the transplacental passage of immunoglobulins, particularly IgG. As a compensatory adaptation, ungulate colostrum contains very high levels of IgG, even though IgA is the dominant immunoglobulin in external secretions of most mammalian species.

The ability of the neonatal intestine to absorb intact immunoglobulins is limited to the first few hours after birth and progressively decreases, becoming negligible by

Table 10.4 Composition of colostrum in different species

Species	Constituents			References
	lactose (g/100 g)	Fat (g/100 g)	Protein (g/100 g)	
Cow	2.5	6.7	14.9	Bagwe et al. (2015)
Goat	4.7	4.1	3.4	Bagwe et al. (2015)
Sheep	2.4–3.8	4.0–13.7	13.8–22.5	Kessler et al. (2019)
Pig	1.7–5.0	2.5–7.5	5.2–22.3	Nuntapaitoon et al. (2020)
Donkey	5.30	2.08	2.79	Martini et al. (2020)
Dog	27.0	78.0	138.0	Meyer and Kamphues (1990)
Cat	3.6	3.4	4.0	Keen et al. (1982)
Buffalo	2.70	5.44	8.75	Park et al. (2006)
Yak	1.90	14.0	16.1	Park et al. (2006)
Camel	5.90	0.30	19.2	Playford et al. (2001)
Mare	6	1–1.5	2	Mariani et al. (2001)
Llama	4.12	0.75	16.8	Soloshenko et al. (2020)
Elephant	61.8	56.0	21.0	Park et al. (2006)
Alpaca	3.95	0.51	20.4	Mößler et al. (2021)
Rat	2.5	14.7	8.9	Keen et al. (1981)
Rabbit	16.0	147.0	135.0	Meyer and Kamphues (1990)
Human	7.0	3.8	1.2	Ahmadi et al. (2016)

about 24 h. In ungulate species, colostrum synthesis begins approximately 3–4 weeks before parturition and ceases soon after birth. In contrast, in rodents, colostrum production continues throughout the suckling period, with a predominance of IgA. Similarly, human colostrum is also characterized by a high IgA content.

10.4.2 Colostrogenesis

Colostrum synthesis and secretion begin in response to changes in the endocrine environment around parturition. Mammary gland growth and differentiation are stimulated by steroid hormones, particularly estrogen and progesterone, produced by the uterus and the conceptus. During the final week of gestation, elevated progesterone levels trigger colostrogenesis. A key feature of this process is the selective transfer of IgG1 from the bloodstream into the mammary gland through secretory epithelial cells. This IgG1 transport starts approximately 4–6 weeks before parturition and reaches its peak at calving. Following parturition, the rate of IgG1 transfer declines sharply, coinciding with the drop in progesterone levels at calving. These observations suggest that progesterone plays a regulatory role in the selective uptake of IgG1 into the mammary gland. The postpartum decline in progesterone also enables mammary epithelial cells to respond to lactogenic hormones, resulting in the onset of abundant milk secretion. Transmammary transfer of IgG is facilitated by the neonatal Fc receptor (FcRn), an MHC class I–related receptor composed of a heavy α-chain and a light $\beta 2$-microglobulin chain. A histidine residue located in the $\alpha 2$ domain of the α-chain is critical for IgG binding. FcRn exhibits binding specificity for IgG1, IgG2, and bovine serum albumin (BSA), and this interaction is strongly pH dependent, with acidic conditions favoring ligand binding. During colostrogenesis, however, FcRn mediates the preferential transport of IgG1 into colostrum, while IgG2 and BSA are largely recycled. Although IgG1 and IgG2 are present in comparable concentrations in plasma and both enter mammary epithelial cells via pinocytosis, their intracellular fates differ. Within endosomes, FcRn binds both IgG1 and IgG2 as vacuolar H^+-ATPase (V-ATPase) lowers the pH to promote receptor–ligand interaction. The FcRn–IgG1 complexes are then directed toward secretion into colostrum, whereas FcRn–IgG2 complexes are returned to the circulation through recycling pathways. Consequently, despite IgG2 having a higher intrinsic affinity for FcRn, IgG1 accumulates in much greater amounts in bovine colostrum because IgG2 is preferentially recycled. Recent evidence suggests that lactoferrin may facilitate the dissociation of IgG1 from FcRn. As a basic protein with a pKa of approximately 8.7, lactoferrin can increase local pH, thereby promoting the release of IgG1 from FcRn and enhancing its secretion into colostrum. The concentration of lactoferrin is 30- to 100-fold higher than that of milk.

10.4.3 Transition of Colostrum into Milk

A decline in progesterone, accompanied by a rise in prolactin, suppresses the transfer of maternal immunoglobulins (IgG) into colostrum and promotes the onset of abundant milk secretion, leading to dilution of immunoglobulins in the colostrum. The conversion of colostrum to normal milk is variable, typically occurring over a period of 2 to 7 days in cows. In dairy goats and sheep, the transition of colostrum into milk requires 5 days and 3 days, respectively. Colostrum composition changes rapidly, even on an hourly basis, showing a progressive reduction in both its biological activity and nutritional value as its constituents shift (Table 10.5). In parallel, the capacity of calves to absorb immunoglobulins diminishes with time after birth. Studies have demonstrated that the absorptive efficiency of calves declines by approximately one-third within 6 hours postpartum and by nearly two-thirds within 12 h.

10.5 Composition of Milk

Milk is composed of a variety of substances such as water, lactose, proteins, fat, mineral, and vitamins. The mammary gland is a complex machine that is capable of synthesizing new components from those existing in plasma. Table 10.6 depicts the compositional differences (folds) between milk and plasma. The composition of milk varies considerably between species (Table 10.7) as per the requirement to

Table 10.5 Changes in the composition of bovine colostrum over time

Hours after calving	Protein (%)	Fat (%)	Lactose (%)
0	16.8	6.7	2.9
6	11.7	6.1	3.5
12	6.3	4.4	3.9
24	5.5	4.1	4.1
48	4.8	3.9	4.2
120	3.6	3.8	4.5
Milk	3.2	3.8	4.6

Puppel et al. (2019)

Table 10.6 Compositional differences (folds) between milk and plasma

Components	Milk	Blood plasma
Fat	35	3
Lactose	49	0
Caseins	27	0
α-lactalbumin and β-lactoglobulin	4	0
Albumin and globulin	1.5	75
Citric acid	2	0
Chlorides	1.6	6
Phosphates	2.5	0.3

Alais et al. (1985)

Table 10.7 Major constituents of milk of various animals

Species	Fat (%)	Protein (%)	Lactose (%)	Ash (%)	Total solids (%)
Antelope	1.3	6.9	4	1.3	25.2
Ass (donkey)	1.2	1.7	6.9	0.45	10.2
Bear, polar	31	10.2	0.5	1.2	42.9
Bison	1.7	4.8	5.7	0.96	13.2
Buffalo, Philippine	10.4	5.9	4.3	0.8	21.5
Camel	4.9	3.7	5.1	0.7	14.4
Cat	10.9	11.1	3.4	–	25.4
Cow:					
AyrshireBrown SwissGuernseyHolsteinJerseyZebu	4.14.05.03.55.54.9	3.63.63.83.13.93.9	4.75.04.94.94.95.1	0.70.70.70.70.70.8	13.113.314.412.215.014.7
Deer	19.7	10.4	2.6	1.4	34.1
Dog	8.3	9.5	3.7	1.2	20.7
Dolphin	14.1	10.4	5.9	NA	30.4
Elephant	15.1	4.9	3.4	0.76	26.9
Goat	3.5	3.1	4.6	0.79	12
Guinea Pig	3.9	8.1	3	0.82	15.8
Horse	1.6	2.7	6.1	0.51	11
Human	4.5	1.1	6.8	0.2	12.6
Kangaroo	2.1	6.2	Trace	1.2	9.5
Mink	8	7	6.9	0.7	22.6
Monkey	3.9	2.1	5.9	2.6	14.5
Opossum	6.1	9.2	3.2	1.6	24.5
Pig	8.2	5.8	4.8	0.63	19.9
Rabbit	12.2	10.4	1.8	2	26.4
Rat	14.8	11.3	2.9	1.5	31.7
Reindeer	22.5	10.3	2.5	1.4	36.7

(continued)

Table 10.7 (continued)

Species	Fat (%)	Protein (%)	Lactose (%)	Ash (%)	Total solids (%)
Seal, gray	53.2	11.2	2.6	0.7	67.7
Sheep	5.3	5.5	4.6	0.9	16.3
Whale	34.8	13.6	1.8	1.6	51.2

Hurley (2010)
NA no available data

Table 10.8 Major constituents and nutritive values of milk in human, cow, goat, sheep, and buffalo (average values per 100 milliliters of whole milk)

Attributes, unit	Human	Cow	Goat	Sheep	Buffalo
Energy, kcal[a]	71.0	69.0	67.2	106.0	94.8
Water, %	87.8	87.3	87.7	80.7	81.4
Specific gravity	1.03	1.03	1.28	1.02	1.02
Total solids, g	12.4	12.7	17.4	18.3	14.1
Fat, g	3.8	3.7	4.0	6.9	6.7
Cholesterol, mg	1.2	9.6	10.8	26.4	18.4
Fatty acids (total saturated), g	1.5	1.8	2.6	4.5	4.5
Fatty acids (total polyunsaturated), g	1.0	0.2	0.1	0.3	0.1
Lactose, g	7.0	4.8	4.3	5.3	5.1
Protein, g	1.2	3.3	3.5	5.9	3.7
Casein, g	0.4	2.8	2.6	2.9	2.4
Ash, g	0.2	0.7	0.8	0.9	0.8
Calcium, mg	33.0	110.4	130.8	189.2	164.8
Magnesium, mg	4.0	9.6	13.6	17.6	30.4
Potassium, mg	55.0	139.6	199.2	134.4	173.6
Sodium, mg	15.0	39.2	48.8	43.2	50.8
Iron, µg	49.0	42.0	50.0	80.0	62.0
Copper, µg	40.0	30.0	40.0	8.9	21.2
Manganese, µg	0.2	12.0	18.0	10.0	13.0
Phosphorus, mg	15.0	88.8	108.4	154.8	114.0
Selenium, µg	2.0	3.6	1.4	1.7	NA
Zinc, mg	0.2	0.4	0.3	0.5	0.2
Vitamin A, µg	NA	27.2	55.6	43.2	51.6
Thiamin (Vit B_1), mg	0.03	0.01	0.01	0.01	0.01
Riboflavin (Vit B_2), mg	0.3	0.2	0.1	0.3	0.1
Niacin (Vit B_3), mg	0.7	0.1	0.3	0.4	0.1
Pantothenic acid (Vit B_5), mg	0.2	0.4	0.3	0.4	0.2
Pyridoxine (Vit B_6), mg	0.01	0.01	0.01	0.1	0.01
Cobalamin (Vit B_{12}), µg	0.4	0.4	0.1	0.7	0.4
Vitamin C, mg	3.0	0.0	1.3	4.1	2.2
Vitamin D, IU	NA	39.2	11.6	NA	NA

Iyengar (1982), Jensen (1995), Allen (2012), Ren et al. (2015), Bekuma and Galmessa (2018)
[a]Kilocalorie

nourish their young ones. The milk composition of cows, buffaloes, and goats is suitable for human consumption as their composition is close to human (Table 10.8). In general, milk contains 87% water, 4.9% lactose, 3.5% proteins, 3.9% fat, 0.7% minerals, as well as vitamins and other minor constituents.

Milk Constituents

- *Water* (87.2%)
- *Total solids* (12.8%)
  - *Fat* (4%)
    - True fat (3.95%)
    - Other substances associated with fat (0.05%)
      - Phospholipids (like lecithin, cephalin, and sphingomyelin 0.03%)
      - Sterols (0.01%)
      - Carotene (0.005%)
      - Vit A, D, E, K (0.005%)
  - *Solids-not-fat* (8.81%)
    - Carbohydrate (lactose, 4.7%)
    - Total Proteins (3.4%)
      - Casein (2.7%)
      - Whey Proteins 0.7%
        - α-Lactalbumin (0.12%)
        - β- Lactoglobulin (0.33%)
        - Other whey protein fraction (bovine serum albumin immunoglobulins, proteose-peptone) 0.25%
    - Minerals (0.78%), e.g., phosphate, chloride, citrate, calcium, magnesium, etc.
    - Other minor constituents
      - Nonprotein nitrogen substances
        - Ammonia
        - Amino acids
        - Urea
        - Creatine and
        - Creatinine
        - Orotic acid
      - Pigment (riboflavin, carotene, xanthophyll)
      - Soluble gases (CO_2, O_2, N_2)
      - Vitamin C and B complex
      - Enzymes (lipase, phosphatase, lactoperoxidase, catalase, amylase)

10.5.1 Milk Fat

Milk lipids are present in three phases in milk, namely, the fat globule, the membrane surrounding the globule, and the milk serum. Each fat globule in milk is spherical in shape and is surrounded by a specialized surface layer known as the milk fat globule membrane (MFGM). This membrane encloses and protects the nonpolar lipid core of the fat globule and plays a crucial role in stabilizing the globule within the aqueous phase of milk. Because milk fat has a lower density than the surrounding aqueous medium, fat globules tend to rise and can be readily separated from milk by

Table 10.9 Various lipid materials present in milk and their location

Constituents	Location in milk
Triglycerides	Fat globules
Phospholipids (lecithin, cephalin, and sphingomyelin	Fat globule membrane and serum
Sterols (cholesterol)	Fat globule, FGM, and serum
Free fatty acids	Fat globules and serum
Waxes	Fat globule
Squalene	Fat globule
Fat-soluble vitamins	Fat globule

centrifugation. The fat globules are distributed in a continuous aqueous phase as an oil-in-water type emulsion. The average size of milk fat globules is 3 microns. Fat globules are entirely made up of triglycerides coated with FGM containing complex lipids, phospholipids, and proteins (Table 10.9).

The color of milk fat ranges from yellow, mainly because of the presence of carotene, to whitish with a faint bluish tinge, which is attributed to bilirubin. Milk fat melts between 28 and 33 °C and solidifies (sets) in the range of 24 to 29 °C. Its specific gravity lies between 0.936 and 0.946 at 15 °C, while the refractive index ranges from 1.459 to 1.462 at the same temperature.

The milk fat comprises triacylglycerols (95%), diacylglycerol (2%), cholesterol (< 0.5%), phospholipids (1%), and free fatty acids (FFA) (<0.5%).

Triglycerides (TAGs) make up the largest proportion of milk fat, serving as a major source of energy and contributing substantially to flavor characteristics. Each triglyceride molecule consists of a glycerol molecule linked to three fatty acid chains. These fatty acids can be short-, medium-, or long-chain, and their distribution differs among milk from cows, buffaloes, and other species. Such differences in fatty acid composition have a pronounced effect on the functional and physical qualities of dairy products, influencing properties like the whipping performance of cream and the consistency and spreadability of butter.

The fatty acid profile of milk differs among species (Table 10.10). Ruminant milk is typically characterized by a high proportion of saturated fatty acids (SFAs), which constitute around 70% of total fatty acids, and a relatively low level of polyunsaturated fatty acids (PUFAs). The principal SFAs include butyric, caprylic, capric, lauric, and stearic acids. Among these, butyric, caprylic, and capric acids have been reported to possess anticancer properties. Lauric acid exhibits antiviral and antibacterial activity, including the ability to eliminate *Helicobacter pylori*. In addition, both capric and lauric acids can inhibit cyclooxygenase (COX) and therefore have potential anti-inflammatory effects. In goat milk, medium-chain fatty acids predominate, while short-chain fatty acids account for only about 20%. Sheep milk contains higher levels of butyric acid (C4:0) and ω-3 fatty acids compared with other ruminant milks. The major monounsaturated fatty acid in milk is oleic acid, present at approximately 8 g per liter of whole milk. Oleic acid is known for its beneficial effects on lipid metabolism, particularly its ability to reduce blood cholesterol and triglyceride levels.

Table 10.10 Milk fat and fatty acid profiles in ruminant and nonruminant species

Fatty acids profile (% of total fatty acids)	Cow	Buffalo	Sheep	Goat	Horse	Donkey
Saturated fatty acids	55.0–73.0	62.0–74.0	57.0–75.0	59.0–74.0	37.0–55.0	46.0–68.0
Monounsaturated fatty acid	2.0–30.0	24.0–29.0	23.0–39.0	19.0–36.0	18.0–36.0	15.0–35.0
Polyunsaturated fatty acids	2.4–6.3	2.3–3.9	2.6–7.3	2.6–5.6	13.0–51.0	14.0–30.0
Conjugated linoleic acid	0.2–2.4	0.4–1.0	0.6–1.1	0.3–1.2	0.02–0.1	Trace
Omega-3 fatty acid	0.3–1.8	0.2–1.4	0.5–2.3	0.3–1.48	2.2–31.2	4.0–16.3
Omega-6 fatty acid	1.2–3.0	1.74–2.0	1.6–3.6	1.9–4.3	3.6–20.3	6.0–15.2
Cholesterol (mg/100 mL)	13.1–31.4	4.0–18.0	14.0–29.0	10.7–18.1	–	31.3–37.1

Mollica et al. (2021), Stobiecka et al. (2021)

The principal polyunsaturated fatty acids (PUFAs) present in milk are linoleic acid and α-linolenic acid. These fatty acids serve as precursors for eicosanoid synthesis, being converted through intermediates such as arachidonic acid and eicosapentaenoic acid. Phospholipids and glycosphingolipids together account for about 1% of total milk lipids. Despite their small proportion, they play important functional roles, including stabilization of the milk fat emulsion, participation in cell–cell interactions, and involvement in immune recognition. In addition, these lipids can function as receptors for specific hormones and growth factors, contributing to cellular signaling processes.

10.5.2 Milk Sugar (Lactose)

Lactose is the major carbohydrate found in the milk of most mammalian species. In contrast, the milk of rats and mice also contains sialyllactose, an oligosaccharide. Chemically, lactose is a disaccharide consisting of α-D-glucose and β-D-galactose linked through a β-1,4-glycosidic bond. In milk, lactose occurs in both α- and β-anomeric forms, maintaining an equilibrium ratio of β to α of about 1.68 at 20 °C. In liquid milk, lactose remains in true solution, whereas in dairy products it may crystallize in different forms, such as α-lactose hydrate (α-lactose monohydrate), anhydrous β-lactose, or amorphous mixtures of both α- and β-lactose. These crystalline forms impart a gritty texture and are responsible for the sandy texture observed in products like concentrated milk and ice cream. When heated above 150 °C, lactose undergoes yellowing, and at around 175 °C it browns to form caramel, producing the characteristic cooked milk flavor. Microbial fermentation of lactose results in its conversion to lactic acid, leading to souring of milk. Lactose also plays a key role in the colligative properties of milk, contributing to osmotic pressure, lowering the freezing point, and raising the boiling point. In addition to lactose, milk contains small amounts of other sugars, including glucose, fructose, glucosamine, galactosamine, N-acetylneuraminic acid, and various oligosaccharides.

10.5.2.1 Lactose Intolerance

Lactose is digested in the gastrointestinal tract by the enzyme β-galactosidase (lactase), which hydrolyzes it into glucose and galactose. Lactase is located on the microvilli of the intestinal epithelium. In newborn animals, lactase activity is relatively high, but it gradually declines with advancing age. This reduction in enzyme activity can impair the digestion of milk and lactose-containing foods, a condition known as lactose intolerance. Lactose intolerance is typically associated with symptoms such as diarrhea, abdominal pain, bloating, and flatulence following lactose consumption. These symptoms arise due to the accumulation of undigested lactose in the intestine, which draws water from the bloodstream and interferes with normal digestive and fermentative processes. It is estimated that nearly 70% of the global population is susceptible to lactose intolerance, and its prevalence has increased in recent decades, contributing to the growing demand for lactose-free dairy products. Lactose intolerance can be classified into primary and secondary forms. Primary lactose intolerance results from a natural decline in lactase activity after weaning. Secondary, or acquired, lactose intolerance occurs when lactase activity is reduced due to damage to the intestinal mucosa, which may result from intestinal surgery or diseases such as gastroenteritis, inflammatory bowel disease, cow's milk intolerance, or AIDS. In contrast, congenital lactase deficiency is a rare inherited disorder in which lactase activity is absent or markedly reduced from birth and persists throughout life.

Knowledge Corner...

Camel milk has lower lactose and higher mineral content, contributing to better tolerance in lactose-sensitive individuals. It contains no β-lactoglobulin, a major cow milk allergen, and has higher levels of α-lactalbumin.

10.5.2.2 Galactosemia

Galactose is utilized in the body mainly through the Leloir pathway, a metabolic route that ultimately converts galactose into glucose-1-phosphate, allowing it to enter mainstream carbohydrate metabolism. This conversion requires the coordinated action of three key enzymes: galactokinase (GALK), which phosphorylates galactose to galactose-1-phosphate; galactose-1-phosphate uridyltransferase (GALT), which facilitates the exchange of UDP from UDP-glucose to form glucose-1-phosphate; and UDP-galactose-4-epimerase (GALE), which interconverts UDP-galactose and UDP-glucose to sustain the pathway. A deficiency or functional impairment of any one of these enzymes disrupts normal galactose metabolism, leading to the accumulation of galactose and galactose-1-phosphate in tissues and body fluids. These metabolites are toxic, particularly to the liver, kidneys, brain, and eyes. The resulting inherited metabolic disorder is known as galactosemia. Clinically, galactosemia presents with a range of serious manifestations, especially in infants. Common features include hepato-splenomegaly and jaundice due to liver dysfunction, hypoglycemia resulting from impaired glucose metabolism, and renal tubular damage leading to abnormalities in kidney function. Accumulation of galactitol in the lens of the eye causes cataract formation, which is a characteristic finding. If untreated, galactosemia can progress to growth failure, neurological impairment, and even life-threatening complications, highlighting the importance of early diagnosis and dietary restriction of galactose.

10.5.3 Milk Proteins

Milk contains a complex mixture of nearly 200 different proteins with diverse structural and physicochemical characteristics (Table 10.11), accounting for about 95% of the total nitrogen present in milk. Milk proteins are of exceptionally high quality and exhibit a broad range of nutritional, functional, and physiological roles. In bovine milk, the total protein concentration is approximately 3.5% by weight (around 36 g/L), contributing nearly 38% of the solids-not-fat fraction and supplying about 21% of the energy content of whole milk. However, their concentrations vary between humans and different animal species (Table 10.12). Based on their solubility characteristics, milk proteins are broadly classified into two major groups: caseins and whey proteins. Under acidic conditions, caseins lose solubility and precipitate, whereas whey proteins remain soluble at low pH.

10.5.3.1 Casein

Casein is the principal phosphoprotein of milk, present as a calcium caseinate–phosphate complex, and can be isolated from raw milk by acidification to

Table 10.11 Properties of different milk proteins

Property	Average concentration (%)	Molar mass	(Residues/molecule) Amino acid	Phosphoserine	Cysteine	Isoelectric pH
αs1-casein	1.1	23,614	199	7–9	0	4.5
αs2-casein	0.3	25,230	207	10–13	2	5.0
β-Casein	0.9	23,983	209	5	0	4.8
κ-Casein	0.3	19,023	169	1	2	5.6
β-Lactoglobulin	0.32	18,283	162	0	5	5.2
α-Lactalbumin	0.12	4176	123	0	8	4.3
Serum albumin	0.04	66,267	582	0	35	4.8

Mehta (2015)

Table 10.12 Concentrations of different milk proteins in humans and animals

Protein (g/L)	Cow	Goat	Sheep	Buffalo	Camel	Donkey	Human
Total casein	24–28	23–46	42–59	32–49	26	6.4–10.3	2.4–4.2
α_{S1}-casein	9.5–12	3.0–7.0	11–22	9	4–5	1.5	0.77
α_{S2}-casein	1.6–4	3.0–4.0	0–13	5	2–3	0.1	–
β-casein	9–15	11–15	15–36	12–21	12–13	4	3–5
κ-casein	2.0–3.5	2–7	5–12	4–6	0.7	–	1–3
Total whey protein	6–8	3.7–7.0	6–9	5–6	5.9–8.1	4.9–8.0	6.2–8.3
α-Lactalbumin	1.0–1.8	1.7–3.3	1.35	1.4	1.3	1–2	2–3
β-Lactoglobulin	2.8–3.5	3.0	4.6–7.0	3.9	–	3.3–4.0	–
Serum albumin	0.43–0.57	–	0.4–0.6	0.29	0.4	–	0.3
Lactoferrin	0.1–0.2	0.1	0.28	0.03–3.4	0.2	0.08	1–3

Stobiecka et al. (2021)

pH 4.6 at 20 °C. It constitutes nearly 80% of the total milk protein. In milk, casein occurs as micellar particles suspended in a colloidal state. Each micelle is organized into smaller submicellar units that are linked together by colloidal calcium phosphate through ester bonds involving the hydroxyl groups of serine residues. The diameter of casein micelles typically ranges from about 30 to 300 millimicrons.

Chemically, casein contains approximately 52.6–54.0% carbon, 6.75–7.10% hydrogen, 15.51–15.91% nitrogen, 0.71–0.83% sulfur, and 0.71–0.85% phosphorus. Its isoelectric point is around pH 4.6; above this pH, casein carries a net negative charge, while below it becomes positively charged. Consequently, at the natural pH of milk (6.6–6.8), casein is negatively charged and migrates toward the anode when subjected to an electric field.

Casein is composed of four major fractions: αs1-, αs2-, β-, and κ-casein. The αs- and β-caseins are phosphoproteins, whereas κ-casein is glycosylated. β-casein constitutes about 39% of the total casein fraction, followed by αS1-casein at approximately 38%, αS2-casein at around 10%, and κ-casein accounting for about 13% of the total casein content. The properties of different casein fractions are shown in Table 10.11. Both α- and β-caseins are insoluble at their respective isoelectric points (approximately pH 4.7 and 4.9) but become readily soluble at pH values above or below these points. At pH 4.2 and 20 °C, α-casein exhibits lower solubility, whereas β-casein remains more soluble, a property that allows their separation under these conditions.

αS2-casein is present in milk partly in a dimeric form, composed of two polypeptide chains linked by two disulfide bridges. Four genetic variants of αS2-casein—A, B, C, and D—have been identified, of which variant A is the most common. This casein fraction is the most hydrophilic among caseins due to its high level of phosphorylation, with 11 serine residues bearing phosphate groups.

The gene encoding β-casein in cattle is highly polymorphic, and multiple mutations in the bovine β-casein gene have resulted in at least 12 genetic variants, of which A1 and A2 are the most prevalent. These two variants differ at the 67th amino acid position: A1 β-casein contains histidine, whereas A2 β-casein has proline at this position due to a single nucleotide substitution. This amino acid change alters the secondary structure of the β-casein protein. During proteolytic digestion, A1 β-casein can release a bioactive peptide known as β-casomorphin-7 (BCM7). In infants, BCM7 may be more readily absorbed because of an immature digestive system, while in adults it tends to accumulate at the intestinal brush border. BCM7 has been reported to exert biological effects through interaction with opioid receptors in the neuroendocrine and immune systems and has been linked to oxidative modification of low-density lipoproteins (LDL) and arterial plaque formation. Several studies have suggested associations between consumption of A1 β-casein and conditions such as type 1 diabetes, coronary heart disease, arteriosclerosis, autism, and schizophrenia.

The A1 and A2 variants of β-casein are controlled by a pair of alleles located on chromosome 6, with A1 and A2 being the two major forms. Cows that are homozygous A1A1 or A2A2 produce milk containing exclusively A1 or A2 β-casein, respectively, whereas heterozygous A1A2 cows secrete both variants in approximately equal proportions. The A1 β-casein variant is predominantly present in milk from crossbred and European cattle breeds, while A2 β-casein is characteristic of milk from indigenous Indian zebu cattle and buffaloes. Based on these β-casein variants, milk is categorized as A1 or A2 milk: A1 milk contains A1 β-casein either alone or along with A2 (from A1A2 cows), whereas A2 milk contains only the A2 form of β-casein.

κ-Casein is present in cow's milk at a concentration of about 4.4 ± 0.3 g/L and accounts for roughly 13% of the total casein fraction in bovine milk. Among all caseins, it is the least phosphorylated and is unique in being the only casein that is glycosylated across all mammalian species. Structurally, κ-casein displays a distinctive amphipathic (amphipolar) nature: its N-terminal region is predominantly hydrophobic, enabling interaction with other caseins within the micelle, whereas the C-terminal region is hydrophilic and contains carbohydrate moieties. This hydrophilic C-terminal portion extends into the surrounding aqueous phase, contributing to the steric stabilization of casein micelles and preventing their aggregation. κ-Casein has a relatively low affinity for calcium because it possesses only a single phosphorylation site, located at residue 149. This limited calcium-binding capacity plays a crucial role in maintaining micellar stability and solubility in milk. Beyond its structural importance, κ-casein exhibits several biological activities. It has been reported to possess anticoagulant effects, inhibit platelet aggregation, and modulate serotonin release, highlighting its physiological relevance in addition to its functional role in milk stability and dairy processing.

10.5.3.2 Whey Proteins

Whey proteins are the native proteins present in whey or serum and are a constituent of whey, which is prepared after removal of casein through acidification at pH 4.6 or by rennet action during the preparation of cheese. They constitute around 20% of the total milk protein. There are four major classes of whey proteins, such as β-lactoglobulin (50%), α-lactalbumin (25%), immunoglobulins (9%), and bovine serum albumin (6%).

10.5.3.3 α-Lactalbumin

This protein is a metalloprotein composed of 123 amino acid residues and is stabilized by four disulfide bridges formed between Cys6–Cys120, Cys28–Cys111, Cys61–Cys77, and Cys73–Cys91. Its well-defined tertiary structure consists of two distinct domains: a β-domain, made up of β-pleated sheets, and an α-domain composed of four α-helices that together create a compact hydrophobic core. This structural organization contributes to the protein's high stability and functional specificity. The protein is particularly rich in essential amino acids, making it nutritionally valuable. Functionally, it plays a central role in lactose biosynthesis in the mammary gland. It acts as the regulatory subunit of the lactose synthetase complex, where it associates with UDP-galactosyltransferase to alter the enzyme's substrate specificity, enabling the synthesis of lactose from glucose and UDP-galactose. Through this role, the protein is directly involved in determining lactose production and, consequently, milk volume during lactation.

10.5.3.4 β-Lactoglobulin

This protein is a globular whey protein characterized by a well-defined secondary structure consisting of approximately 10% α-helices and 45% β-sheets, stabilized by two disulfide bonds located between Cys106–Cys119 and Cys66–Cys160. It is widely distributed among mammalian species but is notably absent in camelids, rodents, and humans. Functionally, this whey protein serves as an important carrier molecule, facilitating the transport of fatty acids, retinol, and fat-soluble vitamins, particularly vitamins A and D. By binding lipophilic compounds, it also helps protect milk lipids from auto-oxidation, thereby contributing to milk stability and nutritional quality. β-lactoglobulin is also recognized as a major milk allergen and is implicated in food allergy reactions in a substantial proportion of sensitive individuals, accounting for nearly 80% of milk-related allergic responses. Its structural stability and resistance to digestion are considered key factors underlying its allergenic potential.

10.5.3.5 Bovine Serum Albumin (BSA)

It is a minor whey protein that is not synthesized within the mammary gland, but instead enters milk from blood plasma. Structurally, it is a large globular protein composed of 582 amino acids, stabilized by 17 intermolecular disulfide bridges and containing one free thiol (–SH) group at the 34th amino acid residue. Bovine serum albumin (BSA) has a strong capacity to bind free fatty acids, lipids, and various flavor-active compounds, which contributes to its role as a carrier molecule in milk. This binding ability also enables BSA to protect lipids against oxidative deterioration, thereby helping to maintain milk quality and stability. In addition to its functional and nutritional roles, BSA has been reported to exhibit anticancer properties, attributed to its antioxidant activity and its ability to bind and transport bioactive molecules.

Lactoferrin It is an iron-binding glycoprotein with a molecular weight of approximately 80 kDa. The concentration of lactoferrin in bovine milk is relatively low, ranging from 0.02 to 0.35 mg/ml, whereas human milk contains much higher levels (about 4.0 mg/ml). Colostrum is particularly rich in lactoferrin, with concentrations substantially greater than those found in mature milk. Lactoferrin exhibits strong antibacterial activity, primarily because of its high affinity for iron; by sequestering iron, it limits the availability of this essential nutrient to microorganisms, thereby inhibiting their growth. In addition to its antimicrobial role, lactoferrin contributes to innate immune defense within the mammary gland. A detailed discussion of its structure, functions, and immunological significance is presented in the chapter on "Mammary Gland Immunity."

10.5.3.6 Immunoglobulins

The concentration of immunoglobulins is markedly lower in milk (about 0.1%) compared with colostrum, where it reaches approximately 6%. The globulin fraction present in milk is identical to that found in blood, indicating its direct origin from the circulation rather than synthesis within the mammary gland. These immunoglobulins play a crucial role in the transfer of passive immunity, particularly in species where placental transfer of antibodies does not occur. In such species, colostrum and, to a lesser extent, milk serve as the primary sources of maternal antibodies for the newborn, providing early protection against infectious agents. A detailed account of the types, functions, and immunological significance of milk immunoglobulins is presented in the chapter on "Mammary Gland Immunity."

10.5.3.7 Proteose–Peptone (PP)

These proteins represent the heat-stable and acid-soluble fraction of milk proteins. They can be isolated by heat treatment and by adjusting the pH to 4.6, at which most other milk proteins precipitate. Based on their origin and characteristics, they are classified into two main groups. The first group consists of peptides produced by the proteolytic breakdown of β-casein, mediated by indigenous milk proteinases. This group includes component 5, component 8 fast, and component 8 slow. The second group comprises a hydrophobic protein fraction that is not derived from casein hydrolysis, commonly referred to as component 3. In bovine milk, the total proteose–peptone (PP) content is approximately 2.28 mg/mL, of which component 5 (PP5) accounts for about 0.84 mg/mL, while component 8 fast (PP8f) contributes around 0.19 mg/mL. These fractions are important due to their stability and potential functional roles in milk.

10.5.3.8 Nonprotein Nitrogenous (NPN) Substances

The concentration of NPA in cow milk is 25–30 mg/100 ml. These compounds are mainly derived as end products of nitrogen metabolism. Some compounds such as amino acids and peptides are protein degradation products derived from blood.

Table 10.13 Major NPN compounds and their proportion in cow milk

NPN compounds	Amount (mg/100 g of milk)
Urea	14.21
Ammonia	0.88
Creatine	2.55
Creatinine	1.21
Uric acid	0.78
α-Amino N	4.43
Orotic acid N	1.46
Peptide	3.20
Hippuric acid	0.44

Wolfschoon-Pombo and Klostermeyer (1981)

Table 10.14 Amino acid content (g/100 g^{-1}) in milk from various species of animals

Amino acid (g/100 g)	Cow	Goat	Sheep	Buffalo	Camel
Aspartic acid	7.8	7.4	6.5	7.1	6.9
Threonine	4.5	5.7	4.4	5.7	4.1
Serine	4.8	5.2	3.4	4.7	4.3
Glutamic acid	23.2	19.3	14.5	21.4	18.1
Proline	9.6	14.6	16.2	12.0	12.0
Cysteine	0.6	0.6	0.9	0.6	1.9
Glycine	1.8	2.1	3.5	1.9	2.1
Alanine	3.0	3.6	2.4	3.0	2.1
Valine	4.8	5.7	6.4	6.8	4.1
Methionine	1.8	3.5	2.7	0.9	2.0
Isoleucine	4.2	7.1	4.6	5.7	4.9
Leucine	8.7	8.0	9.9	9.8	6.1
Tyrosine	4.5	4.8	3.8	3.9	3.1
Phenylalanine	4.8	6.0	4.3	4.7	4.0
Histidine	3.0	5.0	6.7	2.7	2.1
Lysine	8.1	8.2	7.8	7.5	–

Stobiecka et al. (2021)

Major NPN compounds and their proportion in cow milk have been described in Table 10.13. Amino acid content in milk from various species of animals is presented in Tables 10.13 and 10.14.

10.5.3.9 Bioactive Peptides in Milk

Milk is a rich source of bioactive peptides that exhibit a broad range of physiological and health-promoting activities, including antihypertensive, antidiabetic, antioxidant, and antimicrobial effects. Because of these beneficial properties, milk-derived bioactive peptides are increasingly exploited in the development of nutraceuticals, functional foods, and natural therapeutic agents. In native milk proteins, these peptides generally remain biologically inactive and are embedded within the primary structure of larger protein molecules. They are released and become functionally active only after proteolytic cleavage, which may occur during gastrointestinal digestion by gut enzymes, through the action of milk-derived proteases, or as a result of enzymes produced by microorganisms during fermentation and food processing. Some important bioactive compounds of milk in different species are presented in Table 10.15.

10.5.4 Minerals

Milk contains minerals and salts collectively referred to as "ash," which represent the noncombustible fraction of milk and account for approximately 0.7% of its composition. The overall mineral concentration of milk remains relatively stable, and any marked deviation from this level usually suggests an abnormal physiological or pathological condition. The principal minerals present in milk ash include calcium, phosphorus, magnesium, sodium, potassium, chloride, citrate, and sulfur. Among these, milk is especially valued as an excellent dietary source of calcium. Calcium in milk is largely associated with casein micelles, a relationship that significantly enhances its bioavailability and absorption in the gastrointestinal tract. A detailed account of the mineral composition of milk is provided in Table 10.16.

10.5.5 Vitamins

Milk is a valuable source of both fat-soluble and water-soluble vitamins (Table 10.17). The fat-soluble vitamins present in milk include vitamins A, D, E, and K, while the water-soluble group comprises vitamins B_1, B_2, B_6, B_{12}, pantothenic acid, niacin, biotin, folic acid, and vitamin C. During milk processing and separation, these vitamins are distributed according to their solubility. Fat-soluble vitamins are predominantly concentrated in the cream fraction, whereas water-soluble vitamins remain largely in the whey portion.

10.5.6 Enzymes

Milk contains a wide array of enzymes—approximately 60 different types—which originate from multiple sources. These enzymes are either synthesized by the mammary secretory cells, transferred from the blood, or, in some cases, are of microbial origin. Milk enzymes can exert both beneficial and undesirable effects, influencing milk quality, shelf life, processing characteristics, and safety. Certain enzymes, such as plasmin, catalase, and N-acetyl-β-D-glucosaminidase, are released in increased amounts during mammary gland infections (mastitis) and therefore serve as important biochemical markers of udder health. Elevated levels of these enzymes are commonly associated with tissue damage and increased somatic cell

Table 10.15 Major bioactive compounds of milk in different species

Sequence of bioactive peptide	Source	Species	Therapeutics properties
DKIHP	*β*-CN f (47–51)	Cow	Angiotensin-converting-enzyme (ACE) inhibitory
FFVAP	*α*s1-casein f (23–27)	Cow	ACE-inhibitory
VAPFPE & LPVPQ	Bovine milk	Cow	ACE-inhibitory
YQEPVLGPVRGPFPI	*β*-CN f (208–222)	Cow	Antimicrobial
LLY	*β*-CN f (191–193)	Cow	Antioxidative
MAIPPKKNQDK	k-casein f (106–116)	Cow	Antithrombic
TAQVTSTEV	κ-CN f (154–162)	Cow	Antithrombotic
LVYPFPGP	*β*-CN f (58–65)	Goat	ACE-inhibitory
TVDQHQ	*α*S2-CN f (182–187)	Goat	Antidiabetic activity
SDIPNPIGSE	*α*S1-casein f (195–204)	Goat	Antidiabetic activity
QEPVLGPVRGPFP	*β*-casein f (207–219)	Goat	Antidiabetic activity
LHSMKEGNPAHQKQP	*α*s1-CN f (120–134)	Goat	Antioxidant activity
PLRVYVEELKP	*β*-Lg f (38–48)	Goat	Antioxidant activity
ATTLEGKLVEL	Lactophorin B, f (79–89)	Camel	Antioxidant activity
KADAVTLDGGL	Lactoferrin f (53–63)	Camel	Antioxidant activity
LSLSQFKVLPVPQ	*β*CN f (178–191)	Camel	ACE-inhibitory activity
KDLWDDFKGL MPSKPPLL	–	Camel	Anti-obesity
PYVRYL	*α*s2-CN f (203–208)	Sheep	ACE-inhibitory
HPHPHLSF	κ-CN f (98–105)	Sheep	ACE-inhibitory
VMFPPQSVL	*β*-CN f (155–163)	Sheep	Antimicrobial
PPEIN	κ-CN f (156–160)	Yak	ACE-inhibitory
YQNPRLGPTGELDPATQPIVAVHNPVIV	*β*-CN f (217–241)	Mare	ACE-inhibitory
LNVSSETVES	*β*-CN	Donkey	Antioxidant activity
VAPFPQPVVP	*β*-CN f (176–185)	Donkey	ACE-inhibitory activity

Table 10.16 Mineral content in milk

Macro-minerals	*Amount (g/100 ml)*
Sodium	0.048
Potassium	0.143
Calcium	0.117
Magnesium	0.011
Chloride	0.110
Phosphate	0.230
Citrate	0.175
Sulfate	0.0100
Trace elements	*Amount (μg/liter)*
Zinc	4000
Aluminum	500
Iron	400
Copper	120
Molybdenum	60
Manganese	30
Nickel	25
Silicon	1500
Bromine	1000
Boron	200
Fluorine	150
Iodine	60

Mehta (2015)

Table 10.17 Vitamins present in milk of different species

Vitamin (mg /100 g)	Cow	Goat	Sheep	Buffalo	Camel
Vitamin A	37–46	55–185	64–146	35–69	20.1
Vitamin E	0.21	0.03	Not detected	0.19	0.32
Vitamin D	2	1.33	2	2	3
Vitamin B6	0.04–0.06	0.045	0.08	0.33	–
Vitamin B12	0.36–0.45	0.66	0.71	0.40	–
Vitamin C	1.94	1.29	4.16	2.2	3.3

Stobiecka et al. (2021)

counts in milk. Other enzymes, including alkaline phosphatase, lactoperoxidase, and γ-glutamyl transpeptidase, are widely used as indicators of the thermal stability and heat treatment adequacy of milk. Their presence or inactivation provides valuable information regarding the effectiveness of pasteurization and other heat-processing methods. Activities of milk enzymes can be altered in response to heat, light, and pH changes. Milk enzymes are present in four phases: water-soluble, casein-bound, lipid-bound, and associated with microsomal particles. Important enzymes present in bovine milk and their specificity are described in Table 10.18.

Table 10.18 Enzymes present in bovine milk and their specificity

Enzymes	Distribution	Specificity	Substrate	Optimum pH	Optimum temperature (°C)
Aldolase	Cream fraction	Ketose mono- and diphosphates	Fructose, 1,6- diphosphate	7.0	35
α-Amylase	Lactoglobulin fraction of skim milk	α-l, 4-D glucan linkages in polysaccharides with 3 or more consecutive α-l, 4-D glucan linkages	Starch, glycogen, polysaccharide, and oligosaccharides	7.4	34
β-Amylase	Lactoglobulin fraction of skim milk	α-l, 4-D glucan linkages in polysaccharides to remove successive maltose units from nonreducing end	Starch, glycogen, polysaccharide and oligosaccharides	–	–
Carbonic anhydrase	–	Carbonic acid-CO_2 interconversion	Carbonic acid	–	–
Catalase	Milk microsomes, lactoglobulin	Hydrogen peroxide	Hydrogen peroxide, ethanol	7.0	–
Cytochrome C	Fat globules	–	$NADH^+$	7.3	18
Diaphorase	Fat globules	–	$NADH^+$	7.3	18
A-esterase	–	Aryl esters	Phenyl acetate	8.0	37
B-esterase	Aqueous phase	n-methyl esters of fatty acids and triglycerides	Tributyrin	8.0	37
C-esterase	–	Choline esters tributyrin	Phenyl propionate	8.0	37
Lactose synthetase	Aqueous phase	UDP-galactose and α-D-glucose	UDP-galactose and α-D-glucose	7.2	37
Lipase	Skim milk	Glycerol esters	Milk fat, tri-butyrin, and glycerides	9.0–9.2	37
Lysozyme	Whey	*B*- l, 4 linkage between N-acetylglucosamine and N-acetylmuramic acid	Cell walls	7.9	37
Alkaline phosphatase	Cream, skim milk	Phosphate mono esters, serine-P, β-glycerol-P	Phosphate esters	9.8	37
Peroxidase	Whey	Hydrogen peroxide		6.0–7.0	20

(continued)

Table 10.18 (continued)

Enzymes	Distribution	Specificity	Substrate	Optimum pH	Optimum temperature (°C)
			Hydrogen peroxide and reducible agent		
Protease	Casein	–	Tryptic and/or chymotryptic specificity	6.5–8	37
Xanthine oxidase	Fat globules	–	Aldehydes, oxypurines, pterin, DPN, and xanthine	6–9	37

Shahani et al. (1973)

Exercises

Objective Questions

1. In milk, protein remains as ____________________ and lactose is present in the form of__________________.
2. In cow's milk, the pH typically falls between __________________.
3. Predominant immunoglobulin present in the colostrum is __________________.
4. The major fat component of milk is __________________.
5. The principal polyunsaturated fatty acids (PUFAs) present in milk are________________ and ______________________.
6. The sandy texture observed in products like concentrated milk and ice cream is due to which milk component? __________________.
7. Lactose intolerance is developed due to deficiency of __________________ enzyme.
8. A2 β-casein is characteristic of milk from __________________ breeds of cows.
9. The major milk allergen is ___________________.
10. The freezing point of cow's milk is largely determined by its ________________ content.

Subjective Questions

1. Briefly describe the chemical properties of milk.
2. Write down the differences between A1 and A2 milk.
3. Write a short note on galactosemia.
4. Write in brief about the bioactive peptides in milk and their role in health and diseases.
5. Describe in brief the formation of colostrum.

Answer to Objective Questions

1. Colloidal Suspension, True solution
2. 6.5–6.7
3. IgG1
4. Triacylglycerols
5. Linoleic acid and α-linolenic acid
6. Lactose
7. β-galactosidase or lactase
8. Indigenous Indian zebu cattle and buffaloes.
9. β-lactoglobulin
10. Lactose

References

Books

Mehta BM (2015) Chemical composition of milk and milk products. In: Cheung PCK, Mehta BM (eds) Handbook of food chemistry. Springer-Verlag, Berlin Heidelberg

Park YW (2006) Minor species milk. In: Park YW, Haenlein GFW (eds) Handbook of milk of non-bovine mammals, 1st edn. Blackwell Publishing, Ames, pp 393–406

Research Articles

Ahmadi M, Boldura O, Milovanov C, Dronca D, Mircu C, Hutu I, Popescu S, Padeanu I, Tulcan C (2016) Colostrum from different animal species—a product for health status enhancement. Bulletin UASVM Animal Science and Biotechnologies 73:95–100

Alais C, Alais C, Godina AL (1985) Ciencia de la leche: principios de técnica lechera. Editorial Reverté, Barcelona

Allen LH (2012) B vitamins in breast milk: relative importance of maternal status and intake, and effects on infant status and function. Adv Nutr 3(3):362–369

Bagwe S, Tharappel LJP, Kaur G, Buttar HS (2015) Bovine colostrum: An emerging nutraceutical. J Complement Integr Med 12:175–185

Bekuma A, Galmessa U (2018) Review on hygienic milk products practice and occurrence of mastitis in cow's milk. Agric Res Technol 18(2):556053

Guthrie AH (1989) Introductory nutrition. Times Mirror/Mosby College Publishing, St. Louis

Hariyani AS, Hazra T, Thesiya AJ, Ahuja KK (2024) Composition of milk: a comparative analysis on goat, cow and buffalo milk from Amreli region of Gujarat. Ind J Animal Health 63(1):41–49

Hurley WL (2010) Milk composition and synthesis. University of Illinois [Online]

Iyengar GV (1982) Elemental composition of human and animal milk: a review. In: IAEA-TECDOC-269. International Atomic Energy Agency, Vienna

Jensen RG (1995) Handbook of milk composition. Academic Press

Keen CL, Lonnerdal B, Clegg MS, Hurley LS, Morris JG, Rogers QR, Rucker RB (1982) Developmental changes in composition of cats' milk: trace elements, minerals, protein, carbohydrate and fat. J Nutr 112:1763–1769

Keen L, Lönnerdal B, Clegg M, Hurley LS (1981) Developmental changes in composition of rat milk: trace elements, minerals, protein, carbohydrate and fat. J Nutr 111:226–230

Kessler EC, Bruckmaier RM, Gross JJ (2019) Immunoglobulin G content and colostrum composition of different goat and sheep breeds in Switzerland and Germany. J Dairy Sci 102:5542–5549

Leseur R, Melik N (1990) Lait et produits laitiers. Edition: Cedex, Paris, pp 2–7

Mariani P, Summer A, Martuzzi F, Formaggioni P, Sabbioni A, Catalano AL (2001) Physicochemical properties, gross composition, energy value and nitrogen fractions of Haflinger nursing mare milk throughout six lactation months. Anim Res 50:415–425

Martini M, Licitra R, Altomonti I, Salari F (2020) Quality of donkey mammary secretion during the first ten days of lactation. Int Dairy J 109:104781

Meyer H, Kamphues J (1990) Grundlagen der Ernährung von Neugeborenen. In: Walser K, Bostedt H (eds) Neugeborenen- und Säuglingskunde der Tiere. Ferdinand Enke Verlag, Stuttgart, pp 55–71

Mollica MP, Trinchese G, Cimmino F, Penna E, Cavaliere G, Tudisco R, Musco N, Manca C, Catapano A, Monda M (2021) Milk fatty acid profiles in different animal species: focus on the potential effect of selected PUFAs on metabolism and brain functions. Nutrients 13:1111

Mößler M, Aichner J, Müller A, Albert T, Wittek T (2021) Concentrations of fat, protein, lactose, macro and trace minerals in alpaca colostrum and milk at different lactation stages. Animals 11: 1955

Nuntapaitoon M, Juthamanee P, Theil PK, Tummaruk P (2020) Impact of sow parity on yield and composition of colostrum and milk in Danish landrace × Yorkshire crossbred sows. Prev Vet Med 181:105085

Ontsouka CE, Bruckmaier RM, Blum JW (2003) Fractionized milk composition during removal of colostrum and mature milk. J Dairy Sci 86:2005–2011

Park YW (2007) Rheological characteristics of goat and sheep milk. Small Rumin Res 68(1–2): 73–87

Playford RJ (2001) Peptide therapy and the gastroenterologist: Colostrums and milk-derived growth factors. Clin Nutr 20:101–106

Puppel K, Gołębiewski M, Grodkowski G, Slósarz J, Kunowska-Slósarz M, Solarczyk P, Łukasiewicz M, Balcerak M, Przysucha T (2019) Composition and factors affecting quality of bovine colostrum: a review. Animals 9:1070–1084

Ren X, Yang Z, Shao B, Yin S, Yang X (2015) B-vitamin levels in human milk among different lactation stages and areas in China. PLoS One 10(7):e0133285

Shahani KM, Harper WJ, Jensen RG, Parry RM Jr, Zittle CA (1973) Enzymes in bovine milk: a review. J Dairy Sci 56(5):531–543

Soloshenko KI, Lych IV, Voloshyna IM, Shkotova LV (2020) Polyfunctional properties of goat colostrum proteins and their use. Biopolymers and Cell 36:197–209

Stelwagen K, Carpenter E, Haigh B, Hodgkinson A, Wheeler TT (2009) Immune components of bovine colostrum and milk. J Anim Sci 87:3–9

Stobiecka M, Król J, Brodziak A, Wajs J (2021) Characteristics of milk from different species of farm animals with special emphasis on health-promoting ingredients. Acta Scientiarum Polonorum Zootechnica 20(3):85–96

Walstra P, Jenness R (1984) Dairy chemistry and physics. John Wiley, New York

Wolfschoon-Pombo A, Klostermeyer H (1981) The NPN fraction of cow's milk. Milchwissenschaft 36:598

Yoganandi J, Mehta BM, Wadhwani KN, Darji VB, Aparnathi KD (2014) Comparison of physico-chemical properties of camel milk with cow milk and buffalo milk. J Camel Practice Res 21(2): 253–258

Zahoor T, Riaz AH (1991) Comparative study of milk composition and fat globule size in various mammals. Pak J Agril Sci 28(2):144–147

Mammary Gland Disorders

11

Contents

Abstract

The mammary gland is prone to a wide variety of disorders that affect the quality and quantity of milk. The mammary gland disorders can be categorized into congenital disorders (supernumerary teats, nonfunctional quarters), physiological disorders (udder edema, precocious mammary development, failure of milk

J. Mukherjee et al., *Veterinary Lactation Physiology*,
https://doi.org/10.1007/978-3-032-21123-1_11

ejection, agalactia, galactorrhea), diseases of teats and skin (ulcerative mammillitis, fibropapillomas, hyperkeratosis at teat-end, necrotic dermatitis, udder impetigo, udder cleft dermatitis), and inflammatory (mastitis) and traumatic disorders (laceration of the bovine udder, teat obstructions, breakdown of udder support apparatus, hemolactia, teat sphincter inadequacy). The present chapter encompasses all these disorders, their predisposing factors, treatment, and prevention.

Graphical Abstract

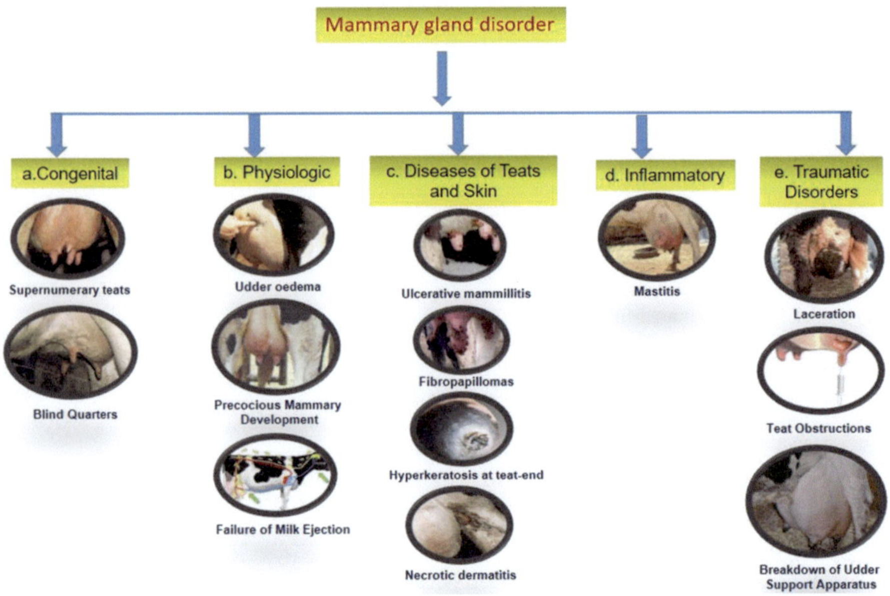

Description of the graphic: The mammary gland disorders can be categorized into congenital disorders (**a**), physiological disorders (**b**), diseases of teats and skin (**c**), inflammatory (**d**), and traumatic (**e**). The major congenital anomalies include supernumerary teats and blind quarters. Udder edema, precocious mammary development, and failure of milk ejection are grouped under physiological disorders. Common diseases of teat and udder skin are ulcerative mammilitis, fibropapilloma, hyperkeratosis at teat-end, necrotic dermatitis, udder impetigo, and udder cleft dermatitis. Mastitis is the inflammation of mammary gland which causes severe economic loss due to decreased production. Traumatic injuries are caused by barbed wire, thorns, or cow's own hooves that include laceration, teat stenosis, breakdown of udder support apparatus, hemolactia, and teat sphincter inadequacy

Keywords

Congenital diseases · Mastitis · Diseases of teat and udder skin · Udder edema · Traumatic injury

Inside the Chapter

- *Congenital Disorders*
  - Supernumerary Teats
  - Nonfunctional (Blind) Quarters
- *Physiologic Disorders of the Udder*
  - Udder edema
  - Precocious Mammary Development
  - Failure of Milk Ejection
  - Agalactia
  - Galactorrhea
- *Diseases of Teats and Skin*
  - Ulcerative mammillitis
  - Fibropapillomas (Warts)
  - Hyperkeratosis at Teat-End
  - Necrotic Dermatitis (Udder Seborrhea)
  - Udder Impetigo
  - Udder Cleft Dermatitis (Udder Sores)
- *Inflammatory*
  - Mastitis
- *Traumatic and Structural Disorders*
  - Laceration of the Bovine Udder
  - Teat Obstructions
  - Breakdown of Udder Support Apparatus
  - Hemolactia (Blood in Milk)
  - Teat Sphincter Inadequacy

Learning Objectives

- Common disorders of the mammary gland, their classification, and etiology.
- Diagnosis and treatment of different mammary gland disorders.
- Prevention and control of mammary gland disorders.

The quality and quantity of milk production depend on the udder health, and thus it is obviously the main determinant of successful dairy farming. The diseases of udder and teats (Table 11.1) lead to severe economic loss in terms of quality and quantity of milk production, together with food safety and animal well-being. The economic losses are due to decreased milk production, treatment costs, and increased early culling of animals. The deterioration in the quality of milk affects the processing and shelf life of milk and milk products, together with customer safety. Being external organs, the udder and teats are vulnerable to trauma or injury. The major causes of udder injuries are inappropriate milking, injury by the teeth of calves, wound by the wire fencing around the farms, lying down over sharp objects, and accidental stepping on the teat by untrimmed claws of other cows. The cows may also exhibit congenital udder and teat anomalies that lead to structural defects. The most severe form of the udder diseases is mastitis or the inflammation of the mammary gland,

Table 11.1 Diseases of the udder and teats

Type	Diseases
Congenital disorders	Supernumerary teats Nonfunctional (blind) quarters
Physiologic disorders of the udder	Udder edema Precocious mammary development Failure of milk ejection Agalactia Galactorrhea
Diseases of teats and skin	Ulcerative mammillitis Fibropapillomas (warts) Hyperkeratosis at teat-end Necrotic dermatitis (udder seborrhea) Udder impetigo Udder cleft dermatitis (udder sores)
Inflammatory	Mastitis
Traumatic and structural disorders	Laceration of the bovine udder Teat obstructions Breakdown of udder support apparatus Hemolactia (blood in milk) Teat sphincter inadequacy

which is infectious in origin. Sometimes the external injury and congenital defects also interfere with milk outflow and may predispose to mastitis.

11.1 Congenital Disorders

11.1.1 Supernumerary teats (Webbed or "Siamese" Teats)

Supernumerary teats are the most common congenital abnormalities of the mammary gland in cows, sheep, and goats. The supernumerary teats can be attached either to fore and rear teats or can be seen in different locations, such as between the fore and rear teats or behind the rear teats. The size of the supernumerary teats is smaller than the normal teats and can be easily distinguished. Supernumerary teats can be categorized into nonsecreting supernumerary teats (hyperthelia) and secreting supernumerary teats (hypermastia). The term "polythelia" is used to describe hyperthelia in humans. In the case of hypermastia, the teat possesses its own streak canal and sphincter and secretes a small amount of milk during suckling. The hyperthelia on the other hand is nonfunctional or vestigial. Another form of supernumerary teats is fused teats, in which two teats are fused at the base by the skin without involvement of the teat canal or muscle. These are seen in buffaloes and rarely in cows. The supernumerary teats should be removed at the age of two to six weeks, as the young calf has little blood circulation around the area of extra teats, so little bleeding will occur. The extra teats are surgically removed with scissors at the point of teat skin and udder skin after restraining the animal. A suitable antiseptic solution is applied to prevent secondary infections.

11.1.2 Blind Quarters

The blind quarter refers to the quarter that produces no milk. This condition may be congenital or acquired. The congenital blind quarter is of two types. Sometimes there is a total absence of the teat canal, or there may be a persistent membrane between the teat cistern and the base of the teat. In the acquired form of blind quarter, the gland cistern is degenerated due to infections or trauma caused by the suckling calf. The typical signs of a blind quarter include less or complete absence of milk flow, flabby and fibrosed teat, and diffuse obstruction that can be palpated externally toward the gland cistern. The diagnostic modalities include ultrasonography of the teat and teat cannulation. The USG is less effective if there is no milk in the teat cistern. Probing of the teat cistern with a sterile teat cannula (7.5–10.0 cm) helps to detect the integrity of the streak canal and the detection of fibrous or membranous obstructions of the gland cistern. Surgical intervention to treat a blind quarter caused by fibrosis is generally not very effective. In rare cases, fenestration at the base of the gland cistern may show good results. Teat implants (temporary or permanent) could be a good option to treat blind quarters with 50% success rate. The stenosis at the teat end can be corrected by slow dilation of streak canal with a sharp 14-gauge needle directed into the teat lumen. After the needle puncture, the stenosis can be opened.

11.2 Physiologic Disorders of the Udder

11.2.1 Udder Edema

It is the excess accumulation of lymphatic fluid in and around the interstitial space of the udder. The udder edema occurs several weeks before calving. It has been reported that 97% of high-yielding cows suffer from udder edema around the time of parturition. During this period, mammary gland undergoes extensive growth and morphological changes that contribute to the development of udder edema.

The causes of udder edema are unclear, but reduced mammary blood flow and increased cranial intravenous pressure due to fetal pressure in the pelvic cavity during late gestation may be the primary causes of udder edema in cows. There is threefold increase in the mammary blood flow from 2 weeks pre-partum, and it has been reported that the cows that suffered from udder edema had 17% lower mammary blood flow than the healthy animals. Increased formation of lymph due to high mammary gland metabolism around calving leads to accumulation of lymph, which may also cause udder edema. The stasis of milk due to failure of milk let-down is also a predisposing factor for udder edema. Increased oxidative stress and production of reactive oxygen species may contribute to udder edema. Selection of animals for more milk production increases the incidence of udder edema, and a high positive correlation exists between milk yield and incidence of udder edema. It has been reported that heifers are more prone to udder edema than older cows. Excess intake of sodium, potassium, and grains during the pre-partum period leads to the occurrence of udder edema in cows. A significant positive correlation also exists between udder edema and the incidence of metritis and cystic ovarian diseases. The other predisposing factors of udder edema are calf gender, calving season, and height at parturition. The heifers containing male fetuses are more susceptible to udder edema as the male calf is heavier and exerts more fetal pressure. The udder edema is most likely to occur during the winter season due to increased feed intake and higher consumption of sodium and potassium. The fodder such as alfalfa and fodder harvested with manure contain high potassium, and excessive consumption may develop udder edema. Hypoproteinemia (especially hypoalbuminemia) decreases colloidal osmotic pressure of plasma and may contribute to udder edema. Heifers with larger size are more susceptible to udder edema than smaller heifers. Some studies showed that the plasma concentration of estrogen and progesterone had a significant effect on udder edema. It was thought that estrone and estradiol-17α promote the development of udder edema, whereas progesterone and estradiol-17β decreased the severity of udder edema.

The udder edema is of two types: physiological (acute) and pathological (chronic). The physiological udder edema is usually non-painful generally and generally occurs around calving and gradually subsides over 2 to 4 weeks. It occurs in two stages. Initially, there is gradual congestion under the skin, which gradually leads to pitting edema and the udder becomes turgid. Chronic or pathological edema persists for a longer duration than physiological udder edema and may persist throughout the lactation. It is generally caused by the breakdown of the udder supporting structure.

The udder edema leads to milking problems, increased risk of mastitis and reduced production. The udder edema causes alterations in the intra mammary pressure interfere with milk let-down and causes reduced milk production. The discomfort due to udder edema also leads to production loss.

The diagnosis of udder edema is easier and can be made by visual observations and palpation of the udder with pitting on pressure. The edema is symmetrical and involves all the quarters. The udder edema should be differentiated from udder abscess, hematoma, abdominal hernia, and mastitis. The microbiological evaluation of milk samples is desirable to rule out mastitis.

Most of the cases of udder edema do not require any treatment and gradually subside after calving. A massage three times daily for 20 min, along with the application of hot and cold water, gives fruitful results. Udder rubbing with 200 mg of diethylstilbestrol in 10 ml of corn oil over the edematous area on first and third day after calving helps to reduce the swelling. In some cases, surgical interventions by stabbing the skin near edematous area at 2 days post-partum can give a good prognosis, but hygiene should be maintained to avoid infections. The use of diuretics in bovine udder edema is not very effective due to slower responses.

11.2.2 Precocious Mammary Development

It refers to the premature development of the udder in heifers and calves, and the affected animal may secret milk before parturition. It may involve a single gland or a symmetric development of the whole udder. Single udder involvement occurs due to suckling by a herdmate. The premature symmetrical development results from chronic estrogenic stimulation, either due to cystic ovaries or consuming feedstuff containing phytoestrogens or mycotoxin zearalenone. Some studies reported that feeding of mulberry leaves containing a flavonoid called astragalin, which is structurally similar to estrogen, can cause precocious mammary development. Estrogen stimulates mammary duct growth, and the combined effect of estrogen and progesterone induces lobulo-alveolar growth. Estrogen-induced pre-mature mammary gland development is sometimes associated with vulvar swelling. The precocious mammary development does not require any treatment and usually resolves after the removal of feedstuffs containing phytoestrogen.

11.2.3 Failure of Milk Ejection

This condition is characterized by bimodal milk flow, where the milk flow rate is reduced or absent transiently at the beginning of milking and the milk flow rate is below the threshold level at the end of milking. It has a negative impact on milk production and udder health as well. The failure of milk ejection can also occur when the cisternal fraction of milk is filled only when the alveolar pressure forces the milk to reach into the cisternal compartment (elastic limit). In this case, the delayed milk ejection does not follow a bimodal pattern. The milk ejection is a neuroendocrine reflex, and pre-milking tactile teat stimulation is essential to induce the release of oxytocin, which causes expulsion of the alveolar milk fraction into the gland cistern. The time from tactile stimulation to milk ejection varies from 40 s to 2 min, and inappropriate pre-stimulation for younger cows may result in failure in milk ejection. Older cows on the other hand require longer pre-stimulation for appropriate milking. Stress and anxiety due to unfamiliar surroundings results in beta-endorphin release, which hampers milk ejection. The release of adrenaline also causes vasoconstriction and prevents oxytocin from reaching the mammary gland. The condition can easily be overcome by making the heifers accustomed to the milking parlor, careful handling, and adequate tactile stimulation (>20 s) before milking. In some cases, the injection of oxytocin (20 U, IM) can be given to induce milk ejection.

11.2.4 Agalactia

The complete loss of milk production in a lactating animal due to failure of milk let-down or failure in milk production is called agalactia. It can be seen in cows of all age but the young cows are mostly susceptible. It is generally caused by system diseases and udder infections. Agalactia is common in peri-parturient sows in combination with mastitis and metritis; hence, the disease is called MMA syndrome (mastitis, metritis, and agalactia). In small ruminants, contagious agalactia (CA) is caused by *Mycoplasma agalactiae*, *Streptococcus agalactiae*, and *Streptococcus dysgalactiae* and may cause significant mortality of their offspring. The etiology of agalactia is congenital mammary gland anomalies, reduced feed intake in systemic diseases that cause nutritional deficiency, failure in milk down, severe heat stress, udder edema, mastitis, endocrine disturbances, endometritis, ingestion of toxins (endophyte-infected fodder), and ergot alkaloids that lead to suppression of prolactin secretion. The physiological agalactia can be seen during estrus. The treatment of agalactia is dependent on the etiology. In the majority of the cases, the suckling by the litter is encouraged to induce the normal milk down process. In nervous dams, sedatives such as acepromazine (0.125 to 0.5 mg/kg PO BID to TID) can be given to increase milk production. The treatment with oxytocin can also be applied to induce milk let-down. Agalactia due to nutritional deficiencies can be treated by supplementing feed additives (mineral mixtures, vitamins). Intramammary antibiotic infusion can be applied in the case of contagious agalactia. In inflammatory conditions, fomentation with magnesium sulfate is recommended.

11.2.5 Galactorrhea

It is the condition characterized by spontaneous milk flow irrespective of pregnancy and lactation. The premature mammary secretion is popularly known as witch's milk. It usually results from increased prolactin or decreased progesterone concentrations. It is most common in bitches, but young foals and ruminants are also susceptible. It is most common during pseudo pregnancy in bitches at the end of the luteal phase (nearly 60 days after estrus bitch and 40 days after induced ovulation without conception in a queen). It is also seen after ovariohysterectomy that mimics the luteal regression. The exogenous progesterone withdrawal can also lead to galactorrhea in dogs and cats. In foals and ruminants, the most common cause of galactorrhea is abortion. The mammary gland starts secreting milk before the expulsion of dead fetuses. Multiple fetuses, ovarian tumors, and placentitis may also lead to galactorrhea. Pseudopregnancy-induced galactorrhea is recovered spontaneously and does not require any treatment. The self-licking of teats can be prevented by the application of an Elizabethan collar in bitches. Administration of progesterone (Megestrol acetate: 2 mg/kg PO, SID for 5 days, Proligestone: 20 to 30 mg/kg SC, Delmadinone acetate: 1.0 to 1.5 mg/kg SC, Medroxyprogesterone acetate: 5 to 11 mg/kg SC, IM) can give good results. Prolactin antagonists (Cabergoline: 5 mg/kg PO SID for 5 to 10 days) can also be applied in bitches.

11.3 Diseases of Teats and Skin

11.3.1 Ulcerative Mammillitis

Ulcerative mammillitis is an infectious skin condition of the teats and udder caused by bovine herpesvirus-2 (BoHV-2). It typically appears as outbreaks in first-calving heifers shortly after giving birth, often associated with mastitis. This condition does not occur in dry cows, likely because the virus remains dormant and is reactivated when the immune system weakens around the peri-partum period. Infected cows can transmit the virus to suckling calves, which may then develop ulcers on the muzzle, tongue, and inside the mouth. The disease initially presents as fluid-filled blisters on the teat tips, which eventually rupture to form painful ulcers. These ulcers may merge and become covered with thick scabs, making milking painful and difficult. The fluid from the blisters contains a high concentration of virus particles. Disinfecting the teats with iodophor solution has been found effective. Additionally, applying emollients and glycerin helps soften the affected skin and ease milking. Once recovered, cows typically develop lifelong immunity to the disease.

11.3.2 Fibropapillomas (Warts)

Teat warts are caused by various strains of papovaviruses and are commonly found on the lower part of the teat, particularly in pregnant and first-lactation heifers. Transmission typically occurs through flies, making cows raised near fly-prone areas such as rivers and streams more vulnerable to infection. These warts present as fleshy nodules or feathery growths. There are five distinct strains of papovaviruses, each producing warts with unique characteristics—ranging from feathery and keratinized to papilliform appearances. However, the most frequently observed type is fibropapillomas, which include both fleshy nodules and feathery warts. Feathery warts can often be pulled off easily, while the more solid types tend to be firmly attached to the skin. Warts typically develop near the teat orifice and around the teat sphincter, which can hinder the milking process and sometimes lead to milk leakage. This leakage increases the risk of udder infections. Painful warts can disrupt milking and cause teat injuries, further predisposing the animal to secondary infections.

11.3.3 Hyperkeratosis at Teat-End (Teat End Callosity, Canal Eversion)

This condition is one of the most common lesions caused by machine milking, marked by the formation of a protruding mass of keratinized tissue around the teat sphincter. It typically begins as a swelling in the sphincter area and gradually develops into a dry, creamy, brown or white protrusion. The lesion is more frequently observed in teats with a pointed shape compared to cylindrical ones. It tends to occur more often in high-yielding animals, particularly during early to mid-lactation, and usually regresses during the dry period. However, the damage can be cumulative, meaning teats affected in one lactation are likely to suffer more severe lesions in subsequent lactations. Since the condition results from improper machine milking, effective milking management practices are key to its prevention.

11.3.4 Necrotic Dermatitis (Udder Seborrhea)

Excess udder edema sometimes leads to ischemia in the skin, followed by necrosis. It is usually seen in heifers during the first 1–2 weeks after calving. The lesions are characterized by moist and foul-smelling superficial dermatitis, which later on turns into reddish purple with serous exudate. In some animals, the dermatitis leads to extensive thickening of the teats that makes milking very difficult. The treatment modalities include cleaning of the lesions, removal of debris, and topical application of antiseptics.

11.3.5 Udder Impetigo

It is a diffuse miliary folliculitis or pustular dermatitis of the udder of cattle and buffaloes, characterized by the formation of pustules at the base of the teat, which may spread to the whole udder. It is generally caused by staphylococci and streptococci. The disease initially appears as vesicles surrounded by erythema, which subsequently develops into pustules. The disease spreads quickly in the herd during milking. The predisposing factors for udder impetigo are poor hygienic conditions, trauma or injury, and high temperature and humidity. Applications of topical or systemic antibiotics give good results. Regular teat dipping is useful to prevent the disease.

11.3.6 Udder Cleft Dermatitis (Udder Sores)

It is a kind of foul-smelling moist dermatitis located between the junction of the medial thigh and the dorsal attachment of lateral udder skin, on the ventral midline adjacent to the median septum of fore quarter or between the two forequarters. Initially, it appears as a mild skin infection characterized by erythema, papules, and pustules, which later become more severe necrosis with open wounds, pus, and blood. The oozing of pus, coupled with skin hair, develops moist dermatitis, which is further aggravated by infections with anaerobic bacteria such as *Fusobacterium necrophorum* and *T. pyogenes* to form crusts and scabs. These organisms cause foul smell, hence it is also called "udder rot." The exact cause of udder cleft dermatitis is unknown, but studies have shown that the lesions are associated with mange mites, treponemes, and secondary bacterial infection. The cow-related factors such as udder confirmation, parity, and environmental factors are also predisposing to udder sores. The udder confirmations that are vulnerable to udder sores are poor udder attachment, internal milk pressure, and udder edema. Udder sores are more frequent during the summer months. High-producing cows are mostly susceptible to udder cleft dermatitis during mid to late lactation. The udder sores are usually treated with an astringent aerosol spray. The hygienic practice should be followed. The prognosis of udder sore is good, but a long time is required if the case is untreated.

11.3.7 Mastitis

It is a multi-etiological disease characterized by inflammation of the udder that affects the milk quality and production potential of the dairy animals and causes severe economic loss in the dairy sector. The inflammation is caused by the invasion of different bacterial, viral, and fungal agents into the mammary gland. The general symptoms of mastitis includes hot, painful, swollen udder with decreased milk secretion and altered milk composition. The infected cows can also have fever, depression, and anorexia. Mastitis can be categorized into clinical and subclinical forms based on the degree of inflammation. The clinical form of mastitis can be identified by visible clinical signs, but the subclinical forms are difficult to diagnose as it does not have any characteristic udder abnormalities. From the economic point of view, the subclinical form is most fatal as it remains undiagnosed and causes severe production loss.

11.3.7.1 Predisposing Factors

The prevalence of mastitis is associated with the cow and environmental factors. Among the cow factors, breeds, age, parity, stage of lactation, and production potentials are the important determinants of mastitis occurrence. The older animals are susceptible to subclinical mastitis at the beginning or end of lactation. The peri-parturient immune suppression causes a higher incidence of mastitis during early lactation. The nutritional stress around the peri-partum period may also lead to immune suppression and mastitis occurrence. The milk yield is positively correlated with the incidence of mastitis. The mastitis occurrence increases with parity due to alterations in the morphology of the udder and teat canals.

11.3.7.2 Causative Agents

Mastitis is primarily caused by bacterial infections, particularly from *Staphylococcus* and *Streptococcus* species, though other pathogens such as mycoplasmas, fungi, algae, protozoa, and viruses can also be involved. In addition to infections, inflammation of the udder can result from physical injury, exposure to irritating chemicals that trigger an immune reaction, or other forms of physiological damage. Bacterial mastitis is of major concern due to its impact on both animal health and economic productivity. According to the National Mastitis Council, around 200 different microorganisms have been identified as causative agents of mastitis in cattle, although only a limited number are frequently isolated in practice. The mastitis-causing pathogens are classified into contagious pathogens in the udder or environmental pathogens found in the cow's surroundings, such as soil, utensils, and bedding materials. The common contagious pathogens include *Streptococcus agalactiae, Streptococcus dysgalactiae, Staphylococcus aureus, and Mycoplasma* spp. Environmental pathogens include *Escherichia coli, Enterobacter aerogenes, Klebsiella pneumoniae, Serratia* spp., *Proteus* spp., *Pseudomonas* spp., other Gram-negative bacteria, coagulase-negative *staphylococci* (CNS), yeasts and fungi such as *Prototheca*, environmental streptococci, *Trueperella pyogenes*, and *Corynebacterium bovis*. Although yeasts are an uncommon cause of mastitis, they have been identified in herds with poor milking hygiene, frequent udder injuries or irritation, and excessive or repeated use of antibiotics or intramammary treatments. In such cases, infections have been linked to various yeast species, including those from the genera *Candida*, *Cryptococcus*, *Rhodotorula*, and *Trichosporum*. Additionally, mastitis can be caused by two species of *Prototheca* algae, namely *Prototheca zopfii* and *Prototheca blaschkeae*. Importantly, among the two known genotypes of *P. zopfii*, only genotype 2 has been isolated from animals showing clinical signs of the disease.

11.3.7.3 Mode of Transmission

Contagious pathogens can spread from infected udders to healthy ones via contaminated milking equipment, milkers' hands, teat cup liners, paper or cloth towels used during milking, or even by flies. Environmental pathogens, such as *Streptococcus dysgalactiae* and coliforms (*Escherichia coli* and *Klebsiella*), are also transmitted through milking equipment. Coliforms are typically linked to poor hygiene, such as manure contamination or dirty, wet conditions. *Klebsiella*, in particular, is commonly found in sawdust bedding that contains bark or soil. The *S. aureus* can spread from infected cows to sucking calves after feeding contaminated milk. The fly-borne *S. aureus* infection can also occur in heifers.

11.3.7.4 Pathogenesis

The udder defense system is compromised around the peri-partum period (3 weeks pre-partum to 3 weeks post-partum). Different components of innate and adaptive immune responses like anatomical, cellular, and humoral defense factors are less effective in resisting the infection during this period, and the mastitis pathogens enter the mammary and colonize there. The toxins, enzymes, and cell-wall components of the microorganisms initiate inflammatory responses. Phagocytes, such as polymorphonuclear neutrophil (PMN) leukocytes, migrate from bone marrow to the site of infection in response to chemotactic agents from damaged tissues. During their migration, PMNs pass between mammary epithelial cells by breaking the epithelial cell barrier and enter the lumen of mammary gland alveoli and increase the somatic cell count (SCC) as well as damaging secretory cells.

The phagocytes engulf the organisms and destroy them. The migrated leukocytes also release some mediators that attract more leukocytes to the area to fight the infections. The aggregation of leukocytes and blood clotting factors blocks the small ducts and prevents complete milk evacuation. After the resolution of inflammation, the tissue repair starts and the mammary gland returns to its normal function. In some severe cases, damaged epithelium forms scar tissue that results in permanent loss of the tissue and the function of the mammary gland.

11.3.7.5 Signs and Symptoms

Based on the signs and symptoms, mastitis can be classified into clinical and subclinical forms. The occurrence of clinical mastitis is sudden with characteristic signs of inflammation such as redness and swelling of the udder. General symptoms include lethargy, anorexia, and fever. In subclinical forms, there are no visible signs

Table 11.2 Alterations in the milk composition due to mastitis

Constituent	Normal milk	Milk with high SCC
Fat	3.5	3.2
Lactose	4.9	4.4
Total protein	3.61	3.56
Total casein	2.8	2.3
Whey protein	0.8	1.3
Serum albumin	0.02	0.07
Lactoferrin	0.02	0.10
Immunoglobulins	0.10	0.60
Sodium	0.057	0.105
Chloride	0.091	0.147
Potassium	0.173	0.157
Calcium	0.12	0.04

National Mastitis Council (1996)

except decreased milk production and increased milk SCC. Mastitis causes considerable changes in the milk composition (Table 11.2). The milk SCC increases considerably. The quality of milk casein and whey proteins declines, which negatively affects the quality of milk products such as paneer and cheese. Due to an increase in the vascular permeability, different serum proteins such as immunoglobulins, albumin, and transferrin increase in milk. The proteolytic enzymes such as plasmin derived from somatic cells increase more than twofold and cause protein breakdown. The conductivity of the milk increases along with an increase in sodium and chloride concentration. The potassium and calcium concentrations also decline during mastitis.

The signs and symptoms vary with the nature of causative agents and severity of infections (Table 11.3).

11.3.7.6 Diagnosis of Mastitis

Clinical mastitis is easy to detect due to visible clinical signs and symptoms. The subclinical form is difficult to diagnose as it does not manifest clinical signs. The early detection of subclinical mastitis is essential not only to ensure therapeutic interventions but also to prevent the spread of infection and minimize the tissue damage. The diagnostic modalities for subclinical mastitis include cow-side tests like the California mastitis test (CMT) and laboratory tests such as somatic cell count (SCC) and milk bacteriological culture.

Cow-Sides Tests

Strip Cup Test

This test is designed to identify clinical mastitis by detecting visible particles in milk. As previously noted, mastitis leads to noticeable changes in milk composition, including discoloration, a watery texture, and the presence of clots or flakes. In this procedure, the initial few drops of milk are collected on an enamel plate divided

Table 11.3 Clinical signs of mastitis caused by different types of pathogens

Causative agents	Clinical signs
Streptococcus agalactiae	The majority of mastitis cases are subclinical, accounting for over 50% of infections. In contrast, clinical mastitis occurs less frequently, with an incidence of about 2% to 4%. When clinical signs are present, they typically include abnormal milk, which may or may not be accompanied by udder swelling. Systemic symptoms such as fever, loss of appetite, and depression are rare but can appear in the early stages of infection.
Streptococcus dysgalactiae	In contrast to *Streptococcus agalactiae, Streptococcus dysgalactiae* typically causes clinical mastitis, with symptoms confined to the affected mammary gland. The condition is characterized by abnormal milk containing clots or flakes, and may be accompanied by noticeable inflammation and swelling in the affected quarter
Streptococcus uberis	It can cause both clinical and subclinical mastitis, infecting a wide range of lactating and non-lactating. The infection initially appears in clinical form, which subsequently develops chronic subclinical form. General signs include mild illness with abnormal milk containing flakes or clots, decreased appetite, reduced rumination, lethargy, and high milk SCC
Staphylococcus aureus	In most cases, the infection remains subclinical; however, acute and recurrent episodes are also frequently observed. Spontaneous recovery from *Staphylococcus aureus*mastitis is uncommon. The affected mammary glands often suffer irreversible parenchymal damage, characterized by the formation of microabscesses and fibrosis
Coagulase-negative *staphylococci*	No visible clinical signs except elevated SCC
Mycoplasma mastitis	Mycoplasma mastitis typically presents as an acute condition characterized by a swollen, warm, and firm udder. In the early stages, the milk appears watery and contains sandy particles, which later progress to a serous discharge with clots, flakes, and pus. Common systemic signs include fever and a reduction in milk yield. In certain herds, mycoplasma mastitis may also be linked to arthritis, lameness, respiratory illness in adult cows, and pneumonia in calves
Trueperella pyogenes	Acute infection is marked by a firm or hard, painful swelling of the affected quarters. Common systemic signs include fever and loss of appetite. In sub-acute or chronic stages, the udder becomes very hard and contains thick, foul-smelling pus with a consistency similar to toothpaste
Coliform mastitis	In acute mastitis, the affected udder quarters become swollen and firm. In peracute cases, the swelling may be mild and can be obscured by the normal peri-parturient edema. The milk or secretions from the affected quarters often appear watery or resemble serum. Systemic signs may include fever, musculoskeletal injuries, laminitis, and metabolic imbalances such as hypocalcemia, hypokalemia, and lactic acidosis. In severe instances, these may progress to multi-organ failure. *Klebsiella* infections are frequently linked with endotoxemia

(continued)

Table 11.3 (continued)

Causative agents	Clinical signs
Other gram-negative bacteria	Pseudomonas species induce acute, endotoxic mastitis, which is marked by a hard and swollen udder along with blood-tinged, serum-like secretions containing clots
	Serratia liquefaciens and *Serratia marcescens* cause chronic subclinical or clinical mastitis without visible clinical signs. Secretion may be serous with clots
	Pasteurella spp. or *Mannheimia* spp. cause acute or chronic mastitis. The mammary secretion becomes thick, creamy yellow with a foul smell
Yeast mastitis	The udder develops a doughy consistency as a result of edema and mild inflammation. Since the mammary parenchyma remains unaffected in this form of mastitis, udder hardness is not observed. The milk appears watery and may contain clots or flakes
Fungal agents	Fungal mastitis is marked by subcutaneous edema of the udder and enlargement of the supramammary lymph nodes. The mammary secretions typically appear watery or clear yellow, often containing strands of cloudy material. In cases of cryptococcal mastitis, the secretions may be stringy, grayish-white, and have a mucilaginous consistency
Prototheca spp.	The subclinical form is characterized by alterations in the milk quality and increased milk SCC. The mammary secretions become watery with flakes. The chronic form is characterized by decreased milk yield and increased SCC
Clostridium perfringens type A	The typical sign of this form of mastitis is the discoloration of the udder with a crepitant appearance. It should be differentiated from gangrenous mastitis

into four strip cups with a smooth black surface. The milk is then carefully examined by tilting the cups to observe any abnormalities. The test is straightforward and can easily be performed by a layperson. In large-scale milking parlors, the floors are intentionally constructed with smooth black surfaces to allow for quick evaluation of foremilk strips.

California Mastitis Test (CMT)

CMT is one of the most reliable and rapid screening tests to detect mastitis based on the presence of somatic cells. The herd milk SCC above 400,000 cells/mL and individual cow SCC >200,000 cells/mL indicate the presence of subclinical mastitis, as specified by the European Union. The CMT qualitatively estimates the concentrations of DNA in milk as an indirect method to detect SCC in milk. The test is performed by mixing 2 mL of milk sample with 2 mL of the CMT detergent, which dissolves cell walls to release deoxyribonucleic acid (DNA) and forms DNA gels. The degree of gel formation is directly proportional to the SCC in milk. The test can be read as negative, trace, +1, +2, and + 3, which approximate SCC as per Table 11.4.

Table 11.4 Relationship between CMT score and SCC in milk

CMT score	Approximate somatic cell count
Negative	0–200,000
Trace	150,000–500,000
+1	400,000–1 million
+2	800,000–5 million
+3	>5 million

The California Mastitis Test (CMT) has a lower accuracy rate (ranging from 87.4% to 90.8%) and is less sensitive than Somatic Cell Count (SCC) analysis. However, it offers higher specificity (between 48.1% and 87.1%) compared to SCC. A notable drawback of the CMT is that it is time-consuming and not ideal for processing a large volume of samples.

Wisconsin Mastitis Test (WMT)

This test is a modified form of CMT where milk viscosity is measured after the formation of gel. Unlike CMT, the results are not approximated, but rather measured by the height of the gel in a tube and expressed in millimeters. It gives more precise results than CMT and is utilized as an on-farm or cow-side test for the detection of subclinical mastitis.

Somatic Cell Count (SCC)

Somatic cell count (SCC) is considered the gold standard for diagnosing subclinical mastitis. Somatic cells are body-derived cells comprising leukocytes (75%) and mammary epithelial cells (25%). The leukocyte population includes neutrophils, lymphocytes, and macrophages. During intramammary infections, the number of leukocytes increases, leading to elevated SCC levels. Therefore, a higher SCC is indicative of subclinical mastitis. However, SCC values can also be influenced by factors such as milk yield, parity, stage of lactation, season, breed, and physiological stress. A threshold SCC value of $\geq$200,000 cells/mL is generally recognized as indicative of subclinical infection.

Somatic cells in milk can be measured using various techniques. One method involves direct microscopic counting after removing fat with xylene and staining the cells with suitable dyes. Additionally, portable automatic cell counters are available that assess SCC using either esterase-based enzymatic reactions or by staining cell nuclei with a DNA-specific fluorescent dye like propidium iodide. These automatic counters are faster and more cost-effective, though their sensitivity decreases at lower SCC levels.

Electrical Conductivity Test

The basic principle of this test is that the electrical conductivity of milk is increased in mastitis due to increased Na^+ and Cl^- concentration and decreased in lactose and K^+ levels. The electrical conductivity is compared with an established threshold value obtained from the maximum value for each healthy quarter and time-series analysis using historical information. The electrical conductivity of normal cow's

Table 11.5 Electrical conductivity values (means ± standard errors) in milk for healthy, subclinically and clinically infected quarters

Electrical conductivity	Normal	Subclinical	Clinical
Average of the 20 highest electrical conductivity quarter values (mS/cm)	4.87 ± 0.01 (n = 10,431)	5.37 ± 0.02 (n = 2122)	6.44 ± 1.53 (n = 599)

Norberg et al. (2004)

milk ranged between 4.0 and 5.5 mS/cm (milliSiemens/centimeter) at 25 °C. A significant increase in the electrical conductivity of milk is reported in Table 11.5. The electrical conductivity can be measured by practical hand devices or by an in-line indicator in automated milking systems. The method is cheap and less time-consuming, but its usefulness is still under investigation.

Culturing

Bulk tank cultures serve as indicators of milking hygiene and are particularly valuable for identifying specific mastitis-causing organisms such as *Streptococcus agalactiae* and *Mycoplasma* species. Various culturing techniques can be applied to bulk tank milk, including the standard plate count (SPC), laboratory pasteurized count (LPC), *Mycoplasma* culturing, coliform counts, and testing for other contagious mastitis pathogens. Before collecting samples, the milk must be properly agitated and drawn using a sterile dipper to avoid contamination from environmental bacteria. SPC results from bulk tank cultures do not accurately reflect coliform levels, as milk from infected cows may be discarded or the cows may no longer produce milk. However, elevated coliform counts in bulk tank milk usually point to inadequate hygiene practices, improper milking procedures, or contamination from milking equipment. Ideally, coliform levels should remain below 50 CFU/mL. The LPC assesses the presence of heat-resistant bacteria in milk after pasteurization, and values exceeding 200 CFU/mL suggest issues with equipment sanitation. The interpretive criteria for bulk tank culturing are depicted in Table 11.6.

11.3.7.7 Treatment and Control of Mastitis

The National Institute for Research in Dairying (NIRD) has outlined a Five-Point Plan to control mastitis in dairy cows, which includes identifying and treating clinical cases, disinfecting teats after milking, implementing dry cow therapy (DCT), culling cows with chronic infections, and regularly maintaining milking equipment. However, these measures are not very effective against environmental pathogens, indicating the need to explore alternative or additional strategies for effective control.

Treatment of Clinical Cases

Antibiotics

The most common approach to treating mastitis is through the use of antimicrobials. However, identifying antibiotics that are not only effective, safe, and economical but

Table 11.6 The interpretive criteria for bulk tank culturing

Bacterial count	Normal range (cfu/mL)	Interpretive criteria
SPC	<5000	>5000 = milking system needs attention
Staphylococcus aureus	0	If detected in 2/4 bulk tank samples, suggests cows with *S.* aureus infection
Group B streptococci	0	If detected in 2/4 bulk tank samples, suggests cows with *S.* aureus infection
Enterobacterales	<50	>50 = check teat and teat end cleanliness, and check milking system cleaning
Non-enterobacterales	<200	>200 = check teat and teat end cleanliness, and check milking system cleaning
Staphylococcus sp. not aureus	<1000	>1000 = check teat end cleanliness, teat dipping, bedding, and cows with mastitis
Environmental streptococci	<1000	>1000 = check teat end cleanliness, teat dipping, bedding, and cows with mastitis
Mycoplasma	0	Growth = cows with Mycoplasma infection
Prototheca	0	Growth = cows with *Prototheca* infection

National Milk Council (2020)

Table 11.7 Targeted routes for antimicrobial therapy in mastitis

Causative agents	Milk/ducts	Udder tissue	Cow
Streptococcus agalactiae	+++	–	–
Other streptococci	+++	+	–
Staphylococcus aureus	+	+++	–
Coagulase-negative staphylococci	+++	–	–
Arcanobacterium pyogenes (summer mastitis)	–	++	+++
Coliforms	+	–	+++

Erskine (2003)

also pose minimal risk to public health remains a challenge. A major limitation in treating intramammary infections with antibiotics—whether administered parenterally or via intramammary (IMM) infusion (Table 11.7)—is the ability of the drug to adequately penetrate the udder tissue. The pharmacokinetic characteristics of antibiotics, such as lipid solubility, ionization rate, binding affinity to serum or udder proteins, and the type of carrier used, play a crucial role in their effectiveness. Additionally, the pharmacodynamic properties, particularly the degree to which milk interferes with drug activity, must be taken into account. For instance, the efficacy of antibiotics like tetracyclines, macrolides, and trimethoprim-sulphonamides is known to diminish in the presence of milk. Therefore, ideal antibiotics for mastitis treatment should have a low minimum inhibitory concentration (MIC) against the causative pathogens.

Table 11.8 Food and Drug Administration–approved intramammary antibiotics for lactating dairy cattle

Active ingredient	Drug type	Milk withholding time (hr)	Meat withholding time (days)	Frequency of treatments and number of treatments
Amoxicillin	Prescription	60	12	q12 hr/3
Ceftiofur hydrochloride	Prescription	72	2	q24 hr/2–8
Cephapirin	Over the counter	96	4	q12 hr/2
Cloxacillin	Prescription	48	10	Hetacillin
Hetacillin	Prescription	72	10	q24 hr/3
Penicillin G	Over the counter	60	3	q12 hr/3
Pirlimycin	Prescription	36	9	q24 hr/2–8

Table 11.9 Food and Drug Administration–approved injectable antibiotics for mastitis in lactating dairy cattle

Active ingredient	Drug type	Milk withhold time (hr)	Meat withhold time (days)	Dose
Ampicillin trihydrate	Prescription	48	6	2–5 mg/lb. body weight once daily (not to exceed 7 days)
Ceftiofur crystalline-free acid	Prescription	None	13	1.5 mL/100 lb. body weight SC at base of ear
Ceftiofur hydrochloride	Prescription	None	4	0.5–1.0 mg/lb. body weight for 3 to 5 days SC
Ceftiofur sodium	Prescription	None	4	0.5–1.0 mg/lb. body weight for 3–5 days IM
Oxytetracycline	Over the counter	96	28	Doses and routes of administration vary with formulations
Penicillin G	Over the counter	48	4–10	3000 units/lb. body weight

Another important aspect of mastitis therapy is the route of administration of drugs. Some studies showed that the route of therapy should be planned according to the degree of penetration of the causative agents into the mammary gland. The intramammary route is usually preferred because it ensures high concentrations of the drugs, particularly into the infected quarters, thus reducing low consumption.

Food and Drug Administration–approved intramammary and injectable antibiotics for lactating dairy cattle are presented in Tables 11.8 and 11.9.

In recent years, antimicrobial resistance has been a matter of great concern. The studies have confirmed that nearly 62% of mastitis-causing pathogens are resistant to at least one antibiotic. The highest levels of resistance have been observed against streptomycin, cephalexin, neomycin, and penicillin. The condition is more severe in the case of *Str. agalactiae* where 100% isolates were resistant to at least one antibiotic (amoxicillin, cloxacillin, penicillin, cephalexin, ceftiofur, tetracycline, streptomycin, neomycin, lincomycin, rifaximin, sulfamethoxazole/trimethoprim, and enrofloxacin). Similar reports were found in 86% of *Str. uberis* and 79% of *E. coli* isolates.

Alternative therapy for mastitis other than the use of antibiotics is the need of the hour to reduce antimicrobial resistance and to combat public health issues.

Plant-Derived Compounds

Different plant-derived bioactive compounds have been shown to exert antimicrobial and anti-inflammatory effects by different pathways. They have advantages over antibiotics in terms of minimal resistance, even after prolonged use and limited toxicity. Different plant-derived anti-inflammatory and antimicrobial compounds, along with the mechanism, are summarized in Table 11.10.

Plant-derived essential oils are also reported to act as antimicrobial agents against *Staph. aureus, Staph. chromogenes, Staph. warneri, Staph. xylosus*, and *E. coli* (Table 11.11).

Table 11.10 Plant-derived anti-inflammatory and antimicrobial compounds

Compounds	Mechanism of action	References
Baicalein	Anti-inflammatory	He et al. (2015)
Baicalin	Inhibits apoptosis	Guo et al. (2014)
Thymol	Inhibits *Staph. aureus* internalization	
Citral and linalool	Inhibits *Staph. aureus* growth and biofilm formation	Federman et al. (2016)
Limonene	Antimicrobial activity against *Strep. uberis*	Wei et al. (2014)
Liquidambar orientalis leaf extracts	Antimicrobial activity against *Staph. aureus* and coagulase negative stapylococci	Ökmen et al. (2017)
Thalictrum minus root extract	Antimicrobial activity against *Staph. xylosus, Staph. lentus, Staph. equorum, Enterococcus faecalis,* and *Pantoea agglomerans*	Mushtaq et al. (2016)
Terminalia chebula fruit extracts	Antimicrobial activity against *Staph. aureus, E. coli, Pseudomonas aeruginosa*, and *Bacillus megaterium*	Kher et al. (2019)

Table 11.11 Plant-derived essential oils against mastitis-causing pathogens

Origin of essential oil	Mechanism of action	References
Satureja montana L., *Thymus vulgaris* L. ct. thymol, and *Origanum majorana* L.	Antimicrobial activity against *Staph. aureus*	Fratini et al. (2014)
Origanum vulgare and *Leptospermum scoparium*	Antimicrobial activity against *Staph. aureus, Staph. chromogenes, Staph. warneri, Staph. xylosus* and *E. coli*	Fratini et al. (2017)
Origanum vulgare	Inhibits *Staph. aureus* and *E. coli*	Cho et al. (2015)
Valencia orange	Inhibits *Staph. aureus* growth and biofilm formation	Federman et al. (2016)
Minthostachys verticillata and Citrus	Antimicrobial activity against *Strep. uberis*	Montironi et al. (2016)
Minthostachys verticillata	Antimicrobial activity against *Staph. aureus, Staph. epidermidis, Staph. hyicus, Staph. xylosus*, and *E. coli*	Montironi et al. (2019)

Animal-Derived Products

Some animal-derived compounds have also been shown to induce anti-inflammatory and antimicrobial properties. Melittin and propolis are the active compounds of bee venom was reported to have anti-inflammatory properties by suppressing cyclooxygenase-2 (COX-2) protein and pro-inflammatory cytokines like TNF-α and IL-6. Immunomodulators such as lactoferrin can also be used as non-antibiotic antimicrobial agents to treat mastitis in cows. Lactic acid bacteria (LAB) of the *Lactobacillus* and *Bifidobacterium* genera isolated from honey were reported as new antibacterial agents. Intramammary infusion of probiotics like *Lactococcus lactis* subp. Lactis CRL 1655 and *L. perolens* CRL 1724 have the ability to adhere to the teat canal, thus preventing mastitis during the dry period. Another antimicrobial peptide, bacteriocins, produced by bacteria has shown promising results against mastitis in cows. Bacteriophages and their derivatives, such as endolysin, exolysin, and depolymerase, can also be used as an alternative to antibiotics.

Vaccination

The development of a vaccine against mastitis is difficult, as mastitis involves multiple etiological factors. Some experimental studies have been conducted to develop vaccines against *Staph. aureus*, *Strep. agalactiae*, and *E. coli*. The vaccines for *Staph. aureus* and *Strep. agalactiae* utilize either the whole organisms (attenuated vaccines, inactivated high encapsulated or unencapsulated cells) or sub-units (polysaccharides, toxins, surface extract). For *E coli* mutant core antigen, J5 was used for the preparation of vaccines.

Disinfecting Teats After Milking

The teat disinfection is one of the important preventive measures to control mastitis for a long time. The teat disinfection can be done either pre-milking or post-milking. Pre-milking teat disinfection is effective against environmental mastitis (*Strep uberis*), whereas post-milking teat disinfection controls contagious mastitis (*Staph aureus*). Teat disinfection can be done either by teat dipping using a cup or by spraying disinfectant from below. There are several compounds available for teat disinfection, such as iodine, chlorhexidine, hydrolyzed fatty acids, quaternary ammonium compounds, hypochlorite, and acid anionic compounds. Emollients such as glycerine, sorbitol, lanolin, and propylene glycol are added with disinfectants to improve skin health.

Dry Cow Therapy

The dry period is characterized by a series of changes in the mammary gland, which influences the immune function of the udder. High concentration of lactoferrin and leukocyte infiltration in the udder during the dry period decreases the chances of clinical mastitis, but subclinical infections are 10 times more common in lactating animals, and the most common pathogens are *E. coli* or *Strep. uberis.* Dry cow therapy refers to the application of an intramammary antibiotic immediately after the last milking of lactation to control the occurrence of mastitis during the dry period. These intramammary antimicrobial preparations eliminate existing Gram-positive bacteria, particularly *Staphylococcus aureus* and streptococcal infections, and also prevent new infections during the early dry period. However, these products are less effective against Gram-negative environmental bacteria such as coliforms. Internal sealant infusions are another effective method for dry cow therapy. In this process, the teat canal is sealed by natural keratin plug throughout the dry period to prevent new intramammary infections. The artificial teat sealants are also available alone or in combination with antibiotic infusion. The artificial teat sealant without antibiotic infusion is recommended only in an uninfected quarter. The external teat sealant can also be applied by dipping the teat. However, they don't have long-lasting protection.

Knowledge Corner...

Treatment with allogeneic mesenchymal stem cells (MSCs) led to a decrease in the overall bacterial count, including *Staphylococcus aureus* and bacteria from the *Enterobacteriaceae* family, along with a consistent reduction in somatic cell count (SCC) in milk. The therapeutic effect was obtained through either combined intravenous and intramammary administration or intramammary administration alone.

11.4 Traumatic and Structural Disorders

11.4.1 Laceration of the Bovine Udder

This is the traumatic injury caused by barbed wire, thorns, or a cow's own hooves. These injuries are characterized by superficial to deep wounds affecting the teat canal and increasing the chance of mastitis. Immediate therapeutic interventions are recommended for proper prognosis. Proper cleaning with antiseptic lotion and application of topical antibiotics are recommended for a superficial wound. In the case of deeper wounds, atraumatic manipulation of the wound is usually recommended to reconstruct the tissue with small-diameter absorbable suture material. Proper antibiotic and anti-inflammatory preparations should be applied along with a fly repellent. The hand milking should be restricted for 10 days to ensure proper healing. Ultrasound evaluation can be applied to find out internal injury. The compression and ligation are recommended for severe hemorrhage in large vein lacerations.

11.4.2 Teat Obstructions (Teat Stenosis)

This condition is characterized by narrowing of the streak canal. It usually occurs due to swelling, clots, or scab formation. In some cases, granulation tissue following injury may result in milk flow obstruction, commonly referred to as "teat peas.". Intermittent milk flow obstruction can occur due to the presence of small masses or the accumulation of butterfat and minerals within the milk ducts. Lactoliths (milk stones) may form in milk rich in minerals and can also interfere with normal milk flow.

These obstructions may be removed using a teat cannula inserted through the streak canal; however, this procedure increases the risk of mastitis. Membranous obstructions are particularly difficult to treat.

11.4.3 Breakdown of Udder Support Apparatus

The suspensory apparatus of the udder includes lateral and medial suspensory ligaments. Any stretch or rupture of these supporting structures results in a pendulous udder along with a hematoma between the forequarters and the ventral body wall. The teat displacement and udder engorgement result in difficulty during milking. Rupture of the supporting structures is generally incurable.

11.4.4 Hemolactia (Blood in Milk)

The presence of blood in milk may result from several causes. Blood-tinged milk is commonly observed soon after calving in freshly calved cows due to the passage of blood cells from capillaries into mammary tissue during diapedesis. However, if it persists more than two weeks, it may be considered as hemolactia. Common causes include trauma or injury to the udder, such as bruising from the hind limbs due to an abnormal gait, udder oedema, a pendulous udder being kicked by the legs, or rupture of the anterior udder ligaments. Hemolactia is characterized by milk tinged with blood clots or fresh blood coming from all four quarters, often leading to the discarding of large quantities of milk. The hemorrhage from the major veins results in dark brown mammary secretions like venous blood without clotting properties. Systemic infections caused by some bacteria (*Leptospira* spp., *Serratia marcescens*, *Micrococcus cerasinus*, *Lactorubefaciens gruber*, *Brevibacterium erythrogenes*), viruses, and red yeast (*Monascus purpureus*) may cause intravascular hemolysis, resulting in blood in milk. The ingestion of certain plants—particularly those belonging to the family Rubiaceae—moldy sweet clover causing dicoumarin poisoning, *Euphorbia*, and shave grass containing red pigments, may also lead to reddish discoloration of milk. Thrombocytopenia and deficiency of vitamin C also result in hemolactia. The therapeutic management of hemolactia includes administration of intravenous calcium borogluconate, magnesium, and phosphorus (300–450 ml) as a coagulant. Parenteral (tranexamic acid, adrenochrome monosemicarbazone) and intramammary (adrenaline) infusion of coagulants also give good results. Vasoconstrictors such as adrenaline, ergot alkaloids (ergonovine maleate), or methylergometrine hydrogen maleate can also be applied locally or through the parenteral route. Antibiotics such as lincomycin and spiramycin can also be applied if the hemolactia is of infectious origin. In cases of leptospiral infection, streptomycin (25 mg/kg b.wt. intramuscular for 3–5 days) is the drug of choice. Supplementary therapy includes vitamin C and antioxidants.

11.4.5 Teat Sphincter Inadequacy ("Leakers" or Incontinentia Lactis)

This condition usually occurs in high-producing cows with a small udder cistern. When the udder cistern is full, milk leakage may occur due to the inability of the teat sphincter to close the teat meatus tightly. Predisposing factors for teat sphincter inadequacy include a high milk flow rate, short teats, and inverted teat ends. Cows that leak milk are more prone to mastitis. The condition is generally incurable, and culling of affected cows from the herd is often recommended.

Knowledge Corner...

In the future, bioengineering techniques could be utilized to restore mammary gland function. Among the various strategies in tissue bioengineering, the decellularized extracellular matrix (dECM) is particularly promising, as it supports cell proliferation, migration, and differentiation. The dECM is produced by removing cellular material from an organ while retaining the extracellular matrix (ECM) components. Because its structure and biomechanical characteristics closely resemble those of the native organ, it serves as an excellent biomaterial for replicating natural tissue and providing essential biochemical and physical cues for new cell growth and tissue integration.

Exercises

Objective Questions

1. The supernumerary teats should be at the age of ________________ in cows.
2. Cows suffering from udder edema have 17% higher mammary blood flow. (True/False).
3. Premature symmetrical development results from chronic stimulation of _____________ hormone.
4. The complete loss of milk production in a lactating animal is called ___________________.
5. MMA syndrome is most common in ______________________ species.
6. Spontaneous milk flow irrespective of pregnancy and lactation is called ________________________.
7. Teat warts are caused by various strains of ________________ viruses.
8. *Fusobacterium necrophorum* is the causative agent for ______________________.
9. The discoloration of the udder with a crepitant appearance is seen in ______________________ infection.
10. Somatic cells are body-derived cells comprising ______________ % leukocytes and _______________ % mammary epithelial cells.
11. Red yeast (*Monascus purpureus*) causes intravascular hemolysis that results in _________________.

Subjective Questions

1. Write in brief about the alternative therapy of mastitis to combat antibiotic resistance.
2. Write down the pathophysiology of udder edema.

3. Write down the diagnostic modalities of mastitis in cows.
4. Describe in details about dry cow therapy to prevent mastitis.

Answers to Objective Questions

1. Two to six weeks
2. False
3. Estrogen
4. Agalactia
5. Sow
6. Galactorrhea
7. Papovaviruses
8. Udder cleft dermatitis
9. *Clostridium perfringens* Type A
10. 75%, 25%
11. Hemolactia

References

Books

National Mastitis Council (1996) Current concepts of bovine mastitis, 4th edn, Arlington

National Milk Council (2020) Laboratory Handbook on Bovine Mastitis, 3rd edn

Research Articles

Cho B-W, Cha C-N, Lee S-M, Kim M-J, Park J-Y, Yoo C-Y, Son S-E, Kim S, Lee H-J. (2015). Therapeutic effect of ore gano essential oil on subclinical bovine mastitis caused by *Staphylococcus aureus* and *Escherichia coli*. Korean J Vet Res 2015;55:253–257 https://doi.org/10.14405/kjvr.2015.55.4.253

Erskine RJ (2003) Antibacterial therapy of clinical mastitis –part I. Drug selection. Part II Administration. North Am Vet Conf, Proc, pp 13–16

Federman C, Ma C, Biswas D (2016) Major components of orange oil inhibit Staphylococcus aureus growth and biofilm forma tion, and alter its virulence factors. J Med Microbiol 65:688–695. https://doi.org/10.1099/jmm.0.000286

Fratini F, Casella S, Leonardi M, Pisseri F, Ebani VV, Pistelli L, Pistelli L (2014) Antibacterial activity of essential oils, their blends and mixtures of their main constituents against some strains supporting livestock mastitis. Fitoterapia 96:1–7. https://doi.org/10.1016/j.fitote.2014.04.003

Fratini F, Mancini S, Turchi B, Friscia E, Pistelli L, Giusti G, Cerri D (2017) A novel interpretation of the fractional inhibitory concentration index: the case Origanum vulgare L. and Leptospermum scoparium J. R. et G. Forst essential oils against Staphylococcus aureus strains. Microbiol Res 195:11–17. https://doi.org/10.1016/j.micres.2016.11.005

Guo M, Cao Y, Wang T, Song X, Liu Z, Zhou E, Deng X, Zhang N, Yang Z (2014) Baicalin inhibits Staphylococcus aureus-induced apoptosis by regulating TLR2 and TLR2 related apoptotic factors in the mouse mammary glands. Eur J Pharmacol 723:481–488. https://doi.org/10.1016/j.ejphar.2013.10.032

He X, Wei Z, Zhou E, Chen L, Kou J, Wang J, Yang Z (2015) Baicalein attenuates inflammatory responses by suppressing TLR4 mediated NF-κB and MAPK signalling pathways in LPS-induced mastitis in mice. Int Immunopharmacol 28:470–476. https://doi.org/10.1016/j.intimp.2015.07.012

Kher MN, Sheth NR, Bhatt VD (2019) In vitro antibacterial evaluation of Terminalia chebula as an alternative of antibiotics against bovine subclinical mastitis. Anim Biotechnol 30:151–158. https://doi.org/10.1080/10495398.2018.1451752

Montironi ID, Cariddi LN, Reinoso EB (2016) Evaluation of the antimicrobial efficacy of Minthostachys verticillata essential oil and limonene against Streptococcus uberis strains isolated from bovine mastitis. Rev Argent Microbiol 48:210–216. https://doi.org/10.1016/j.ram.2016.04.005

Montironi ID, Reinoso EB, Paullier VC, Inés Siri M, Pianzzola MJ, Moliva Melina, Campra N, Bagnis G, LaRocque-de-Freitas IF, Decote-Ricardo D, Freire-de-Lima CG, Raviolo JM, Cariddi LN. (2019). *Minthostachys verticillata* essential oil activates macrophage phagocytosis and modulates the innate immune response in a murine model of *Enterococcus faecium* mastitis. Res Vet Sci 125: 333–44. https://doi.org/10.1016/j.rvsc.2019.07.015

Mushtaq S, Rather MA, Qazi PH, Aga MA, Shah AM, Shah A, Ali MN (2016) Isolation and characterization of three benzylisoquinoline alkaloids from Thalictrum minus L. and their antibacterial activity against bovine mastitis. J Ethnopharmacol 193:221–226. https://doi.org/10.1016/j.jep.2016.07.040

Norberg E, Hogeveen H, Korsgaard IR, Friggens NC, Sloth KHMN, Løvendahl P (2004) Electrical conductivity of milk: ability to predict mastitis status. J Dairy Sci 87(4):1099–1107

Ökmen G, Cantekin Z, Alam MI, Türkcan O, Ergün Y (2017) Anti bacterial and antioxidant activities of Liquidambar orientalis mill. Various extracts against bacterial pathogens causing mastitis. Turkish J Agric-Food Sci Technol 5:883–887. https://doi.org/10.24925/turjaf.v5i8.883-887.1163

Wei Z, Zhou E, Guo C, Fu Y, Yu Y, Li Y, Yao M, Zhang N, Yang Z (2014) Thymol inhibits Staphylococcus aureus internalization into bovine mammary epithelial cells by inhibiting NF-κB activation. Microb Pathog 71:15–19. https://doi.org/10.1016/j.micpath.2014.01.004

Biotechnological Interventions to Augment Milk Production 12

Contents

J. Mukherjee et al., *Veterinary Lactation Physiology*,
https://doi.org/10.1007/978-3-032-21123-1_12

Abstract

Milk is an essential food of high biological value. The global demand for milk and dairy products continues to rise, while the resources available for animal rearing remain limited. Conventional methods of breeding, feeding, and management have improved milk production but are now reaching a plateau. Biotechnology provides modern scientific tools that help to increase milk yield, improve quality, and ensure sustainability in dairy farming. Advances in molecular genetics, genomics, and reproductive biology have transformed dairy science. Marker-assisted selection, genomic selection, and genome editing techniques such as CRISPR/Cas9 allow precise improvement of traits related to milk yield, composition, and disease resistance. Reproductive biotechnologies, including artificial insemination, embryo transfer, in vitro fertilization, and sexed semen, enable rapid multiplication of superior germplasm. Nutritional biotechnology focuses on nutrigenomics, probiotics, and enzyme supplementation to enhance nutrient utilization and reduce methane emissions. Molecular and hormonal interventions such as recombinant bovine somatotropin (rBST), growth hormone-releasing factors, and oxytocin analogs further support efficient milk synthesis. Recent innovations in mammary gland biology, stem cell research, and omics-based tools have deepened the understanding of lactation control. Digital technologies such as biosensors, precision dairy systems, and artificial intelligence now integrate biotechnological data into farm management. These approaches together improve productivity, animal health, and economic returns. Although biotechnology offers great promise, it must be used with care to address bioethical, environmental, and welfare concerns.

Graphical Abstract

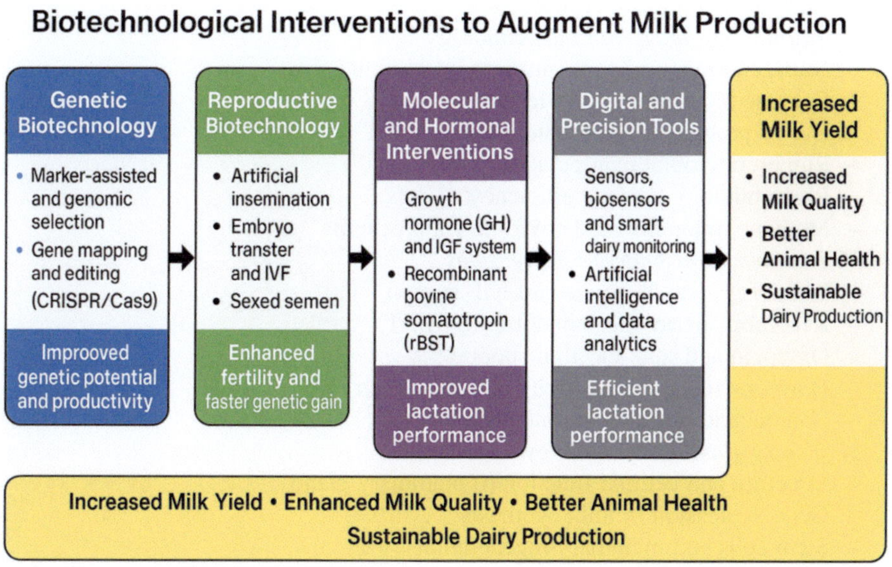

Description of the graphic: Biotechnology enhances dairy farming by improving milk yield, quality and sustainability through advanced tools. Techniques like marker-assisted and genomic selection, along with CRISPR/Cas9, enable precise genetic improvement. Reproductive technologies such as artificial insemination, embryo transfer, IVF and sexed semen accelerate multiplication of superior animals. Nutritional approaches including nutrigenomics, probiotics and enzymes improve feed efficiency and reduce methane emission. Hormonal and molecular tools like rBST and oxytocin analogs further support efficient milk production

Keywords

Biotechnology · Milk production · Genomic selection · Reproductive biotechnology · Nutrigenomics · Recombinant hormones · Precision dairy farming · Sustainability

Inside the Chapter

- *Genetic improvement*
  - Marker-assisted selection
  - Genomic selection
  - Gene mapping and QTL analysis
  - Genetic engineering and transgenic animals
  - Genome editing (CRISPR/Cas9)
  - Cloning and conservation of elite animals
- *Reproductive biotechnology*
  - Artificial insemination
  - Embryo transfer technology
  - In Vitro fertilization

  - Oocyte maturation and cryopreservation
  - Sexed semen
  - Hormonal control of reproduction
- *Nutritional and microbial biotechnology*
  - Nutrigenomics and gene–nutrient interaction
  - Enzyme biotechnology in feed utilization
  - Use of probiotics and prebiotics
  - Rumen microbial manipulation
  - Biotechnology for feed efficiency
  - Methane mitigation and environmental benefits
- *Molecular and hormonal interventions*
  - Role of growth hormone and IGF system
  - Recombinant bovine somatotropin (rBST)
  - Oxytocin and milk ejection support
  - Hormone receptor sensitivity and regulation
  - Nanotechnology in hormone delivery
- *Mammary gland biotechnology*
  - Structure and cellular function of mammary gland
  - Gene expression in milk synthesis
  - Stem cells and mammary regeneration
  - Molecular regulation of lactation genes
  - Genetic control of milk protein synthesis
- *Diagnostic and monitoring tools*
  - Biomarkers of milk yield and quality
  - Proteomics and metabolomics in dairy science
  - Biosensors and rapid detection kits
  - Molecular diagnosis of mastitis
  - Smart dairy monitoring systems

Learning Objectives
- Application of biotechnology to enhance milk yield and genetic potential in dairy animals.
- Understanding of reproductive, nutritional, microbial, molecular, and hormonal interventions in dairy production.
- Identify modern diagnostic, monitoring, and digital tools in dairy systems.
- Assessment of ethical, economic, and environmental impacts of dairy biotechnology.
- Evaluate emerging technologies and future challenges in dairy biotechnology.

Milk is an important source of food for humans. It gives protein, fat, sugar, minerals, and vitamins that are needed for growth and health. The demand for milk and milk products is rising day by day. Population growth, urban life, and better living standards have increased milk consumption. Traditional breeding, feeding, and management practices helped to improve milk production in the past. However, these methods are now slow and not enough to meet the present demand. Limited land, feed shortage, and diseases reduce milk yield in many countries.

Biotechnology gives new and powerful tools to solve these problems. It uses the science of biology, genetic and molecular techniques to improve animals, feeds, and farm management. It helps to make dairy farming more productive, profitable, and environmentally friendly. Biotechnology offers many useful solutions for improving milk production. Genetic biotechnology helps to select animals with better milk-producing genes using marker-assisted and genomic selection. Reproductive biotechnology, such as artificial insemination, embryo transfer, and in vitro fertilization, allows faster multiplication of elite animals. Nutritional biotechnology uses enzymes, probiotics, and nutrigenomics to improve digestion and feed use. Molecular and hormonal biotechnology applies growth hormones, recombinant proteins, and oxytocin to improve milk secretion and let-down. Digital and precision technologies use sensors and computer data to monitor animal health and milk yield in real time. Together, these methods increase milk yield, improve quality, reduce disease, and make dairy farming more sustainable.

12.1 Genetic Improvement

Genetic improvement means changing or improving the genetic makeup of animals to make them more productive and efficient. In dairy science, it focuses mainly on improving milk yield, milk composition, udder health, and disease resistance. The genetic potential of an animal is controlled by many genes that are passed from one generation to the next. Biotechnology provides advanced tools to identify, test, and select these genes accurately. Traditional breeding programs take many years to achieve progress because animals must reach maturity before their performance can be measured. Modern genetic technologies reduce this time by allowing early selection, more precise prediction, and faster multiplication of superior animals. Genetic improvement through biotechnology combines molecular biology, genomics, and reproductive techniques. It ensures that the next generation of dairy animals carries the best possible genes for high milk yield, efficient feed use, and better adaptability.

Knowledge Corner...
In 2008, genomic selection was first implemented in Holstein cattle breeding programs in the United States and Europe. It reduced the generation interval from 5–6 years to about 2–3 years and dramatically increased the accuracy of predicting milk production traits.

12.1.1 Marker-Assisted Selection (MAS)

Marker-assisted selection (MAS) is one of the earliest applications of biotechnology in animal breeding. It uses genetic marker-specific segments of DNA that are closely linked to important traits such as milk yield, fat percentage and protein percentage, fertility, and disease resistance. Each animal carries a unique set of DNA markers, like a genetic fingerprint. Scientists identify which markers are associated with desirable traits. Once these markers are known, animals carrying them can be selected for breeding without waiting for them to complete a lactation cycle. The process begins with the collection of biological samples, such as blood, hair, or tissue, from individual animals. DNA is then extracted from these samples, and specific genetic markers are identified using molecular techniques like Polymerase Chain Reaction (PCR) or DNA sequencing. These genetic profiles are compared with production records to identify associations between particular markers and desirable traits, such as milk yield, disease resistance, or fertility. Animals carrying favorable markers are subsequently selected for breeding, accelerating genetic improvement by targeting specific traits more efficiently than conventional selection methods. Marker-assisted selection is faster and more accurate than traditional selection. It increases the rate of genetic progress, especially for traits that are hard to measure like disease resistance or fertility. In many countries, MAS has been used successfully to improve milk protein content and mastitis resistance in cattle and buffalo breeds.

12.1.2 Genomic Selection

Genomic selection is an advanced form of marker-based breeding that studies the entire genome instead of a few markers. The complete set of genes (DNA) in an animal is called the genome. This method uses thousands of Single Nucleotide Polymorphisms (SNPs)-tiny variations in DNA to estimate an animal's genetic potential for multiple traits. Using genomic selection, scientists calculate a Genomic Estimated Breeding Value (GEBV) for each animal. This value predicts how well the animal will perform in milk yield, fat percentage, and health traits of animals. The process begins with the establishment of a reference population, consisting of a large number of animals with both detailed performance records and genotypic data. Statistical models are then applied to analyze the relationship between genetic markers and traits of interest, such as milk yield, fertility, or disease resistance. Using these models, genomic estimated breeding values (GEBVs) are predicted for young animals that have only genotype data, without needing full performance records. Finally, animals with high GEBVs are selected as breeding parents, enabling faster and more accurate genetic improvement compared to traditional selection methods. Genomic selection helps to shorten the generation interval from 5–6 years to about 2–3 years. It allows selection of the best young bulls and heifers even before they start producing. It also reduces the cost of progeny testing and improves accuracy for low-heritability traits like fertility and health. Many dairy breeding programs worldwide, such as Holstein genomic evaluation, have adopted this system, leading to rapid improvement in milk yield and udder health.

12.1.3 Gene Mapping and Quantitative Trait Loci (QTL) Analysis

Many traits in dairy animals, like milk yield, fat percentage, and somatic cell count, are quantitative traits. They are controlled by many genes, each contributing a small effect. The regions on chromosomes that influence such traits are called Quantitative Trait Loci (QTL). QTL mapping helps researchers locate and identify these important regions on the genome. Once these areas are mapped, the information can be used to select animals carrying beneficial alleles (gene variants). Quantitative trait locus (QTL) mapping is a genetic approach used to identify genomic regions associated with economically important traits in dairy animals. The process starts with collecting data from animals with well-documented performance records. DNA markers, which are distributed across the genome, are then identified and analyzed. Statistical methods are used to find associations between specific markers and the traits of interest. Finally, regions of the genome, known as QTLs, that are linked to desirable traits—such as high milk yield, improved milk composition, or enhanced disease resistance—are located, providing targets for marker-assisted selection and genetic improvement programs. For example, QTLs have been identified on chromosome 14 for milk fat and chromosome 6 for protein content in Holstein cows. QTL information helps in designing better selection programs and developing commercial genetic tests. It also provides insights into the biological pathways that control milk production.

12.1.4 Genetic Engineering and Transgenic Animals

Genetic engineering allows scientists to directly modify or introduce genes into an animal's genome. The goal is to add useful genes or improve existing ones to achieve better performance or disease resistance. Animals that carry and express these new genes are called transgenic animals. In dairy science, transgenic approaches are employed to enhance milk quality, animal health, and overall productivity. These techniques enable the production of milk with improved nutritional profiles, such as higher levels of casein or essential fatty acids, benefiting both processing properties and human nutrition. Transgenic animals can also produce milk containing bioactive human proteins, including lysozyme or lactoferrin, which have antimicrobial and health-promoting effects. Additionally, transgenic strategies are used to develop disease-resistant animals—for example, cows engineered to secrete antibacterial proteins in milk that reduce the risk of mastitis—thereby improving udder health and reducing reliance on antibiotics. A well-known example is the production of transgenic goats that secrete human antithrombin in milk, which is used as a medicine for preventing blood clots. Similarly, research in cattle aims to express lactoferrin or lysozyme in milk to enhance its antibacterial activity. However, the use of transgenic animals requires strict ethical and safety controls. Regulatory authorities evaluate the safety of food derived from such animals before commercial approval. Despite these concerns, transgenic research provides valuable models for studying mammary gland function and milk protein regulation.

12.1.5 Genome Editing (CRISPR/Cas9 and Other Tools)

Genome editing is a more precise and controlled version of genetic engineering. It allows scientists to make exact, small changes in an animal's DNA without adding foreign genes. The most widely used genome-editing system is CRISPR/Cas9 (Clustered Regularly Interspaced Short Palindromic Repeats). It works like molecular scissors that cut DNA at specific sites, allowing targeted modification of genes. Genome editing has significant applications in improving dairy animal productivity, health, and adaptability. It can be used to increase milk yield by modifying genes that regulate mammary gland development and milk synthesis. Fat and protein composition of milk can be enhanced through targeted gene edits, improving its nutritional and processing quality. Genome editing also enables the creation of mastitis-resistant cows by altering genes involved in immune response, reducing disease incidence and antibiotic use. Additionally, genetic modifications can enhance heat and stress tolerance, which is particularly valuable for maintaining productivity in tropical and challenging environmental conditions. Compared to traditional genetic engineering, genome editing is faster, cheaper, and more acceptable because it does not always involve foreign DNA. Research is ongoing to apply genome editing in cattle and buffaloes to improve productivity and adaptability to changing climates. However, ethical, legal, and consumer acceptance issues must be considered before using genome-edited animals for food production.

12.1.6 Cloning and Conservation of Elite Animals

Cloning is a technique used to produce genetically identical animals. It helps to preserve and multiply elite individuals that have high milk yield, excellent conformation, and disease resistance. The most common method of cloning is Somatic Cell Nuclear Transfer (SCNT). In this process, the nucleus from a somatic (body) cell of a genetically superior animal is first extracted. This nucleus is then transferred into an enucleated egg cell, which has had its own nucleus removed. The reconstructed egg is stimulated to begin cell division and develop into an embryo. Once the embryo reaches an appropriate stage, it is implanted into a surrogate mother, resulting in the birth of a clone that is genetically identical to the original donor animal. Cloning allows the rapid multiplication of superior germplasm without losing genetic quality. It is used in cattle, buffalo, sheep, and goats. Apart from SCNT, cryopreservation of semen, embryos, and oocytes is another important biotechnology for conserving valuable breeds. It allows long-term storage of genetic material in gene banks for use in future breeding programs. Although cloning is still expensive and has lower success rates, it is a powerful tool for breed conservation and genetic security. Ethical considerations regarding animal welfare must be respected in all cloning programs.

Knowledge Corner...
Cloning of the sheep Dolly in 1996 marked a revolution in animal biotechnology. The same technique—somatic cell nuclear transfer (SCNT)—is now used in elite dairy cattle and goats to preserve valuable genetics and study lactation biology in identical animals.

12.2 Reproductive Biotechnology

Reproductive biotechnology includes scientific methods that help to control, improve, and speed up the reproductive process in dairy animals. The main aim is to produce more calves from genetically superior parents and to maintain good fertility in the herd. Reproductive biotechnology plays a key role in improving milk production because reproduction is directly linked to lactation. Without regular calving, the cow or buffalo cannot continue to produce milk efficiently. Modern reproductive technologies combine physiology, endocrinology, and molecular biology to improve reproductive performance and shorten the generation interval. These techniques also help in conserving valuable breeds and in producing disease-free animals.

12.2.1 Artificial Insemination (AI)

Artificial insemination is the most common and oldest reproductive biotechnology used in dairy animals. It means placing semen from a selected bull into the reproductive tract of a female animal at the right time of estrus using an artificial insemination gun. Artificial insemination (AI) offers several important advantages in dairy and livestock production. It enables the extensive use of semen from genetically superior bulls, allowing their desirable traits to be disseminated to a large number of females across different herds and regions, thereby accelerating genetic improvement. AI significantly reduces the cost and management challenges associated with maintaining breeding bulls on farms, including expenses related to housing, feeding, health care, and handling. It also plays a crucial role in preventing the transmission of sexually transmitted and other contagious reproductive diseases, as semen is collected, processed, and distributed under hygienic and controlled conditions. In addition, AI facilitates accurate record keeping and effective control of breeding activities, as details related to insemination, pedigree, fertility, and calving can be systematically documented, supporting better reproductive management and herd improvement programs. AI requires proper heat detection and timing. In cow, the best time for insemination is about 12 h after the animal shows standing heat. Semen used in AI can be fresh or frozen. Cryopreservation allows long-term storage of semen at -196 °C in liquid nitrogen. This helps in the transport and use of semen across different regions and even countries.

12.2.2 Embryo Transfer Technology (ETT)

Embryo transfer technology allows the transfer of fertilized embryos from a superior female (donor) to another female (recipient). The donor cow is given hormones to produce multiple eggs (superovulation). After insemination, the fertilized embryos are collected from her uterus after 7 days and placed into synchronized recipient cows. Embryo transfer technology (ETT) involves a series of well-defined steps aimed at maximizing genetic gain in dairy and livestock production. The process begins with the careful selection of a genetically superior donor female and healthy recipient animals with normal reproductive status. The donor is then subjected to hormonal treatment to induce superovulation, stimulating the development and ovulation of multiple follicles instead of a single ovum. Following superovulation, the donor cow is artificially inseminated using semen from a genetically elite bull to ensure high genetic merit of the resulting embryos. After fertilization, embryos are collected from the uterus of the donor by a nonsurgical flushing technique at an appropriate stage of development. The recovered embryos are subsequently examined under a microscope for evaluation and grading based on their morphological quality and viability. Finally, good-quality embryos are transferred into synchronized recipient females whose estrous cycles are matched with the developmental stage of the embryos, allowing normal implantation, pregnancy establishment, and successful calving. Embryo transfer technology (ETT) offers several significant advantages in livestock improvement programs. It enables a single elite cow to produce many calves within a year by generating multiple embryos from one estrous cycle, thereby greatly increasing her reproductive output beyond natural limits. This rapid multiplication of superior genetics accelerates the overall rate of genetic improvement in dairy herds and breeding populations. ETT also facilitates the international exchange and conservation of valuable germplasm, allowing superior genetic material to be preserved, shared, and utilized across regions and countries. Moreover, since embryos can be collected, processed, and transferred under stringent sanitary conditions, the technology permits the movement of disease-free embryos across borders, minimizing the risk of transmitting infectious diseases while supporting global breeding and conservation efforts.

12.2.3 In Vitro Fertilization (IVF)

In vitro fertilization means fertilizing the egg and sperm outside the body, in a laboratory. In dairy animals, IVF helps to produce embryos when normal fertilization in the animal's body does not occur properly. In vitro fertilization (IVF) involves a sequence of controlled laboratory and field procedures to produce embryos outside the animal's body. The process begins with the collection of oocytes (eggs) from the ovaries of donor cows using ultrasound-guided follicular aspiration. These oocytes are then placed in a specialized nutrient medium and allowed to undergo maturation for about 24 h under controlled temperature and atmospheric conditions. After maturation, frozen-thawed semen is added to the culture dishes to achieve fertilization in vitro. The fertilized oocytes develop into embryos, which are subsequently cultured for several days in the laboratory until they reach the blastocyst stage. Finally, healthy and viable embryos are selected and transferred into synchronized recipient cows, where they can establish pregnancy and develop normally to term.

In vitro fertilization (IVF) offers several important advantages in animal breeding and genetic improvement programs. Through IVF, it is possible to produce embryos from elite donor animals that are unable to carry a pregnancy because of advanced age, injury, or reproductive disease, thereby preserving their valuable genetics. IVF also saves time and resources by enabling the production of a large number of embryos from a limited number of superior animals under controlled laboratory conditions. The technology allows the use of sexed semen and facilitates genetic testing of embryos before transfer, helping in the selection of desired traits and improving herd planning. By increasing the number of offspring obtained from genetically valuable animals, IVF accelerates genetic progress. When combined with embryo freezing, IVF is widely applied in genetic improvement programs, conservation of rare and endangered breeds, and research related to early embryonic development and fertility.

Knowledge Corner...
The first bovine calf produced through in vitro fertilization (IVF) was born in the United States in 1981. Since then, IVF has become a major tool in dairy breeding, allowing the rapid multiplication of superior females and conservation of valuable germplasm worldwide.

12.2.4 Oocyte Maturation and Cryopreservation

Oocyte maturation is a key step for successful fertilization. In laboratory conditions, immature eggs can be matured in special nutrient solutions that contain hormones and growth factors. Mature oocytes are then fertilized by sperm to produce embryos.

Cryopreservation is the process of freezing biological materials like semen, embryos, and oocytes at very low temperatures (-196 °C). It is an essential biotechnology for storing valuable genetic resources. Cryopreservation provides significant benefits in animal reproduction and genetic resource management. It allows the long-term storage of genetic material such as semen, oocytes, and embryos from genetically superior animals without loss of viability. The technique facilitates easy and safe transport of germplasm across different regions and countries, supporting breeding programs and international genetic exchange. Cryopreservation plays a vital role in the conservation of endangered breeds by preserving valuable genetic diversity for future use. In addition, the availability of frozen oocytes and embryos supports research, training, and advancement in reproductive biotechnology by providing reliable biological material when needed. Recent developments such as vitrification (ultra-fast freezing) have improved the survival rate of frozen oocytes and embryos. These methods ensure that genetic resources are preserved safely for future breeding and research.

12.2.5 Sexed Semen Technology

Sexed semen technology allows the selection of sperm cells carrying either the X or Y chromosome before insemination. Since the X chromosome produces female calves and the Y chromosome produces male calves, farmers can plan the desired sex of offspring. The most common method of sperm separation is flow cytometry, where sperm are stained with a fluorescent dye and sorted by laser based on their DNA content. Sexed semen offers several important advantages, particularly in dairy farming systems. By increasing the proportion of female calves born, it helps expand the population of future milk-producing animals, thereby enhancing long-term milk yield and productivity. The use of sexed semen also reduces the economic burden associated with rearing unwanted male calves, lowering costs related to feeding, housing, and management. In addition, it improves herd structure and overall breeding efficiency by allowing farmers to plan replacements more accurately, accelerate genetic progress, and optimize the use of resources within the dairy enterprise. However, sexed semen is more expensive and has slightly lower conception rates than conventional semen. With better sorting techniques and semen handling, conception rates are improving. Many dairy farms now use sexed semen for heifers to produce more female replacements.

12.2.6 Hormonal Control of Reproduction

Reproductive hormones play an important role in regulating the estrous cycle, ovulation, pregnancy, and lactation. By using hormone-based protocols, reproduction can be controlled and synchronized to improve fertility and calving rate.

Commonly used hormones include:

Gonadotropin-releasing hormone (GnRH): stimulates the release of LH and FSH for follicular development.

Prostaglandin $F_{2}\alpha$ *(*$PGF_{2}\alpha$*)*: used to induce heat by regressing the corpus luteum.

Progesterone: used in synchronization protocols like CIDR (Controlled Internal Drug Release) devices.

Equine Chorionic Gonadotropin (eCG): used to induce superovulation.

Hormonal applications play a crucial role in the reproductive management of dairy animals. They are widely used for heat synchronization to enable fixed-time artificial insemination (FTAI), reducing the need for estrus detection and improving conception rates. Hormonal treatments are also essential for inducing superovulation in donor animals for embryo transfer programs, thereby increasing the number of embryos produced per cycle. In anestrous or postpartum cows, hormones help induce estrus and restore normal ovarian activity, improving fertility and reproductive efficiency. Additionally, controlled hormonal interventions allow regulation of calving intervals, ensuring more uniform and predictable calving patterns that support continuous and sustained milk production. Proper use of hormonal protocols increases reproductive efficiency and ensures that animals calve regularly, leading to sustained milk production.

12.3 Nutritional and Microbial Biotechnology

Nutrition plays a major role in determining milk yield, composition, and animal health. A well-fed animal can express its full genetic potential, while poor nutrition limits production even in high-yielding breeds. Traditional feeding practices are based on general averages and do not account for genetic differences, metabolic needs, and gut microbial balance. Modern biotechnology helps to improve nutrition by studying how feed interacts with genes, how nutrients affect metabolism, and how microbes in the rumen contribute to digestion and milk synthesis. Nutritional and microbial biotechnologies combine molecular biology, microbiology, and animal nutrition to make feeding more scientific, precise, and efficient. These approaches help to reduce feed cost, improve nutrient utilization, lower methane emission, and maintain udder health.

12.3.1 Nutrigenomics and Gene–Nutrient Interaction

Nutrigenomics is the study of how nutrients influence the expression of genes related to milk production, metabolism, and health. It connects nutrition and molecular biology. Every nutrient, such as carbohydrates, proteins, fats, vitamins, and minerals, can affect certain genes. These genes then control milk yield, composition, and animal performance.

For example, energy and protein intake influence the expression of casein and whey protein genes in the mammary gland. Fatty acid composition in the diet regulates genes related to milk fat synthesis. Micronutrients like zinc, selenium, and vitamin E affect immune-related genes and udder health. By studying nutrigenomics, scientists can design feed that activates beneficial genes and suppresses harmful ones. This is called precision feeding. Nutrigenomics also helps identify how different breeds respond to the same diet, allowing region-specific feeding recommendations. This technology is very useful for tropical dairy systems where feed quality varies widely. It ensures that every bite of feed contributes effectively to milk synthesis and animal well-being.

12.3.2 Enzyme Biotechnology in Feed Utilization

Enzymes are biological catalysts that speed up digestion and nutrient absorption. In dairy nutrition, feed enzymes such as cellulase, xylanase, amylase, and protease are used to break down complex feed components. Enzyme biotechnology has important applications in dairy nutrition and production systems. The use of exogenous enzymes improves the digestion of fibrous feeds such as straw, hay, and crop residues by breaking down complex carbohydrates and plant cell wall components. This enhanced digestion increases nutrient availability and overall feed efficiency, allowing animals to utilize feed more effectively. Improved feed utilization helps reduce feed costs and minimizes wastage, contributing to more economical dairy farming. By optimizing rumen fermentation and promoting better microbial activity, enzyme biotechnology also enhances milk yield and can improve milk fat percentage, leading to better productivity and milk quality. For example, adding cellulase and xylanase helps in breaking down cellulose and hemicellulose, which are difficult for animals to digest. Enzyme supplementation is especially useful for buffaloes and crossbred cows that depend on low-quality roughages. New biotechnology-based enzymes are produced using genetically modified microbes that have high activity and stability under rumen conditions. These products are safe, effective, and environmentally friendly.

12.3.3 Use of Probiotics and Prebiotics

The rumen and intestine of dairy animals contain billions of microbes that help in digestion, nutrient absorption, and immune defense. Probiotics are live beneficial microorganisms added to the feed to improve the microbial balance in the gut. Prebiotics are nondigestible food ingredients that promote the growth of good microbes. The probiotics commonly used in dairy animals are *Lactobacillus* species, *Bifidobacterium* species, *Saccharomyces cerevisiae* (yeast), *Bacillus subtilis*, etc. Probiotics and prebiotics offer multiple benefits in dairy production by positively influencing rumen health and animal performance. They improve rumen fermentation and fiber digestion by stimulating beneficial microbial populations, leading to more efficient breakdown of complex feed components. Their use helps stabilize rumen pH, thereby reducing the incidence of acidosis and other digestive upsets. Probiotics and prebiotics also enhance immune function, which contributes to a lower incidence of diseases such as mastitis and diarrhea. By improving gut health and nutrient utilization, they increase feed intake and milk yield. In addition, better rumen efficiency and metabolic balance result in improved milk quality, including higher milk fat percentage. Probiotics also help to reduce methane emissions by balancing rumen microbes. Modern biotechnology helps in selecting and producing specific probiotic strains that work best under local farm conditions.

12.3.4 Rumen Microbial Manipulation

The rumen is the natural fermentation chamber in ruminants where microbes digest fibrous feeds. It contains bacteria, protozoa, fungi, and archaea that work together to break down plant material and produce volatile fatty acids (VFA), which are the main energy source for milk synthesis. Rumen microbial manipulation means changing the population or activity of microbes to improve feed digestion and reduce harmful by-products.

Rumen microbial manipulation involves several strategies aimed at improving fermentation efficiency and animal productivity. One common method is the addition of selected microbial cultures to the diet in order to promote the growth and activity of beneficial rumen microorganisms. Feed additives such as buffers, ionophores, and plant extracts are also used to suppress harmful microbes, stabilize rumen pH, and improve fermentation patterns. The inclusion of rumen-protected fats and amino acids helps optimize rumen fermentation by supplying essential nutrients without disturbing microbial balance. In advanced applications, genetic modification of rumen microbes is explored to enhance enzyme production, thereby improving the breakdown of fibrous feeds and overall feed utilization efficiency. Modern molecular tools such as metagenomics and metatranscriptomics help scientists identify the structure and function of rumen microbial communities. These studies help design diets that favor efficient fermentation, reduce methane release, and increase energy availability for milk synthesis.

Knowledge Corner...

Recent nutrigenomic studies show that balanced high-energy diets activate genes responsible for casein and fat synthesis in the mammary gland. Supplementation with probiotics and enzymes improves rumen health and enhances milk yield, especially during heat stress.

12.3.5 Biotechnology for Feed Efficiency

Feed cost forms about 60–70% of the total cost of milk production. Improving feed efficiency is therefore one of the main goals of dairy biotechnology. Feed efficiency means how effectively an animal converts feed nutrients into milk. Biotechnological strategies to improve feed efficiency in dairy animals integrate genetic, nutritional, and molecular approaches. Molecular markers are used to identify and select animals with superior feed conversion efficiency, enabling more precise breeding decisions. Genetic selection for lower residual feed intake (RFI) helps develop animals that require less feed for the same level of production, thereby improving efficiency and reducing costs. Nutritional interventions such as the use of enzymes, probiotics, and rumen-protected nutrients enhance digestion, nutrient utilization, and rumen function. Nutrigenomics-based feed formulation tailors diets according to gene–nutrient interactions, optimizing metabolic responses and productivity. In advanced systems, nano-delivery technologies enable controlled and targeted release of nutrients, further improving nutrient utilization and overall feed efficiency. For example, genetically efficient cows can produce more milk with the same amount of feed. Molecular markers linked to feed efficiency can be used to select such animals for breeding. This reduces the environmental impact of dairy farming by lowering methane production and nutrient waste.

12.3.6 Methane Mitigation and Environmental Benefits

Methane is a greenhouse gas produced during rumen fermentation. It represents a loss of feed energy and contributes to global warming. Biotechnological interventions help reduce methane production without affecting milk yield.

Several biotechnological and management approaches are used to reduce methane production in ruminants. The inclusion of feed additives such as essential oils, tannins, and nitrates helps inhibit methane-producing microbes (methanogens) in the rumen and alters fermentation pathways. The use of genetically selected or engineered rumen microbes that generate less methane further contributes to lowering enteric emissions. Supplementation with specific probiotics can redirect hydrogen away from methane formation toward more efficient end products such as propionate. Improving feed digestibility through enzyme supplementation or microbial treatments enhances fermentation efficiency and reduces the amount of hydrogen available for methanogenesis. In addition, selective breeding of animals with inherently lower methane emissions supports long-term and sustainable reduction of greenhouse gas output from dairy systems. Reducing methane also improves energy efficiency because less feed energy is lost as gas. This approach makes dairy farming more climate-friendly and supports global goals for sustainable livestock production.

12.4 Molecular and Hormonal Interventions

Molecular and hormonal biotechnology focuses on understanding and controlling the biological processes that regulate milk synthesis and secretion. Milk production is mainly governed by endocrine signals, cellular activity in the mammary gland, and molecular pathways inside mammary epithelial cells. By using biotechnology, scientists can study these processes in detail, identify key regulatory molecules, and apply hormonal or molecular agents to enhance milk yield, improve milk quality, and support udder health. These interventions must be carefully managed to maintain animal welfare, milk safety, and long-term productivity.

12.4.1 Role of Growth Hormone and the IGF System

Growth hormone (GH), also called somatotropin, is a peptide hormone secreted by the anterior pituitary gland. It plays an important role in regulating growth, metabolism, and lactation. GH does not act directly on the mammary gland; instead, it stimulates the production of Insulin-like Growth Factor-1 (IGF-1) in the liver and other tissues. IGF-1 acts as a mediator of GH action on cells. In dairy animals, the growth hormone–insulin-like growth factor (GH–IGF) system plays a central role in enhancing milk production by regulating nutrient partitioning and mammary gland function. It increases the uptake of nutrients such as glucose, amino acids, and fatty acids by mammary tissue, ensuring an adequate supply of precursors for milk synthesis. The GH–IGF axis promotes mammary cell growth, proliferation, and differentiation, thereby increasing the secretory capacity of the gland. It also improves the efficiency of energy utilization by directing available energy preferentially toward milk production rather than other metabolic processes. In addition, the system modulates body tissue metabolism by reducing excessive body fat mobilization and channeling nutrients toward milk formation, ultimately supporting sustained and higher milk yield. During early lactation, natural GH levels are high, which supports maximum milk yield. Modern biotechnology allows controlled use of recombinant GH to maintain optimal hormone levels during lactation, provided ethical and safety guidelines are followed.

12.4.2 Recombinant Bovine Somatotropin (rBST)

Recombinant bovine somatotropin (rBST) is a biotechnologically produced form of growth hormone. It is made using recombinant DNA technology, where the bovine GH gene is inserted into bacteria such as *E. coli*. These bacteria produce large amounts of the hormone, which is purified for use.

12.4.2.1 Mechanism of Action

When injected into lactating cows, rBST increases milk production by improving the efficiency of nutrient utilization. It enhances the supply of glucose, amino acids, and fatty acids to the mammary gland. This increases milk yield by 10–20% in well-fed cows. The use of recombinant bovine somatotropin (rBST) in dairy cows offers several benefits, primarily by increasing milk yield per cow and improving feed conversion efficiency, allowing more milk to be produced from the same amount of feed. This enhanced productivity can also reduce the environmental footprint per liter of milk by lowering resource use and greenhouse gas emissions relative to production volume. However, the effectiveness of rBST is limited to healthy, well-nourished cows, and improper management can increase metabolic stress and health risks. Additionally, strict adherence to withdrawal periods and animal welfare standards is essential to ensure milk safety and maintain ethical farming practices. Many countries allow rBST use under veterinary supervision, while others have restricted it due to consumer perception. Nevertheless, rBST remains an excellent example of applied biotechnology in dairy production.

12.4.3 Oxytocin and Milk Ejection Support

Oxytocin is a natural hormone produced by the hypothalamus and released from the posterior pituitary gland. It is essential for milk ejection or let-down during milking or suckling. Oxytocin causes contraction of myoepithelial cells surrounding the alveoli, which pushes milk into the ducts and teat cistern. Oxytocin has significant biotechnological applications in dairy and veterinary practice. Synthetic oxytocin can be administered to support milk let-down in animals with a weak reflex, such as stressed or first-time lactating cows, ensuring efficient milk flow. Its use also promotes complete milk removal from the udder, which helps prevent residual milk accumulation and reduces the risk of mastitis. Beyond lactation, oxytocin plays a vital role in reproductive management by assisting parturition and promoting uterine involution, thereby supporting overall reproductive health and productivity in dairy herds.

Precautions Continuous or excessive use can lead to dependency and reduced natural reflex sensitivity. Therefore, oxytocin should be used responsibly, only under veterinary advice.

Biotechnology research is now exploring oxytocin analogs and slow-release formulations to ensure safer and longer-lasting effects.

12.4.4 Hormone Receptor Sensitivity and Regulation

Hormones act on target tissues through specific receptors located on cell membranes or inside the cells. The response depends not only on hormone concentration but also on receptor number, sensitivity, and binding affinity. In the mammary gland, receptors for prolactin, oxytocin, estrogen, progesterone, and growth hormone play key roles in lactation. Biotechnology allows the study of receptor structure and function through molecular cloning, receptor assays, and immunohistochemistry.

Biotechnological applications related to hormone receptor regulation in dairy animals focus on improving productivity and reproductive efficiency. Genetic analysis can identify variants that affect the efficiency of hormone receptors, providing insights for selective breeding programs. Strategies can then be developed to enhance receptor sensitivity using natural compounds or targeted feed supplements, optimizing the animal's physiological response to hormones. Additionally, studying receptor function helps in understanding hormonal imbalances that may limit milk yield, enabling interventions to restore normal endocrine function and improve overall lactation performance. For example, long-term stress reduces oxytocin receptor expression in the mammary gland, resulting in poor milk ejection. Balanced nutrition, gentle handling, and hormonal support can restore receptor activity. Receptor-based studies also guide breeding programs for better hormonal responsiveness in dairy animals.

12.4.5 Nanotechnology in Hormone Delivery

Nanotechnology is an emerging tool in animal biotechnology. It involves designing nanoparticles, i.e., very small particles that can carry and deliver hormones or drugs efficiently in the body. Nano-hormone delivery systems offer several advantages in dairy animal management by improving the efficiency and safety of hormonal treatments. These systems provide controlled and sustained release of hormones such as rBST or oxytocin, ensuring consistent physiological effects over time. They enable targeted delivery to specific tissues, like the mammary gland, minimizing systemic side effects. Sensitive hormonal molecules are protected from degradation in the body, maintaining their bioactivity and effectiveness. Additionally, the technology reduces the frequency of injections, lowering stress and handling requirements for the animals while enhancing overall welfare and productivity. For example, growth hormone can be encapsulated in biodegradable nanoparticles to enable slow and uniform release. Nano-lipid carriers can be used to deliver reproductive hormones such as GnRH or progesterone. Nano-formulated minerals and vitamins are used to improve reproductive efficiency and udder health. Nanotechnology makes hormone therapy safer and more efficient. It represents the future of veterinary biotechnology, combining precision delivery with improved animal comfort and welfare.

Knowledge Corner...
Slow-release nano-formulations of recombinant bovine somatotropin (rBST) are being developed to maintain steady hormone levels. These new delivery systems increase milk yield while reducing injection frequency and stress in dairy animals.

12.5 Mammary Gland Biotechnology

The mammary gland is the organ responsible for milk synthesis and secretion. Understanding its structure, development, and molecular control is essential for improving milk yield and quality. Biotechnology helps in studying the mammary gland at the cellular, molecular, and genetic levels. It provides new tools to explore how genes, hormones, and nutrients interact to regulate milk production. Mammary gland biotechnology focuses on gene expression, cell culture, stem cells, and molecular regulation of milk protein synthesis. The knowledge gained from this field is directly applied to improve lactation efficiency, udder health, and milk composition in dairy animals.

12.5.1 Structure and Cellular Function of the Mammary Gland

The mammary gland is a complex secretory organ made up of alveoli, ducts, connective tissue, and blood vessels. The alveoli are small sacs lined by mammary epithelial cells (MECs) that synthesize milk. Around these alveoli lie myoepithelial cells, which contract under oxytocin influence to eject milk. Biotechnological studies of the mammary gland focus on understanding its cellular structure and functional organization to improve lactation management. Microscopic examination combined with histochemical staining is used to study different cell types and the overall tissue architecture. Molecular markers help identify specific cell populations, including epithelial, myoepithelial, and immune cells, providing insights into their roles in milk synthesis and glandular defense. Advanced imaging techniques, such as confocal and electron microscopy, allow detailed visualization of milk secretion pathways and intracellular processes, enhancing our understanding of mammary physiology at the cellular and subcellular levels. Understanding the cellular organization helps in identifying factors that control milk secretion, cell turnover, and mammary gland health. In dairy research, mammary tissue biopsies are often used to analyze gene activity related to milk proteins, enzymes, and fat synthesis.

12.5.2 Gene Expression in Milk Synthesis

Milk synthesis depends on the expression of specific genes that code for milk proteins (casein, whey proteins), milk fat enzymes, and lactose synthesis enzymes.

Biotechnology allows precise measurement of these gene expressions using tools such as RT-PCR (Reverse Transcription Polymerase Chain Reaction), microarray analysis, and RNA sequencing (RNA-Seq).

Key genes involved in milk synthesis include:

- CSN1S1, CSN2, CSN3: code for casein proteins.
- LALBA (α-lactalbumin): essential for lactose synthesis.
- BTN1A1 and XDH: related to milk fat globule formation.
- ACACA and FASN: control fatty acid synthesis.

By studying these genes, scientists can identify which genes are active during different stages of lactation and how they are influenced by hormones such as prolactin, growth hormone, and insulin. This knowledge helps in improving milk yield and composition through selective breeding or nutritional manipulation.

12.5.3 Stem Cells and Mammary Regeneration

Stem cells are undifferentiated cells that can develop into specialized cells and regenerate tissues. In the mammary gland, mammary stem cells (MaSCs) are responsible for the growth and renewal of alveolar and ductal cells during lactation cycles.

Stem cell biotechnology has important applications in the study and improvement of the mammary gland. It is used to investigate mammary development and involution processes, providing insights into growth, differentiation, and tissue remodeling. Stem cells can also be applied for the regeneration of damaged mammary tissue following infection or injury, supporting udder health and lactation recovery. In genetic improvement programs, specific genes can be introduced into mammary stem cells to produce high-yielding transgenic animals with enhanced milk production or desired traits. Additionally, stem cells enable the in vitro growth of mammary tissue, facilitating research on milk synthesis, secretion, and the molecular mechanisms underlying lactation. Researchers can isolate stem cells from mammary tissue, culture them in laboratory media, and study their differentiation under various hormonal and nutritional conditions. Stem cell research in dairy animals provides valuable information on lactation biology and may help restore milk production in animals affected by mastitis or gland damage.

12.5.4 Molecullar Regulation of Lactation Genes

The activity of milk-producing genes is controlled by complex molecular mechanisms. These include transcriptional regulation, epigenetic modification, and hormonal signaling.

- *Transcriptional Regulation:* Proteins called transcription factors bind to DNA regions (promoters) near lactation genes to turn them on or off. Examples include STAT5, C/EBP, and ELF5, which are activated by prolactin and growth hormone.

- *Epigenetic Control:* Epigenetic changes such as DNA methylation and histone modification affect gene expression without altering the DNA sequence. Nutritional and environmental factors can modify these patterns, influencing milk yield and composition.
- *Hormonal Regulation*: Prolactin, cortisol, and insulin interact to activate genes involved in milk synthesis. Prolactin mainly stimulates casein gene expression, while cortisol enhances fat synthesis.

Using molecular biotechnology, scientists can measure changes in these regulatory mechanisms and identify how management, nutrition, and stress alter milk gene activity. Understanding molecular regulation is important for designing feeding strategies, hormonal interventions, and genetic selection programs that optimize lactation.

Knowledge Corner...
Scientists have created three-dimensional mammary organoids from bovine cells to study milk synthesis and mastitis. These lab-grown models help researchers test hormones, nutrients, and drugs without using live animals.

12.5.5 Genetic Control of Milk Protein Synthesis

Milk proteins, mainly caseins and whey proteins, are synthesized in mammary epithelial cells. Their production depends on both genetic and hormonal factors. Different animals have different casein gene variants that affect milk yield, cheese-making quality, and nutritional value.

Casein genes (CSN1S1, CSN2, CSN3):

- Determine total protein content and milk quality.
- Some variants improve curd formation in cheese production.
- Selection for favorable variants can improve milk processing traits.

Whey proteins (α-lactalbumin, β-lactoglobulin): Contribute to the nutritional value and immune properties of milk.

Variations in these genes can influence milk allergenicity and digestibility.

Molecular techniques such as SNP genotyping and DNA sequencing help identify these genetic variations. Breeding animals with superior milk protein genotypes is now a common goal in dairy improvement programs. Biotechnology also supports the production of transgenic animals expressing special milk proteins for pharmaceutical and nutritional use.

12.6 Diagnostic and Monitoring Tools

Diagnosis and monitoring are important parts of modern dairy biotechnology. They help to identify diseases, monitor milk quality, and evaluate the health and productivity of dairy animals. Traditional diagnostic methods are often slow and may require laboratory culture or manual examination. Biotechnology provides faster, more sensitive, and accurate diagnostic tools based on molecular, biochemical, and sensor technologies. These tools help in early detection of problems such as mastitis, metabolic disorders, and reproductive failures, allowing quick treatment and improved milk production. Diagnostic biotechnology also plays a major role in the quality control of milk and dairy products. Molecular tests, biosensors, and digital monitoring systems are now widely used to ensure food safety and animal welfare.

12.6.1 Biomarkers of Milk Yield and Quality

A biomarker is a biological substance that can indicate the physiological or health status of an animal. In dairy science, biomarkers are used to monitor milk yield, composition, and udder health. They can be found in blood, milk, urine, and tissue samples.

Biomarkers play a crucial role in monitoring health, reproduction, and productivity in dairy animals. Progesterone levels are commonly used to assess pregnancy status and ovarian activity, helping manage breeding programs effectively. Somatic cell count (SCC) serves as an indicator of udder health, with elevated levels signaling subclinical mastitis. Enzymes such as lactate dehydrogenase (LDH) and N-acetyl-β-D-glucosaminidase (NAGase) increase in response to mammary gland inflammation, providing early detection of mastitis. Milk urea nitrogen (MUN) reflects protein utilization and energy balance, guiding nutritional management. Additionally, the fat-to-protein ratio in milk can indicate overall nutritional adequacy and help identify animals at risk of metabolic disorders such as ketosis. Modern biotechnology allows measurement of these biomarkers through ELISA kits, immunoassays, and biosensors. Monitoring biomarkers helps farmers detect early metabolic stress, mastitis, and feeding problems before they affect milk yield.

12.6.2 Proteomics and Metabolomics in Dairy Science

Proteomics is the large-scale study of proteins in cells, tissues, and milk. Metabolomics studies the small chemical compounds (metabolites) that result from metabolism. Together, they provide a detailed picture of how the animal's body functions during lactation, disease, or stress. Proteomics and metabolomics have valuable applications in dairy production by providing detailed insights into milk composition and animal metabolism. Proteomic studies help identify milk proteins that influence yield, flavor, and nutritional quality, enabling selection for improved dairy traits. They also allow the detection of specific protein markers associated with mastitis, facilitating early diagnosis and better udder health management. Metabolomic analyses are used to study metabolic changes during lactation, heat stress, or other physiological conditions, helping optimize nutrition and management strategies. Additionally, these approaches support the development of functional foods and nutraceutical milk products by characterizing bioactive components and enhancing the health benefits of dairy products. Commonly used techniques in proteomics and metabolomics for dairy research include two-dimensional gel electrophoresis (2D-GE), which separates proteins based on their isoelectric point and molecular weight, allowing detailed protein profiling. Mass spectrometry methods, such as MALDI-TOF and LC–MS, are widely employed for precise identification, quantification, and characterization of proteins and peptides. Nuclear Magnetic Resonance (NMR) spectroscopy is used for metabolite profiling, providing comprehensive information on the chemical composition and metabolic changes in milk and other biological samples. These techniques together enable a deeper understanding of milk quality, animal health, and physiological status. For example, proteomic studies have identified casein variants and whey proteins that differ between breeds and lactation stages. Metabolomic analysis of milk has revealed biomarkers of energy balance, ketosis, and mastitis. These technologies help improve milk quality and animal health through better management and nutrition.

12.6.3 Biosensors and Rapid Detection Kits

A biosensor is an analytical device that combines a biological element (enzyme, antibody, nucleic acid, etc.) with an electronic detector. It converts a biological response into a measurable signal. Biosensors provide quick, on-farm testing for various milk and animal health parameters.

Biosensors are valuable tools in dairy production for rapid and precise monitoring of animal health and milk quality. They are used to detect the presence of antibiotics, hormones, and adulterants in milk, ensuring safety and compliance with regulatory standards. Biosensors also measure milk composition, including fat, protein, and lactose content, supporting quality control and nutritional assessment. They play a crucial role in mastitis management by detecting somatic cell count or specific enzymes indicative of udder infection. Additionally, biosensors can monitor metabolic indicators such as urea, ketone bodies, and glucose levels in blood and milk, aiding in herd health management and early detection of metabolic disorders. Biosensors are portable, easy to use, and give results within minutes. They reduce the need for laboratory testing and help farmers make immediate decisions. Newer biosensors use nanomaterials, microfluidics, and wireless technology to improve accuracy and connectivity. Rapid detection kits based on lateral flow assays (similar to pregnancy tests) are now available for field use. They detect diseases like mastitis, brucellosis, foot-and-mouth disease, etc., quickly and affordably.

12.6.4 Molecular Diagnosis of Mastitis

Mastitis is one of the most common and costly diseases in dairy animals. Early detection is essential to prevent production loss and reduce antibiotic use.

Biotechnology has made mastitis diagnosis faster and more accurate through molecular tests that detect the pathogen's DNA or RNA directly.

Common molecular techniques for detection of mastitis are

(i) Polymerase Chain Reaction (PCR): It amplifies bacterial DNA for detection.
(ii) Real-Time PCR (qPCR): It quantifies bacterial load and identifies multiple species simultaneously.
(iii) Loop-Mediated Isothermal Amplification (LAMP): It is a rapid, field-friendly test that does not require complex equipment.
(iv) DNA microarrays: It can detect several mastitis-causing bacteria in one test.

Molecular tests can identify pathogens such as *Staphylococcus aureus*, *Streptococcus agalactiae*, *E. coli*, etc. within a few hours instead of the days required by culture methods. These tests also detect antibiotic resistance genes, helping veterinarians choose the most effective treatment. Such rapid and precise diagnostics improve udder health, reduce milk discard, and increase farm profitability.

Knowledge Corner...

Portable PCR and LAMP (loop-mediated isothermal amplification) kits can now detect mastitis-causing bacteria on farms within an hour. Smart milk analyzers instantly measure fat, protein, and lactose, helping farmers maintain milk quality and detect udder problems early.

12.6.5 Smart Dairy Monitoring Systems

Smart dairy monitoring systems combine biotechnology with information technology to record and analyze animal data in real time. They use sensors, wearable devices, and computer software to monitor the physiological and behavioral parameters of dairy animals.

Smart systems in modern dairy farming integrate sensors and digital technologies to monitor animal health, productivity, and management in real time. Wearable sensors track parameters such as body temperature, activity, rumination, and estrus behavior, providing early indicators of health or reproductive status. Milking parlor sensors record milk yield, conductivity, and flow rate, enabling precise monitoring of udder health and milk quality. Automated feeding systems adjust feed allocation based on individual milk output and body condition, optimizing nutrition and efficiency. IoT (Internet of Things) platforms connect all these devices to cloud-based systems, allowing comprehensive data analysis, decision-making, and herd management on a digital platform. These systems alert farmers to early signs of disease, heat, or stress. For example, changes in milk conductivity or cow activity can indicate mastitis or estrus before visible symptoms appear. Integration of artificial intelligence (AI) helps predict health events, optimize milking schedules, and improve reproductive efficiency. Smart dairy technologies make farms more efficient, reduce labor, and support better decision-making for milk production and animal welfare.

Overall, biotechnology provides an integrated, science-based approach to achieving higher milk yield, better animal health, and environmental sustainability—the foundation of future dairy development.

Exercise

Objective Questions

1. Technique that involves identifying animals with desirable genes is called ________________.
2. The type of growth hormone used to augment milk production is ____________________.
3. Enzyme helps to digest fibrous feed materials is ____________________________.
4. Techniques for gene editing is ________________________.
5. Live beneficial microorganisms are called _________________.
6. Most common biomarker for mastitis detection is ____________________.
7. Precision dairy farming mainly uses ______________________________
8. The full form of IoT in dairy farming is ____________________________.

Subjective Questions

1. Describe in detail the biotechnological methods used for genetic improvement in dairy animals.
2. Explain the process and advantages of embryo transfer technology (ETT) and in vitro fertilization (IVF).
3. Discuss the role of nutritional and microbial biotechnology in improving milk production.
4. Write an account of molecular and hormonal interventions used to enhance milk yield.
5. Describe the structure and functions of the mammary gland and explain how biotechnology is applied in mammary research.
6. Explain the principles and applications of genomic selection and genome editing tools (like CRISPR/Cas9) in dairy animal breeding.
7. Explain how nanotechnology is applied in dairy science for hormone delivery, disease control, and nutrient supplementation.
8. Describe the major genes influencing milk synthesis and discuss how gene mapping and QTL analysis contribute to their identification.

Answer to Objective Questions

1. Marker-assisted selection
2. rBST
3. Cellulase
4. CRISPR/Cas9
5. Probiotics
6. Somatic cell count
7. Sensor and data-based monitoring
8. Internet of things

Additional Resources for Further Reading

Bauman DE, Vernon RG (1993) Effects of exogenous bovine somatotropin on lactation. Annu Rev Nutr 13:437–461

Bionaz M, Loor JJ (2008) Gene networks driving bovine mammary protein synthesis during the lactation cycle. Bioinform Biol Insights 2:85–97

Collier RJ, Bauman DE (2014) Physiology and management adaptations to heat stress in dairy cattle. J Dairy Sci 97:7565–7579

De Vries A (2020) Economic considerations of precision dairy farming technologies. Anim Front 10(1):14–21

Dhakal IP, Nair SG (2018) Advances in bovine reproduction and embryo biotechnology. Indian J Anim Sci 88(10):1120–1132

Garcia M, Singh K (2021) Nutrigenomic approaches in ruminant nutrition: a review. Anim Nutr Feed Technol 21(3):487–499

Gera S, Pandey N (2022) Nanobiotechnology in animal health and milk production. Vet World 15(9):2238–2246

Khatri P, Kumar S (2023) Applications of CRISPR/Cas9 technology in livestock improvement. Front Genet 14:1156764

Kumar H, Yadav MC (2021) Immunomodulators and probiotics for dairy animal health. J Vet Sci Biotechnol 10(2):78–90

National Dairy Development Board (NDDB) (2020) Indian dairy sector report: emerging technologies and sustainability. Anand, India

Sharma N, Singh RK, Pandey A (2019) Molecular diagnostics for mastitis management in dairy cows. J Anim Health Prod 7(2):63–70

Singh K, Ganguly I (2023) Omics integration for milk production enhancement in dairy animals. Indian J Biotechnol 22(4):314–327

Tucker HA (2020) Hormonal control of lactation: advances in molecular endocrinology. Domest Anim Endocrinol 75:106619

Wiggans GR, VanRaden PM, Cooper TA (2017) Genomic evaluation of U.S. dairy cattle: history, progress, and future outlook. J Dairy Sci 100(12):10014–10027

World Organisation for Animal Health (WOAH) (2024) Animal welfare and biotechnology guidelines. WOAH Publications, Paris

Appendix

Table A.1 Leading countries in milk and dairy product production (milk equivalent basis)

Rank	Country	Approximate production 2024 (MT)
1	India	245.0
2	United States	102.5
3	Pakistan	66.3
4	China	43.2
5	Brazil	38.2
6	Germany	34.4
7	Russian Federation	34.1
8	France	26.2
9	Turkey	22.0
10	New Zealand	21.5

Table A.2 Ten leading countries in cattle population

Rank	Country	Approximate cattle population (million)
1	Brazil	238.6
2	India	194.5
3	United States	88.8
4	China	73.6
5	Ethiopia	70.9
6	Pakistan	55.5
7	Argentina	54.2
8	Tanzania	37.9
9	Chad	37.6
10	Mexico	37.6

J. Mukherjee et al., *Veterinary Lactation Physiology*,
https://doi.org/10.1007/978-3-032-21123-1

Table A.3 Five leading countries in buffalo population

Rank	Country	Approximate population (million)
1	India	109.85
2	Pakistan	41.19
3	China	23.27
4	Egypt	3.68
5	Nepal	3.50

Table A.4 Five leading countries in goat population

Rank	Country	Approximate population (millions)
1	India	148.88
2	China	132.4
3	Nigeria	88.0
4	Pakistan	82.5
5	Ethiopia	49.3

Table A.5 Five leading countries in sheep population

Rank	Country	Approximate population (millions)
1	China	193
2	India	77.4
3	Australia	72.1
4	Iran	52.0
5	Nigeria	51.4

Table A.6 Physical properties of milk in different species

Species	Specific gravity	Viscosity (cPas)	Surface tension (dyne/cm)	Refractive index
Cow	1.0258	1.7	51.77 ± 0.184	1.3459 ± 0.000
Buffalo	1.0288	2.2	50.78 ± 0.259	1.3464 ± 0.000
Sheep	1.0318	2.48	–	–
Goat	1.0256	2.12	–	–
Camel	1.0297	2.8	58.39 ± 0.421	1.3423 ± 0.001

Table A.7 Composition of colostrum in different species

Species	Constituents		
	Lactose (g/100 g)	Fat (g/100 g)	Protein (g/100 g)
Cow	2.5	6.7	14.9
Goat	4.7	4.1	3.4

(continued)

Table A.7 (continued)

Species	Constituents		
	Lactose (g/100 g)	Fat (g/100 g)	Protein (g/100 g)
Sheep	2.4–3.8	4.0–13.7	13.8–22.5
Pig	1.7–5.0	2.5–7.5	5.2–22.3
Donkey	5.30	2.08	2.79
Dog	27.0	78.0	138.0
Cat	3.6	3.4	4.0
Buffalo	2.70	5.44	8.75
Yak	1.90	14.0	16.1
Camel	5.90	0.30	19.2
Mare	6	1–1.5	2
Llama	4.12	0.75	16.8
Elephant	61.8	56.0	21.0
Alpaca	3.95	0.51	20.4
Rat	2.5	14.7	8.9
Rabbit	16.0	147.0	135.0
Human	7.0	3.8	1.2

Table A.8 Major constituents of milk of various animals

Species	Fat (%)	Protein (%)	Lactose (%)	Ash (%)	Total solids (%)
Antelope	1.3	6.9	4	1.3	25.2
Ass (donkey)	1.2	1.7	6.9	0.45	10.2
Bear, polar	31	10.2	0.5	1.2	42.9
Bison	1.7	4.8	5.7	0.96	13.2
Buffalo, Philippine	10.4	5.9	4.3	0.8	21.5
Camel	4.9	3.7	5.1	0.7	14.4
Cat	10.9	11.1	3.4	–	25.4
Cow:					
Ayrshire	4.1	3.6	4.7	0.7	13.1
Brown Swiss	4.0	3.6	5.0	0.7	13.3
Guernsey	5.0	3.8	4.9	0.7	14.4
Holstein	3.5	3.1	4.9	0.7	12.2
Jersey	5.5	3.9	4.9	0.7	15.0
Zebu	4.9	3.9	5.1	0.8	14.7
Deer	19.7	10.4	2.6	1.4	34.1
Dog	8.3	9.5	3.7	1.2	20.7
Dolphin	14.1	10.4	5.9	NA	30.4
Elephant	15.1	4.9	3.4	0.76	26.9
Goat	3.5	3.1	4.6	0.79	12
Guinea Pig	3.9	8.1	3	0.82	15.8
Horse	1.6	2.7	6.1	0.51	11
Human	4.5	1.1	6.8	0.2	12.6

(continued)

Table A.8 (continued)

Species	Fat (%)	Protein (%)	Lactose (%)	Ash (%)	Total solids (%)
Kangaroo	2.1	6.2	Trace	1.2	9.5
Mink	8	7	6.9	0.7	22.6
Monkey	3.9	2.1	5.9	2.6	14.5
Opossum	6.1	9.2	3.2	1.6	24.5
Pig	8.2	5.8	4.8	0.63	19.9
Rabbit	12.2	10.4	1.8	2	26.4
Rat	14.8	11.3	2.9	1.5	31.7
Reindeer	22.5	10.3	2.5	1.4	36.7
Seal, gray	53.2	11.2	2.6	0.7	67.7
Sheep	5.3	5.5	4.6	0.9	16.3
Whale	34.8	13.6	1.8	1.6	51.2

NA no available data

Table A.9 Major constituents and nutritive values of milk in human, cow, goat, sheep, and buffalo (average values per 100 milliliters whole milk)

Attributes, unit	Human	Cow	Goat	Sheep	Buffalo
Energy, kcal[a]	71.0	69.0	67.2	106.0	94.8
Water, %	87.8	87.3	87.7	80.7	81.4
Specific gravity	1.03	1.03	1.28	1.02	1.02
Total solids, g	12.4	12.7	17.4	18.3	14.1
Fat, g	3.8	3.7	4.0	6.9	6.7
Cholesterol, mg	1.2	9.6	10.8	26.4	18.4
Fatty acids (total saturated), g	1.5	1.8	2.6	4.5	4.5
Fatty acids (total polyunsaturated), g	1.0	0.2	0.1	0.3	0.1
Lactose, g	7.0	4.8	4.3	5.3	5.1
Protein, g	1.2	3.3	3.5	5.9	3.7
Casein, g	0.4	2.8	2.6	2.9	2.4
Ash, g	0.2	0.7	0.8	0.9	0.8
Calcium, mg	33.0	110.4	130.8	189.2	164.8
Magnesium, mg	4.0	9.6	13.6	17.6	30.4
Potassium, mg	55.0	139.6	199.2	134.4	173.6
Sodium, mg	15.0	39.2	48.8	43.2	50.8
Iron, µg	49.0	42.0	50.0	80.0	62.0
Copper, µg	40.0	30.0	40.0	8.9	21.2
Manganese, µg	0.2	12.0	18.0	10.0	13.0
Phosphorus, mg	15.0	88.8	108.4	154.8	114.0
Selenium, µg	2.0	3.6	1.4	1.7	NA
Zinc, mg	0.2	0.4	0.3	0.5	0.2
Vitamin A, µg	NA	27.2	55.6	43.2	51.6
Thiamin (Vit B_1), mg	0.03	0.01	0.01	0.01	0.01
Riboflavin (Vit B_2), mg	0.3	0.2	0.1	0.3	0.1

(continued)

Table A.9 (continued)

Attributes, unit	Human	Cow	Goat	Sheep	Buffalo
Niacin (Vit B_3), mg	0.7	0.1	0.3	0.4	0.1
Pantothenic Acid (Vit B_5), mg	0.2	0.4	0.3	0.4	0.2
Pyridoxine (Vit B_6), mg	0.01	0.01	0.01	0.1	0.01
Cobalamin (Vit B_{12}), μg	0.4	0.4	0.1	0.7	0.4
Vitamin C, mg	3.0	0.0	1.3	4.1	2.2
Vitamin D, IU	NA	39.2	11.6	NA	NA

[a]Kilocalorie

Table A.10 Concentrations of different milk proteins in human and animals

Protein (g/ L)	Cow	Goat	Sheep	Buffalo	Camel	Donkey	Human
Total casein	24–28	23–46	42–59	32–49	26	6.4–10.3	2.4–4.2
α_{S1}-casein	9.5–12	3.0–7.0	11–22	9	4–5	1.5	0.77
α_{S2}-casein	1.6–4	3.0–4.0	0–13	5	2–3	0.1	--
β-casein	9–15	11–15	15–36	12–21	12–13	4	3–5
κ-casein	2.0–3.5	2–7	5–12	4–6	0.7	–	1–3
Total whey protein	6–8	3.7–7.0	6–9	5–6	5.9–8.1	4.9–8.0	6.2–8.3
α-lactalbumin	1.0–1.8	1.7–3.3	1.35	1.4	1.3	1–2	2–3
β-lactoglobulin	2.8–3.5	3.0	4.6–7.0	3.9	–	3.3–4.0	–
Serum albumin	0.43–0.57	–	0.4–0.6	0.29	0.4	–	0.3
Lactoferrin	0.1–0.2	0.1	0.28	0.03–3.4	0.2	0.08	1–3

Table A.11 Amino acid content ($g \cdot 100\ g^{-1}$) in milk from various species animals

Amino acid (g/100 g)	Cow	Goat	Sheep	Buffalo	Camel
Aspartic acid	7.8	7.4	6.5	7.1	6.9
Threonine	4.5	5.7	4.4	5.7	4.1
Serine	4.8	5.2	3.4	4.7	4.3
Glutamic acid	23.2	19.3	14.5	21.4	18.1
Proline	9.6	14.6	16.2	12.0	12.0
Cysteine	0.6	0.6	0.9	0.6	1.9
Glycine	1.8	2.1	3.5	1.9	2.1
Alanine	3.0	3.6	2.4	3.0	2.1
Valine	4.8	5.7	6.4	6.8	4.1
Methionine	1.8	3.5	2.7	0.9	2.0
Isoleucine	4.2	7.1	4.6	5.7	4.9
Leucine	8.7	8.0	9.9	9.8	6.1
Tyrosine	4.5	4.8	3.8	3.9	3.1
Phenylalanine	4.8	6.0	4.3	4.7	4.0
Histidine	3.0	5.0	6.7	2.7	2.1
Lysine	8.1	8.2	7.8	7.5	--

Table A.12 Vitamins present in milk of different species

Vitamin (mg/100 g)	Cow	Goat	Sheep	Buffalo	Camel
Vitamin A	37–46	55–185	64–146	35–69	20.1
Vitamin E	0.21	0.03	*Not detected*	0.19	0.32
Vitamin D	2	1.33	2	2	3
Vitamin B6	0.04–0.06	0.045	0.08	0.33	–
Vitamin B12	0.36–0.45	0.66	0.71	0.40	–
Vitamin C	1.94	1.29	4.16	2.2	3.3

Glossary

Acyl-coA synthetase (ACSL) It is an enzyme complex that converts these fatty acids into fatty acyl-CoA through coenzyme-A thioesters formation after internalization of fatty acids through tatty acid translocase. This is called bio-activation of fatty acids that facilitates metabolic trapping of fatty acids entered into the mammary epithelial cells.

Adherens junctions The supra-molecular structure responsible for homophilic intercellular interactions, intracellular signaling, and regulation of the cytoskeleton is called adherens junctions. These junctions are composed of adhesion receptors and associated proteins in the cytoplasm. The major adhesion receptor is E-cadherin, and the associated cytosolic proteins are α-catenin, β-catenin, and p120 catenin.

Adipokines These are the signaling proteins secreted by adipocytes. They act through autocrine, paracrine, and endocrine manner to regulate energy expenditure and obesity. It regulates lipolysis during the period of transition. Examples of adipokines are adiponectin, leptin, resistin, interleukin-6, and tissue necrosis factor.

Adiponectin It is a protein secreted mainly by the white adipose tissue. It promotes lipogenesis in adipocytes and enhances insulin sensitivity. It also induces β-oxidation of fatty acids. The expression of adiponectin is decreased after calving compared to the dry period. The concentration of adiponectin reaches a peak between 40 and 70 days of the lactation cycle.

Afferent pathways Sensory neural routes that transmit tactile and pressure stimuli from teat mechanoreceptors to the spinal cord and hypothalamus. These pathways initiate the activation of oxytocin-secreting neurons. The integrity of afferent signaling is essential for reflex initiation. Disruption may result in delayed or absent milk ejection.

Alanine, serine, cysteine amino acid transport protein (ASCT) They are neutral amino acid transporters belonging to the solute carrier 1 (SLC1) family of proteins. These sodium-dependent transport proteins internalize neutral amino acids like alanine and glutamine in exchange for intracellular amino acids.

Allometric mammary growth When mammary growth is faster than body growth, the phase is termed the allometric growth phase. The allometric phase of growth

J. Mukherjee et al., *Veterinary Lactation Physiology*,
https://doi.org/10.1007/978-3-032-21123-1

lasts up to 9 months in cows. The allometric growth is characterized by the extensive growth and development of mammary ducts invading the surrounding adipose tissue or mammary fat pad.

Alveolar myoepithelial cells Specialized contractile cells forming a basket-like network around mammary alveoli. They respond directly to circulating oxytocin. Contraction of these cells generates pressure for milk expulsion. They represent the final effector component of the reflex.

Alveoli The primary secretory unit of the mammary gland is the alveoli. Mammary alveoli are lined with milk-secreting cuboidal cells surrounding the lumen. The epithelial cells produce milk that accumulate into the lumen. There is a presence of myoepithelial cells in the alveoli that surround the luminal epithelial cells.

Amino acid transporters They facilitate amino acid transport in the basolateral membrane of mammary epithelial cells. There are two different classes of amino acid transporters: Na^+-dependent transporters and Na^+-independent transporters. The Na^+-dependent transport is an energy-dependent process, and it facilitates unidirectional transport of amino acids utilizing electrochemical gradients of Na^+ and other ions. In contrast, Na^+-independent transport is non-energy dependent and favors bidirectional transport of amino acids.

Amniotes Amniotes are a clade of tetrapod vertebrates adapted to lay eggs on land or preserve the fertilized egg within the mother. They are characterized by the presence of an amnion and include reptiles, birds, and mammals.

Amphiregulin (AREG) It is the most abundant EGF ligand in the mammary gland around puberty to regulate estrogen-primed ductal morphogenesis during puberty. AREG was identified in the luminal epithelium, myoepithelial cells, and stroma of the mammary gland.

Antibody-dependent cellular phagocytosis (ADCP) It is a cellular mechanism in which antibody-opsonized particles are engulfed by phagocytes. In this mechanism, pathogens are opsonized by complement factors or antibodies. It is of two types: Fc receptor-mediated phagocytosis or complement receptor-mediated phagocytosis. In Fc receptor-mediated phagocytosis, phagocytes possess Fcγ receptors that bind with the Fc component of the antibodies coating the pathogens. In contrast, in complement receptor-mediated phagocytosis, complement-coated particles directly sink into the cell. The pathogens are killed by the generation of reactive oxygen and nitrogen species (ROS/RNS).

Antimicrobial peptides (AMPs) They are small peptides of the innate immune system involved in the destruction of bacteria, fungi, parasites, and viruses. In the mammary gland, AMPs such as defensins, cathelicidin, Lactoferrin, Phospholipase A2, and lysozyme are released from neutrophils and epithelial cells.

Apical vesicle route In this route, lipid droplets originate in the rough endoplasmic reticulum as microlipid droplets (MLDs) and are transported toward the apical membrane alone or in combination to form cytoplasmic lipid droplets (CLDs). These droplets are enveloped by the apical plasma membrane (APM) and secreted inform of MLDs or CLDs.

Aquaporins (AQP) These are the water channels involved in the transport of water in the mammary gland through the transcellular route. The AQP creates pores in the membrane to facilitate the transport of water influenced by osmotic gradients. The AQPs exist as intracellular vesicles, and arginine-vasopressin mediates their translocation into the membrane. AQP1, AQP2, AQP3, AQP4, AQP5, AQP6, and AQP7 have been identified in the mammary gland of rats, cows, and humans.

Artificial insemination (AI) A reproductive technique in which semen is collected from a male and manually introduced into the reproductive tract of a female to achieve fertilization.

B lymphocytes They are the cells of the adaptive immune system capable of producing antibodies (immunoglobulins, Ig) against specific exogenous antigens. The antigens are recognized by the membrane receptors present in B lymphocytes called B cell receptors (BCR). Soluble antigens, which are proteins, polysaccharides, and lipids in nature, bind with BCR to initiate intracellular signaling pathways to activate them. Activated B lymphocytes are differentiated into long-lived plasma cells and memory B cells. Plasma cells synthesize mainly IgA and IgM.

Biglycan It is a small leucine-rich proteoglycan of the ECM that attaches with chondroitin sulfate/dermatan sulfate side chains and controls the elasticity of the tissue.

Bioactive peptides They are short protein fragments derived from casein and whey proteins that are inactive in their native form but are released during digestion or food processing, such as fermentation or enzymatic hydrolysis. Once released, they can exert hormone-like effects, providing various health benefits including antihypertensive activity, antimicrobial action, immunomodulatory effects, and antioxidant properties. These attributes make milk-derived bioactive peptides valuable components of functional foods and nutritional supplements.

Biomarker A measurable biological substance that indicates the health, productivity, or disease status of an animal.

Biomolecule Molecule produced by the living organism, essential for various biological processes; includes proteins, polysaccharides, lipids, and nucleic acids (DNA and RNA).

Biosensor An analytical device combining a biological element (like an enzyme or antibody) with an electronic sensor to detect and measure substances quickly.

Biotechnology The use of living organisms, cells, and molecular tools to improve animal production, health, and genetic potential.

Body condition scoring (BCS) It is a visual and hands-on method used to evaluate a cow's fat reserves. Using a numerical scale (1–5 in dairy cows, 1–9 in beef cattle), lower scores indicate thin animals and higher scores indicate over-conditioned ones. BCS helps to monitor energy balance and adjust feeding to support health and reproduction, especially around calving. Scores are determined by feeling and observing fat cover over the ribs, spine, hips, and tail head. For dairy cows, an ideal BCS of about 3–3.5 at calving helps avoid problems such as low milk yield and metabolic disorders.

Burst firing Synchronous, rhythmic discharge pattern of magnocellular oxytocin neurons in the hypothalamus. Each burst produces a discrete pulse of oxytocin release. Burst firing ensures coordinated, efficient milk ejection. It is a hallmark of neuroendocrine synchronization.

Candidate gene analysis (for milk production) It focuses on identifying genes that affect milk yield, fat, and protein by associating genetic variations, such as SNPs, with these traits. Techniques like GWAS, expression profiling, and QTL mapping are used in cattle, sheep, and buffalo to detect these associations, supporting marker-assisted selection for improved dairy performance.

Carboniferous Period (359–299 million years ago) It was a late Paleozoic interval marked by extensive humid swamp forests of giant ferns and club mosses that formed major global coal deposits, produced high atmospheric oxygen levels, and supported giant insects such as *Meganeura* and *Arthropleura*.

Casein genes Genes that code for the main milk proteins responsible for milk's nutritional and cheese-making properties.

Casein A phosphorus-containing protein (phosphoprotein), usually present in mammalian milk. The proteins of the cow's milk contain about 80% phosphoproteins.

Catecholamines Stress-associated hormones (epinephrine and norepinephrine) released during fear or pain. They inhibit milk ejection by suppressing oxytocin neuron firing and constricting mammary blood vessels. Their action explains stress-induced let-down failure. Effects are rapid but reversible.

Cationic amino acid transport protein (CAT) It is a Na^+-independent transporter for cationic amino acids such as arginine and lysine in the mammary gland. There are four types of CAT identified in the mammary gland: y + system (detected in humans, cows, pigs, and rats), y^+L system (pigs and cows), $b^{0,+}$ system (pigs), and $B^{0,+}$ system (pigs, humans, rats).

Caveolae-mediated endocytosis (CavME) It is a clathrin-independent mechanism of endocytosis. Myoepithelial cells surrounding the alveolar epithelium contain small vesicles (50–80 nm) called caveoli. Caveolin-1 is the integral membrane protein of caveoli. The phosphorylation of Caveolin-1 facilitates the internalization of caveolae with the cargo materials.

Chemerin This is a chemoattractant cytokine produced by the stromal adipocytes. It is also called retinoic acid receptor responder protein 2 (RARRES2). They are mainly involved in the regulation of lactogenesis in bovine mammary epithelium.

Chemokines These are low-molecular-weight (8- to 12-kDa) chemotactic cytokines. They are mainly produced by a variety of cells, such as endothelial cells, fibroblasts, and lymphocytes. Chemokines act through specific receptors on their target cells. Chemokines facilitate neutrophil trafficking by generating a gradient-guided signal. Examples of chemokines are CXCL1, CXCL2, CXCL3, etc.

Chemotaxis It is the guided movement of neutrophil migration toward the site of infection in response to certain chemoattractants. Chemoattractants are present either within the vasculature or extravascularly. Within the vascular wall, chemoattractants are immobilized by glycosaminoglycans (GAGs) or heparin sulfate on the endothelial membrane. Extravascularly, they can be attached with the extracellular matrix. The chemoattractants for neutrophil chemotaxis are of four types: lipids, N-formylated peptides, complement anaphylotoxins, and chemokines.

Cisternal fraction of milk This is the milk fraction stored in the teat or gland cisterns and larger milk ducts. In cows, the cisternal fraction constitutes 20% of the total milk volume, whereas in ewes and goats, up to 75% of total milk volume can be of cisternal origin. The cisternal milk can be removed easily through the normal milking procedure.

Cisternal milk Milk stored in the gland and teat cisterns before oxytocin-mediated ejection. It is immediately available at milking onset. This fraction is smaller than alveolar milk in ruminants. Complete milk removal requires alveolar emptying.

Cloning A process of producing genetically identical copies of an organism or cell, often used to multiply elite dairy animals.

Colloidal phase (or colloidal state) It describes a heterogeneous mixture where tiny, insoluble particles (1–1000 nm) of one substance (dispersed phase) are suspended evenly in another (dispersion medium), like milk (liquid in liquid).

Colostrogenesis It refers to the physiological process involved in the synthesis and secretion of colostrum. A distinctive feature of this process is the selective movement of IgG_1 from the maternal circulation into the mammary gland via secretory epithelial cells. The transfer of IgG_1 begins about 4–6 weeks prior to parturition and attains its maximum level at the time of calving.

Colostrum It may be described as the initial, energy-dense mammary secretion produced by the dam immediately after parturition, which is rich in immunoglobulins, antimicrobial peptides, and growth factors. Colostrum is often regarded as the "starter kit" for mammals because it supplies essential bioactive components necessary for neonatal survival.

Complement system (CS) Complement system comprises a group of 29 plasma and membrane proteins synthesized from the liver, tissue macrophages, monocytes, and locally by the mammary tissue. They play pivotal roles in innate immunity by inducing inflammation and destruction of pathogens by opsonization, chemotaxis, and intracellular killing. Activation of the complement system leads to a cascade of reactions that sequentially activate other components to exert effector functions. The most important complement proteins in milk are C1q and C5a.

Conditioned reflex Learned anticipatory oxytocin release triggered by repeated sensory cues such as sound or routine. Conditioning shortens reflex latency and improves milk flow. It reflects higher brain involvement in MER. Consistency in milking enhances this response.

Corpora amylacea The hyaline glycoprotein-rich aggregates found in the alveoli and connective tissue as dense bodies are called corpora amylacea. They originate from desquamated epithelial cells. They are present within the alveoli or in the interstitial tissue. However, their number and locations vary with the stage of lactation.

CRISPR/Cas9 A modern genome-editing tool used to precisely modify or repair specific genes in animals.

Cryopreservation The process of freezing and storing biological materials such as semen, embryos, or oocytes at very low temperatures for future use.

Cytokines Cytokines are immunoregulatory peptides synthesized by mammary epithelial cells and leukocytes. They are involved in cell signaling and facilitate the onset, progression, and resolution of inflammation. Cytokines act via specific receptors. Some important cytokines are interleukins, TNF-α, and IFN-γ. Effects of some recombinant cytokines were studied, and their effects on udder defense were explored in different mastitis models and cytokine immunotherapy could be a promising therapeutic intervention in mastitis.

De novo fatty acid synthesis The synthesis of fatty acids in the mammary gland in the cytosol from the basic building block is acetyl-CoA. In ruminants, fatty acids are synthesized from acetate and butyrate, whereas in non-ruminants, the fatty acids are synthesized from glucose. Fatty acid synthesis also requires NADPH as a reducing equivalent, which is derived from the pentose-phosphate cycle and the isocitrate cycle (ruminants) or from the pentose-phosphate cycle and the malate transhydrogenation cycle (non-ruminants). The other co-factors required for de novo synthesis of fatty acids are Mn^{+2}, biotin, and HCO_3^{-}.

Decorin It is a small leucine-rich proteoglycan that binds to collagen I to regulate collagen fibrillogenesis.

Dendritic release Local secretion of oxytocin from dendrites of hypothalamic neurons. It modulates neuronal excitability and promotes synchronization. Dendritic release occurs independently of peripheral hormone secretion. It primes the neural network for burst firing.

Desmosomes These are the adhesive intercellular junctions between mammary epithelial cells and the basal myoepithelial cells. Desmosomes are composed of two main proteins, namely desmoglein (Dsg) and desmocollin (Dsc) of the cadherin family.

Diapedesis It is the passage of blood cells through capillary walls into the tissues. By the process of diapedesis, neutrophils reach the site of infection in response to certain chemoattractants. Diapedesis is mediated by continuous formation of new adhesive contacts at the front and detachment in the rear. During diapedesis, the neutrophils adhere to capillary endothelial cells and subsequently penetrate the endothelial layer to reach subepithelial stromal tissues.

Early mammal A small, shrew-like, warm-blooded vertebrate possessing mammary glands and the ability to produce milk for its young. Early mammals lived alongside dinosaurs during the Late Triassic period (around 210 million years ago).

Eccrine glands These are the most common type of sweat glands, found almost everywhere on the skin, crucial for thermoregulation (cooling the body) by releasing watery sweat (mostly water and salts) directly onto the surface, which cools the body as it evaporates.

Electrical conductivity It measures a material's ability to conduct electric current, indicating how easily electrons flow through it. High conductivity means free charge carriers, while low conductivity means resistance to flow.

Embryo transfer technology (ETT) A technique where embryos from a superior donor female are transferred to recipient females to produce multiple offspring.

Emulsion It is a mixture of two or more liquids that normally don't mix, like oil and water, where tiny droplets of one liquid are dispersed within the other, stabilized by an emulsifier. Common examples include milk (oil-in-water).

Endogenous opioids Neuropeptides (e.g., β-endorphins) released during stress or pain. They inhibit oxytocin neuron activity via opioid receptors. This mechanism contributes to stress-related reflex suppression. Opioid antagonists can experimentally restore MER.

Ephrin This is a paracrine factor secreted by myoepithelial cells that is involved in the adhesion and migration of mammary epithelial cells.

Epidermal growth factors (EGFs) These are the common mitogenic polypeptide involved in the mammary gland growth and differentiation in different species. It induces DNA synthesis in mammary epithelial cells to promote proliferation and duct growth.

Epimorphin This is a paracrine factor released from mammary epithelial cells that helps in branching and tubular morphogenesis.

Epoch A particular phase of a period characterized by a distinguishing development.

Euglycemic–hyperinsulinemic clamp test It is the gold-standard method to assess insulin sensitivity in humans and animals. In this test, insulin is infused at a constant rate to elevate plasma insulin level along with simultaneous glucose administration at different rates to maintain euglycemic state (normal blood glucose). This glucose infusion rate (GIR) is the indicator of insulin sensitivity. High GIR denotes insulin sensitivity, whereas lower GIR indicates resistance to insulin.

Eutheria The placenta-bearing mammals; also called placental mammals.

Fatty acid desaturation It is the process of the dehydrogenation of saturated fatty acids to form monounsaturated fatty acids by the enzyme stearoyl-CoA desaturase (SCD). The enzyme SCD is present in the membrane of the endoplasmic reticulum. In cattle, two forms of SCD are found: SCD1 and SCD5. In the mammary gland and adipose tissue, SCD1 is predominantly expressed.

Fatty acid synthase (FASN) It is a multi-functional enzyme complex involved in fatty acid synthesis. The enzyme complex involves seven enzymes, namely β-ketoacyl synthase (KS), acetyl/malonyl-CoA transferase (MAT), β-hydroxyacyl dehydratase (DH), enoyl reductase (ER), β-ketoacyl reductase (KR), acyl-carrier protein (ACP), and thioesterase I (TE I). The enzyme complex produces a 16-carbon saturated fatty acid from seven malonyl-CoA molecules with one acetyl-CoA.

Fatty acid translocase (FAT) This is a scavenger receptor protein expressed in the immune cells, platelets, adipocytes, enterocytes, myocytes, and retinal and mammary epithelial cells involved in the fatty acid uptake. When the ligand binds with CD36, it internalizes with the ligands and translocates to a lysosome. FAT controls the entry of long-chain fatty acids in collaboration with SLC27A and acyl-CoA synthetase (ACSL).

Feed efficiency The ability of an animal to convert feed nutrients into milk or body weight effectively, reducing feed cost and waste.

Fibromodulin It is a small leucine-rich proteoglycan of the ECM that binds with collagen type I fibrils and regulates collagen fibrillogenesis.

Fibronectin (FN) It is a 500-kDa dimeric glycoprotein of the extracellular matrix that acts as an adhesive for the attachment of the ECM to the basement membrane. It also plays a significant role in ductal morphogenesis and end bud formation during mammogenesis.

Furstenberg's rosette It is the structure made by the mucosal folds at the proximal site of the streak canal. The epithelial lining of the teat canal becomes squamous to columnar epithelium at this point; hence, it is also called the squamocolumnar junction. The rosette acts as a mechanical seal and provides local defense against pathogens.

Furstenberg's rosette-associated lymphoid tissue (FALT) This is the aggregate of lymphoid follicles at the Furstenberg's rosette. It consists of plasma cells and lymphocytes. The plasma cells produce antibodies such as IgG1, IgM, and IgA to provide humoral immunity. The cells of Furstenberg's rosette are reported to produce biquitin, a cationic bactericidal protein.

Galactophore "Galacto" signifies milk, and "Phore" denotes bearing. So, galactophore means the milk-carrying duct, which may also be called the lactiferous duct.

Galactosemia It is a rare inherited metabolic disorder in which the body is unable to properly metabolize galactose, resulting in its toxic accumulation. The condition arises from deficiency or functional impairment of enzymes of the Leloir pathway, such as galactokinase (GALK), which converts galactose to galactose-1-phosphate, and galactose-1-phosphate uridyltransferase (GALT). Common clinical features include hepatosplenomegaly and jaundice, cataract formation, and neurological impairment.

Gap junctions They are specialized conduits between two adjacent epithelial cells that permit the passage of ions and small molecules up to 1500 Da between the cells. Structurally, they are hemichannels made of six connexin molecules.

Genome-wide association studies (GWAS) A study that examines the entire genomes of large groups of individuals to identify genetic variations, such as single-nucleotide polymorphisms (SNPs), linked to specific traits or diseases. By finding markers that are more common in individuals with a particular condition, GWAS helps locate genes and genomic regions involved in the trait, providing insights for improved prevention and treatment strategies.

Genomic selection A method that uses DNA information from across the genome to predict an animal's genetic potential for milk yield and other traits.

Ghrelin It is a hormone produced by the stomach. This hormone regulates energy homeostasis, body weight, and food intake. It is an indicator of negative energy balance and the strongest peripheral stimulator for food intake. Increased concentration of ghrelin during the post-partum period increases the demand for feed during lactation.

Gland cistern (sinus lactiferous or udder cistern) It is the cavities within the udder that store milk between milkings. The capacities of the gland cistern vary considerably between species. In cows, the gland cistern can store 100 to 400 ml of milk.

Glucose-sparing mechanism Ruminants have a well-developed glucose-sparing mechanism in the mammary gland that prevents the use of glucose in the synthesis of milk fatty acids. This is mediated by low activities of key enzymes such as adenosine triphosphate (ATP)-citrate lyase, nicotinamide adenine dinucleotide phosphate (NADP)-malate dehydrogenase, and pyruvate carboxylase required for the citrate cleavage pathway for the generation of extra-mitochondrial acetyl-CoA.

Glucose transporter (GLUT) The GLUT favors facultative glucose transport across the plasma membrane of several epithelial cells. In the mechanism, bidirectional glucose transport occurs down the concentration gradient without the utilization of ATP. Glucose enters the mammary epithelial cells through GLUT1 and GLUT8. These two glucose transporters also favor glucose transport between the cytoplasm and the Golgi apparatus. GLUT8 and GLUT12 help to maintain glucose equilibrium between glucose in MEC and glucose in milk.

Growth hormone (somatotropin) A hormone produced by the pituitary gland that regulates growth and supports milk production by stimulating nutrient use.

Homeorhesis It refers to the alterations in the metabolism of body tissues to support a physiological state. The classical example of homeorhesis is the metabolic changes that occur during the initiation of lactation, such as an insulin-resistant state in which the sensitivity and responsiveness to insulin are decreased in many peripheral tissues that favor the transport of glucose to tissues that are less dependent on insulin, such as the mammary gland.

Hypermastia It is a form of supernumerary teats that can secrete milk. It has a separate teat cistern.

Hyperthelia It is a kind of non-secreting supernumerary teats.

Hypothalamic–pituitary–adrenal (HPA) axis It is the main system for handling stress in the body. It is a coordinated pathway connecting the hypothalamus and pituitary gland with the adrenal glands. When stress occurs, the hypothalamus releases corticotropin-releasing hormone (CRH), which prompts the pituitary to secrete ACTH. ACTH then stimulates the adrenal glands to produce cortisol, a hormone that mobilizes energy and helps the body maintain balance and adapt to stress.

Hypothalamo–hypophyseal axis Functional connection between hypothalamic neurons and posterior pituitary. It enables the rapid conversion of neural signals into hormonal release. This axis is central to oxytocin secretion. It exemplifies neuroendocrine integration.

IGF-binding proteins (IGFBP) They are a group of six structurally similar proteins (IGFBP 1–6) that bind strongly to IGF-1 and IGF-2, and regulate their availability. They transport IGFs, regulate their distribution, and can also influence cells independently of IGFs. By controlling IGF access to its receptors, and sometimes acting through their own signaling pathways or by entering the nucleus, IGFBPs play a key role in regulating growth and metabolism.

Immunoglobulins (Ig) Immunoglobulins (Igs) are the most important humoral defense factors of the mammary gland that link the cellular and humoral immune responses. Major portions of immunoglobulins are transported from the blood via a selective receptor-mediated intracellular route. A small portion is produced from localized plasma cells. The major functions of immunoglobulins include opsonization of bacteria prior to phagocytosis, inhibition of the metabolism of bacteria, activation of complement-mediated bacteriolytic mechanisms, and neutralization of toxins and viruses. There are four important immunoglobulins concerned with mammary gland defense, such as IgG1, IgG2, IgM, and IgA, out of which IgG1, IgG2, and IgM are involved in opsonization and IgA is concerned with toxin neutralization and agglutination of bacteria.

Immunomodulator A substance that enhances or regulates the immune system to improve resistance against diseases.

In vitro fertilization (IVF) A reproductive method where eggs and sperm are combined outside the body to form embryos, which are later transferred into the uterus.

Inhibited milk ejection Functional failure of milk let-down despite normal milk synthesis. It commonly results from stress, pain, or environmental change. Oxytocin release or delivery is impaired. Management focuses on stress reduction rather than milk production.

Insulin-like growth factors (IGF) These are polypeptides produced mainly by the liver and other local tissues having structural similarities with insulin. IGF is produced from stromal cells and mammary epithelial cells under the influence of growth hormone and is involved in mammogenesis to regulate cell growth, cell differentiation, and prevention of apoptosis.

Integrins These are the transmembrane receptors in the mammary epithelial cells that facilitate cell–ECM interaction. These are heterodimers composed of α and β subunits. Integrin receptor has cytoplasmic, transmembrane, and extracellular domains.

Intermammary groove (sulcus intermammaricus) The connective tissue septum between the right and left udder halves forms a groove called the intermammary groove.

Intramammary (IMM) infusion It is the method of application of drugs and other medications directly into the mammary gland through the teat canal. Usually, antibiotics and teat sealants are applied through intramammary infusion. In this method, the medicines are injected through a syringe or applicator into the teat canal.

IP_3-Ca^{2+} pathway Intracellular signaling cascade activated by oxytocin receptor stimulation. IP_3 induces calcium release from intracellular stores. Elevated Ca^{2+} activates contractile machinery. This pathway directly mediates myoepithelial contraction.

Isometric mammary growth The phase of mammogenesis when the mammary growth is proportionate with the body growth is termed isometric mammary growth. The non-epithelial tissues of the mammary gland exhibit isometric growth that lasts for 3 months in cows. The isometric phase of mammary growth is characterized by growth of the mammary fat pad and connective tissue, which increases the udder size.

Keratocan It is a keratan sulfate proteoglycan that helps to maintain mammary gland integrity.

Lactation curve It is a graphical depiction of milk yield across the lactation period. In dairy cows, the curve is typically bell-shaped, showing a steady rise to a peak at about 4–6 weeks, followed by a gradual decline until the cow is dried off before the next calving. The lactation curve indicates overall production efficiency and the factors influencing it. The main phases include early lactation (0–100 days), peak lactation (30–40 days), mid-lactation (100–200 days), and late lactation (200–300 days).

Lactogenesis The initiation of milk secretion is called lactogenesis. The mammary gland undergoes enzymatic and cytological differentiations to produce milk. Lactogenesis occurs in two distinct stages, namely secretory differentiation and secretory activation. Secretory differentiation involves the transformation of mammary epithelial cells into specialized cells (lactocytes) capable of producing milk components such as lactose, casein, α-lactalbumin, and fatty acids. Secretory activation refers to the onset of copious milk secretion.

Lactogenic complex This is a group of hormones of pituitary, ovarian, and placental origin that favors the secretory differentiation of the mammary gland during lactogenesis. The lactogenesis in ruminants is triggered mainly by prolactin and glucocorticoids. However, for the maximum action of these hormones, a declining level of progesterone is essential. Other hormones, like thyroid hormones, act in conjunction with prolactin for the synthesis of α-lactalbumin.

Lactoperoxidase (LPO) It is one of the important enzymes present in the milk that promote killing of pathogens by the production of hypothiocyanite and hypothiocyanous acid from the oxidation of thiocyanate in the presence of hydrogen peroxide. Higher LPO activity was associated with increased SCC in both cows and goats.

Lactose intolerance It is a common digestive condition in which the body is unable to properly digest lactose, the sugar present in milk and dairy products, because of inadequate production of the enzyme lactase. As a result, consumption of lactose-containing foods can cause symptoms such as bloating, gas, abdominal cramps, diarrhea, and nausea.

Lactose synthase (LS) It is the enzyme that catalyzes the synthesis of lactose from UDP-galactose and glucose. It is an enzyme complex that consists of two different proteins, namely β-1,4-galactosyltransferase-1 (B4GALT1) and mammary-specific modifier protein α-lactalbumin (LALBA). B4GALT1 transfers galactose from UDP-galactose, and LALBA acts as an enzyme modifier.

Laminin (LM) It is a glycoprotein released by mammary adipocytes. There are four different LM isoforms in the mammary gland of human like laminin-111 (LM-1; α1, β1, γ1), laminin-322 (LM-5; α3, β3, γ2), laminin-511 (LM-10), and laminin-521 (LM-11). They are involved in the growth and development of the mammary gland.

Latency (reflex) Time interval between teat stimulation and onset of milk flow. It reflects the speed of neuroendocrine activation. Prolonged latency indicates reflex inhibition. Proper pre-stimulation minimizes delay.

Lateral suspensory ligaments The ligament is one of the supporting structures of the udder that originates from the sub-pelvic tendon and enters laterally into the udder. This ligament is non-stretchable. The lateral suspensory ligaments have two layers: the superficial layer of lateral suspensory ligaments and the deep layer of lateral suspensory ligaments.

Leptin It is a hormone secreted primarily by the adipose tissue. It is involved in the regulation of energy metabolism, feeding behavior, and reproductive functions in animals and humans. It links the nutritional status of an animal with reproductive function. Higher concentration of leptin causes diminished feed intake and increased energy expenditure, whereas low concentration of leptin induces feed intake by modulating the activity of the neurons located in the arcuate, ventromedial, and dorsomedial hypothalamic nuclei. The state of negative energy balance is associated with reduced plasma leptin level that induces feed intake and depletion of lipid reserve.

Lipocalins A group of small-sized extracellular proteins chiefly responsible for binding and transporting small hydrophobic molecules. They are involved in immune cell activation, initiation of cellular responses, and pheromone signaling. Example: Retinol-binding protein 4 (RBP4).

Lipolysis It is the metabolic process by which triacylglycerols (TAGs) are broken down by hydrolysis to generate non-esterified fatty acids (NEFA). These NEFAs are oxidized in the liver for energy production. The process of lipolysis is mediated by enzymes lipases such as hormone-sensitive lipase (HSL), adipose triglyceride lipase (ATGL), and monoglyceride lipase (MGL). Lipolysis is of two types, basal lipolysis and demand lipolysis. The basal lipolysis depends on the adipocyte stores and increases throughout lactation. The demand for lipolysis is regulated in response to energy demands and induced by endocrine responses. HSL and MGL play a major role in demand lipolysis.

L-type amino acid transporter-2 (LAT-2) It is an important amino acid transporter system in the mammary gland that facilitates the uptake of branched-chain amino acids (BCAA) in mammary epithelial cells.

Lumican It is a small leucine-rich proteoglycan (SLRP) in the extracellular matrix that interacts with $\alpha 2\beta 1$ integrin to stimulate cell adhesion. It also inhibits cell migration and prevents metastasis.

Lymphocytes Lymphocytes are generally small, round cells containing a large nucleus. In the healthy mammary gland of a cow, the total lymphocyte count was <50,000/mL, which is <20% of the total SCC in milk. Lymphocytes mediate specific responses by recognizing antigens of invading pathogens through membrane receptors. There are two distinct classes of lymphocytes. B-lymphocytes are involved in the production of antibodies against invading pathogens, whereas T-lymphocytes are responsible for cell-mediated immunity.

Lysozyme It is one of the important soluble defense factors under the innate immune system that cleaves β-1,4-glycosidic link between N-acetylmuramic acid and N-acetyl-D-glucosamine residues in peptidoglycans present in the cell wall of Gram-positive bacteria and outer membrane of Gram-negative bacteria. The concentration of lysozyme in milk cow is 0.0004 g/L. A significant increase in lysozyme concentration was reported during mastitis in cows.

Macrophages Macrophages are the predominant leukocytes in the milk, comprising 10–80% of the total cell populations in healthy animals. They are derived from blood and differentiate within the mammary gland. Macrophages perform a dual role both in innate and adaptive immunity. Phagocytosis of the invading pathogens and secretions of pro-inflammatory cytokines are the innate functions of macrophages, while they can also act as antigen-presenting cells to facilitate adaptive immune responses. The macrophages also play a pivotal role in mammary involution by digesting cellular debris and milk components.

Magnocellular neurons Large neurosecretory neurons located in PVN and SON. They synthesize oxytocin and project to the posterior pituitary. Their synchronized activity generates hormone pulses. They form the central motor unit of MER.

Mammalia The warm-blooded higher vertebrates' class that can nurture young with mammary glands that secrete milk. Example: monotremes, marsupials, eutherians, including humans.

Mammary artery The external pudendal artery provides the primary blood supply to the mammary glands; hence, it is called the mammary artery. It originates from the external iliac artery and enters at the dorsal surface of the udder via the inguinal canal.

Mammary bud Knob-shaped structure above the dermis seen around 43 days of embryonic life in cows. It is developed due to continual invagination of the ectodermal layer into the mesenchymal layer. The ectodermal cells are then surrounded by fibroblast-like cells and sink within the collagen of the stroma with a small depression at the outer pole called the mammary pit.

Mammary epithelial cells These are the active secretory cells involved in milk production. They also play a pivotal role in mammary gland immunity. They produce dimeric IgA, antimicrobial peptides, and chemokines. They also act as non-professional phagocytes. They recognize microbe-associated molecular patterns (MAMP) to modulate inflammatory reactions.

Mammary line The transient structures develop from the lower ectodermal layer (Malpighian or germinal layer) around 30, 34, and 10 days of embryonic life, respectively, in cows, buffaloes, and mice. The mammary lines disappear within a short period (35–42 days in cows), and mammary placodes are developed along the mammary lines.

Mammary patch The hair follicles associated with a distinct section of the skin where milk-producing glands are positioned, generally present in the Synapsids. Nipples originated from this region in the Mammalia class.

Mammary placode It is a lens-shaped, minute structure developed as a result of the migration of cells that gives rise to a multilayered columnar cell arrangement inside the mammary lines. There are one pair of mammary placodes in humans and five pairs in mice.

Mammary stem cells (MaSCs) These are multipotent adult stem cells of epithelial origin that give rise to bipotent putative common progenitor cells from which unipotent luminal and basal progenitors are generated. The basal progenitor cells form ductal epithelium and myoepithelial cells, whereas luminal progenitors form secretory epithelial cells. The differentiation of fetal MaSCs into unipotent luminal progenitor cells is mediated by Notch signaling.

Marker-assisted selection (MAS) A breeding approach that uses molecular markers linked to desirable genes to select superior animals.

Marsupials A group of mammals, comprising marsupials (pouch) that have nipples, in the mother's abdomen to nourish the premature young during birth. Example: Kangaroos, Koalas, and Opossums.

Median suspensory ligament This is the main supporting structure of the udder with the greatest tensile strength. It originates as two parallel connective tissue sheaths and runs ventrally to the glandular tissue. It is also divided into abdominal (lamina medialis pars abdominalis) and pelvic (lamina medialis pars pelvinae) parts. This ligament becomes weaker in older cows and leads to a pendulous udder and udder edema.

Metabolomics The study of small molecules (metabolites) in biological samples to understand metabolic changes in animals.

Milk fat globule membrane (MFGM) It is a complex, multilayered biological membrane that envelops milk fat globules and is enriched with bioactive lipids such as phospholipids, sphingolipids, and cholesterol, along with associated proteins. This membrane functions as a protective barrier and plays an essential role in stabilizing the fat–water emulsion in milk.

Milk fat globule membrane (MFGM) It is the membrane that surrounds triacyl glyceride-dense fat globules in milk. It is composed of polar lipids and proteins. The MFGM is derived from either the apical plasma membrane or endoplasmic reticulum. It protects the milk fat globules from digestion and maintains the stability of milk emulsion.

Milk flow curve Graphical representation of milk flow rate during milking. It reflects reflex efficiency and equipment synchronization. Abnormal curves indicate inhibited let-down or pathology. Widely used in dairy diagnostics.

Milk lipid droplets Milk lipids are secreted in the form of milk fat droplets composed of triglycerides (95%) with lesser amounts of sterols, partial glycerides, phospholipids, glycolipids, and hydrocarbons. Milk droplets are of two types: cytoplasmic lipid droplets (CLDs) (size 1–5 μm) and microlipid droplets (MLDs) (size 0.5 μm or less).

Milk vein It is the subcutaneous abdominal vein that extends along the lower side of the abdomen of a cow. This vein exits the mammary gland at the anterior end of the front quarters and runs along the abdominal wall. It is visible under the skin on the cow's abdomen and enters the body cavity through a depression at the xiphoid process, known as the "milk wells," before emptying into the internal thoracic vein.

MMA syndrome (mastitis, metritis, and agalactia) It is mostly seen in sows immediately after farrowing (12 h to 3 days). The disease usually occurs due to bacterial infection and is characterized by udder inflammation and uterine infection, together with vulval discharges and decreased milk production. MMA leads to piglet mortality and reduced weaning weight.

Monotremes The egg-laying, predatory, primitive mammals, with a short gestation and long lactation period, capable of secreting milk from nipple-less mammary patches connected with the abdominal mammolobular-pilo-sebaceous unit (MPSU).

Myeloperoxidase (MPO) It is a lysosomal enzyme (heme protein) present in the primary granules of neutrophils and facilitates oxygen-dependent killing of pathogens. The reaction catalyzed by myeloperoxidase is similar to LPO, but, additionally, it catalyzes chloride oxidation to kill pathogens. The activity of MPO is increased during clinical and subclinical mastitis.

Myoepithelial cells These are modified smooth muscle cells having the characteristics of both smooth muscle and epithelial cells. They are prevalent in both acini and ducts. They have long cytoplasmic projections that form a basket-like network surrounding the luminal epithelial cells. They contain actin and myosin filaments similar to those in smooth muscle and contract in response to oxytocin, thereby facilitating milk let-down. In addition, they are involved in the regulation of tissue polarity, synthesis of basement membrane components, and regulation of ductal morphogenesis.

Myoepithelial contraction Oxytocin-induced shortening of myoepithelial cells surrounding alveoli. It increases alveolar pressure and expels milk. Contraction is rapid and synchronized. Failure leads to milk retention.

Nanobiotechnology The use of nanoscale materials and particles to deliver drugs, hormones, or nutrients efficiently and safely in animals.

Natural selection The evolutionary process for better adaptation to their environment to survive and produce successors. Eventually, divergence of species occurred by this mechanism. The theory was elucidated by Charles Darwin.

Negative energy balance (NEB) It is the state of the body in which the body expends more energy than it consumes, which results in a net loss of energy. During the transition from pregnancy to lactation, the energy requirement exceeds energy consumption, and cows enter a state of NEB. It generally occurs 3 weeks before calving and 3 weeks after calving. During this NEB state, body energy reserves, mainly glycogen, fat, and protein, are mobilized to meet the high energy demands of lactation. If cows fail to adequately compensate for this metabolic challenge, they become predisposed to various metabolic and infectious diseases.

Neogenin This is a paracrine factor secreted by myoepithelial cells that helps in cell clustering during the formation of the terminal end buds.

Neonatal Fc receptor (FcRn) It is an MHC class I–related receptor consisting of a heavy α-chain associated with a light β_2-microglobulin chain. FcRn specifically binds IgG_1, IgG_2, and bovine serum albumin (BSA), with the interaction being highly pH dependent. This receptor plays a crucial role in the selective and preferential transport of IgG_1 into colostrum.

Net energy intake (NEI) It is the amount of usable energy a dairy cow obtains from its feed. It is determined by multiplying the cow's dry matter intake (DMI) by the feed's net energy value. This represents the energy available for body maintenance, milk production, growth, and reproduction after accounting for energy lost as heat and in waste.

N-ethylmaleimide–sensitive fusion (NSF) attachment protein receptor (SNARE) proteins These proteins are involved in the fusion of casein-containing secretory vesicles with the apical plasma membrane prior to exocytosis of milk proteins. There are two classes of SNARE proteins: R-SNAREs present on the membrane of secretory vesicles and Q-SNAREs on the apical membrane. These two classes of SNARE proteins fuse with each other to form the SNARE complex, and exocytosis occurs. The dissociation of the SNARE complex is facilitated by NSF adenosine triphosphatase and its adaptor protein synaptosomal-associated protein (SNAP).

Neuregulins (NRG) They are EGF-like signaling molecules that play a pivotal role in the embryonic development of mammary glands by promoting stem cell renewal and specification of mammary lineage. The epithelial aggregation is stimulated by NRG3 as a mesenchymal paracrine signal during placode formation.

Neuroendocrine reflex Reflex integrating neural input with endocrine output. MER is a classic example. Sensory stimulation leads to hormonal release and peripheral action. It demonstrates brain–gland coordination.

Neutrophil extracellular traps (NETs) It is a novel mechanism intended by neutrophils for non-phagocytic killing of microorganisms. NETs are the large web-like structures made of cytosolic and granular proteins of neutrophils assembled on decondensed chromatin materials that cause immobilization of microorganisms and their elimination.

Nidogen (entactin) It is a 150-kDa sulfated glycoprotein secreted from stromal fibroblasts and helps to form the basal lamina.

Nutrigenomics The study of how nutrients interact with genes to influence milk production, health, and metabolism.

Ontogenetic Development of an entity from its origin (single cell) to a mature or adult (multicellular) state.

Opsonization The process of immune recognition of pathogens by the cells of the immune system is called opsonization. Opsonization is mediated by specific antibodies. Predominant opsonizing antibodies for bovine PMN are IgM and IgG2; however, IgM is the most important for phagocytosis. Other than the antibodies, complement C3b also opsonizes bacteria. The antibody has two sites, one for recognizing the bacterium (Fab regions) and the other to bind with PMN via Fc-receptors (FcR) on the plasma membrane.

Oviparity The reproductive process in which young develop from eggs laid outside the mother's body. Animals that have oviparity are called oviparous.

Oxytocin Nonapeptide hormone synthesized in PVN and SON of the hypothalamus. It induces myoepithelial contraction and milk ejection. Oxytocin also modulates maternal behavior and stress. It is central to lactation physiology.

fvOxytocin receptor (OXTR) G-protein-coupled receptor expressed mainly on myoepithelial cells. Activation triggers PLC–IP_3–Ca^{2+} signaling. Receptor density increases during lactation. Desensitization reduces reflex efficiency.

Oxytocin surge Transient rise in plasma oxytocin concentration during milk ejection. Each surge corresponds to neuronal burst firing. Magnitude determines the strength of contraction. Surges are short-lived due to rapid clearance.

Paracellular transport It refers to the transport of nutrients through leaky tight junctions. This route of transport is usually absent during lactation, but it is functional during pregnancy and late lactation. The hormone prolactin and glucocorticoids are responsible for altering the permeability of mammary epithelial cells and thus the paracellular transport also.

Paraventricular nucleus (PVN) Hypothalamic nucleus housing oxytocin-producing neurons. Works in coordination with SON. PVN neurons synchronize during MER. It integrates sensory and emotional inputs.

Period The basic unit of geologic time, comprising tens of millions of years based on the evolution of a particular rock system. A few periods, in combination, form an era, and a period can be subdivided into an Epoch.

Perlecan This is a complex glycosaminoglycan that comprises a core protein linked with heparin sulfate. It provides structural integrity of the basal lamina.

Persistency of lactation It describes how well a cow maintains milk yield after reaching peak production. It reflects the rate of post-peak decline, with higher persistency shown by a flatter lactation curve. Because cows with high persistency lose milk more slowly, this trait contributes significantly to farm profitability, whereas low persistency leads to a rapid drop in yield.

Phagosomes These are subcellular organelles that generate a hostile environment for the pathogen for its destruction. Phagosomes are formed when opsonized particles are encircled by an invagination of the PMN plasma membrane. The phagosomes are fused with lysosomes to form a phagolysosome that mediates bacterial killing with the help of reactive oxygen species (ROS) and antimicrobial peptides.

Phenolphthalein endpoint It is the point where the solution changes from colorless to a faint, persistent pink, indicating a pH shift to slightly alkaline (around pH 8.2–10.0).

Placentation The formation, type, fashion, and structure of the placenta.

Pleiotrophin (PTN)/heparin affin regulatory peptide (HARP) This is a paracrine factor secreted from mammary epithelial cells that controls tissue morphogenesis by delaying the maturation of epithelial cells.

Polymorphonuclear neutrophils (PMNs) These are the predominant cell type constituting more than 90% of total leukocytes during the early stage of inflammation. Neutrophils constitute 5% to 20% of the total SCC in normal bovine milk. Bovine PMN is characterized by a multilobulated nucleus within the plasma membrane and granular cytoplasm. These granules, present in the cytoplasm of neutrophils, contain several proteins involved in the phagocytic killing of microorganisms. During infection, PMNs usually migrate from the peripheral circulation under the influence of different inflammatory mediators like cytokines, chemokines, complements, and prostaglandins. The primary function of PMN is the phagocytic killing of bacteria. Besides this, they produce antimicrobial peptides and cytokines. They also help in the modification of the extracellular matrix.

Polyunsaturated fatty acids (PUFAs) They are fats characterized by the presence of two or more double bonds and are essential nutrients that must be supplied through the diet. They play vital roles in brain development, maintenance of cell membrane structure, and overall health. PUFAs are mainly classified into two groups: omega-3 and omega-6 fatty acids.

Precision dairy farming A modern management approach using sensors, computers, and data analysis to monitor and optimize animal health and production.

Probiotics Live beneficial microorganisms that improve digestion, rumen function, and immunity in dairy animals.

Proliferator-activated receptor γ (PPARγ) It is a transcription factor that regulates fatty acid synthesis. PPARγ forms a heterodimer with Retinoid X receptor (RXR) and binds with peroxisome proliferator-activated receptor (PPAR) response elements (PPRE), which induces the expression of genes responsible for fatty acid synthesis (fatty acid synthase, acetyl-CoA carboxylase, and stearoyl-coa desaturase) and fatty acid transport (CD36). Long-chain fatty acids (LCFA) are potent agonists of PPARγ. Polyunsaturated fatty acids (PUFAs) are the natural ligands of PPARγ in non-ruminants.

Proteomics The study of all proteins in a biological system to understand cell functions and milk composition.

Proteose-peptone (PP) It is a highly nutritious, heat-stable protein hydrolysate derived from milk or vegetable sources, and is rich in peptides, proteoses, and free amino acids.

QTL mapping (Quantitative Trait Locus mapping) It is a genetic technique used to identify regions of the genome that influence complex traits such as growth, yield, or disease resistance. It links genetic markers with differences in quantitative traits within a designed mapping population. Typically, two genetically distinct parents are crossed to produce offspring (like F2 or backcross generations) with mixed genomes. By comparing marker patterns (such as SNPs) with measured traits and applying statistical analysis, QTL mapping helps uncover the genetic basis and contribution of different genomic regions to complex traits.

Reactive nitrogen species (RNS) These are a family of antimicrobial oxidant molecules derived from nitric oxide. They are generated when nitric oxide reacts with reactive oxygen species like superoxide ($O_2^{\bullet -}$) and hydrogen peroxide (H_2O_2). The examples of RNS are nitrogen dioxide (NO_2) and peroxynitrite (ONOO-). RNS have pivotal roles in phagocytic killing of pathogens, regulation of cell signaling pathways, maintenance of vascular tone, regulation of tight junctions, etc.

Reactive oxygen species (ROS) They are the derivatives of molecular oxygen involved in the respiratory burst activity in phagocytic cells like neutrophils and macrophages. Superoxide anion ($O^{-\cdot}{}_2$), singlet oxygen ($^1O_2$), hypochlorous acid (HOCl), hydrogen peroxide (H_2O_2), and hydroxyl radical ($OH^{\cdot}$) are some important ROS produced by the conversion of molecular oxygen to its univalent reduction products. ROS cause oxidation of DNA, RNA, proteins, and lipids, thus killing the pathogens.

Recombinant bovine somatotropin (rBST) A biotechnologically produced form of growth hormone used to increase milk yield in dairy cows.

Residual milk Milk remaining in alveoli after incomplete ejection. It reduces milk yield and predisposes to mastitis. High residual milk indicates inhibited reflex. Effective stimulation minimizes retention.

Resistin It is a peptide hormone synthesized by the adipose tissue involved in the regulation of insulin action, energy, glucose, and lipid homeostasis. During lactation, resistin promotes lipolysis by inducing the transcription of ATGL and HSL. The concentration of resistin is increased after calving and returns to the pre-partum state by 6 weeks of lactation.

Respiratory burst It is a series of enzymatic events that suddenly increase the oxidative metabolism of a cell and results in the conversion of molecular oxygen to its univalent reduction product, the superoxide anion ($O_2^{-}\bullet$), along with other reactive oxygen species such as hydrogen peroxide (H_2O_2), singlet oxygen ($^1O_2$), hypochlorous acid (HOCl), and hydroxyl radical ($OH\bullet$). This activity is seen in neutrophils and other phagocytic cells during the process of phagocytosis.

Rumen microbial manipulation The process of altering microbial populations in the rumen to improve digestion, reduce methane, and enhance feed efficiency.

Secretory activation It is the process of development of the enzymatic machinery in newly differentiated secretory cells for the synthesis of milk. In cows, the onset of secretory activation starts in parallel with structural differentiation of the mammary gland. In contrast, the enzymatic activation of the mammary gland occurs immediately after parturition in rats and guinea pigs. During this period, enzymes involved in glycolysis, the hexose monophosphate pathway, and the synthesis of milk fat, protein, and lactose are activated, thereby facilitating mammary gland metabolism and the production of milk constituents.

Secretory differentiation The process of secretory differentiation is aimed at developing biochemical and cytological machinery to synthesize milk. The secretory differentiation starts during the peri-parturient period in response to different endocrine factors. The proliferation of mammary epithelium (hyperplasia) occurs during gestation, whereas the cell differentiation (hypertrophy) is the characteristic feature during the post-partum period.

Siamese teats (supernumerary teats) This is the most common congenital anomaly in cows, sheep, and goats of the mammary gland that is characterized by the appearance of small extra teats attached either to fore and rear teats or can be seen in different locations, such as between fore and rear teats or behind the rear teats. The Siamese teat interferes with milking and increases the chances of mastitis; hence, they are usually removed at the age of 2–6 weeks.

Small leucine-rich proteoglycan (SLRP) They are active components of the ECM and bind with growth factors, cytokines, and cell surface receptors to induce signal transduction pathways and regulate biomechanical properties of tissues. Some important SLRPs of the mammary gland are decorin, lumican, biglycan, fibromodulin, and keratocan.

Sodium-coupled neutral amino acid transporter (SNAT) It facilitates the transport of branched-chain amino acids, particularly leucine, into the mammary gland. There are three subtypes of SNAT, namely SNAT 1, 2, and 4. Upregulation of SNAT2 gene expression is induced by estradiol.

Sodium-glucose co-transporters (SGLTs) The SGLTs transport glucose into the mammary gland coupled with Na^+ ions. The SGLT facilitates unidirectional transport of glucose by utilizing the electrochemical gradient of Na^+, which is created by Na^+,K^+ ATPase pump. SGLT1 is present in the brush border membrane of enterocytes and mammary gland, whereas SGLT2 is primarily found in the renal tubular epithelial cells.

Solids-not-fat (SNF) It refers to all components of milk except water and milk fat, primarily comprising protein (casein, whey), lactose (milk sugar), minerals (calcium, phosphorus), and vitamins, which significantly boost milk's nutritional value, texture, and shelf life.

Somatic cell count (SCC) The number of body cells (mainly white blood cells) present in milk; a key indicator of udder health and mastitis.

Somatomedins (insulin-like growth factors, IGFs) They are peptide hormones that carry out many of the growth-promoting actions of growth hormone (GH). IGF-1 and IGF-2 are two important somatomedins. They are essential for cell growth, development, metabolism, and cartilage formation, and are produced primarily in the liver in response to GH stimulation.

Somatotropic axis It is the key hormonal pathway that regulates growth, metabolism, and body composition. It functions through the hypothalamus, releasing GHRH, the anterior pituitary producing growth hormone (GH), and the liver and other tissues generating insulin-like growth factor-1 (IGF-1), the GH receptor (GHR), and IGF-binding proteins (IGFBP).

Spexin (SPX) It is a neuropeptide expressed in the neurons of the hypothalamus and reported to control feed intake during the transition period in cows. The concentration of spexin is negatively correlated with non-esterified fatty acids and ghrelin concentration. It is also inversely related to progesterone and blood metabolites. Spexin is reported to inhibit appetite in mammals. Spexin concentration decreased from 21 days pre-partum to calving and increased during the 14th day of lactation, which could regulate the feed intake during the early lactation period.

Standard plate count (SPC) It is a microbiological technique used to evaluate the number of viable aerobic bacteria in a sample to assess microbial contamination levels for food safety and quality control. In this method, the aliquots of the diluted samples are mixed with a nutrient-rich agar medium in Petri dishes and incubated under aerobic conditions (normally 35 °C for 48 h). The visible bacterial colonies are counted after incubation, and the number of colonies is multiplied by the dilution factor to obtain colony-forming units (CFU) per milliliter or gram of the original sample. SPC >5000 cfu/mL in milk indicates that the milking system is contaminated.

Stem cells Undifferentiated cells capable of developing into specialized cell types; they help regenerate mammary tissue.

Sterol-regulatory element binding protein (SREBP) It is a transcription factor that regulates fatty acid synthesis. It exists in two major isoforms, SREBP-1 and SREBP-2. Both isoforms are synthesized as inactive precursors bound to the endoplasmic reticulum membrane in association with SREBP cleavage-activating protein (SCAP). Decreased cholesterol stimulates SCAP, which facilitates the transport of SREBP to the nucleus and stimulates the expression of acetyl-CoA carboxylase α (ACACA) and fatty acid synthase (FASN) genes to promote fatty acid synthesis and HMG-CoA synthase and HMG-CoA reductase for cholesterol biosynthesis.

Streak canal (ductus papillaris) It is the distal aperture of the teat cistern via which milk is drained outside. The opening of the streak canal is guided by a sphincter made of circular smooth muscles. The sphincter retains the milk and keeps the orifice closed during periods between milking and prevents the entry of pathogens.

Stress-induced inhibition Suppression of MER due to activation of stress pathways. Catecholamines, opioids, and cortisol are involved. It blocks oxytocin release and action. Removal of stress rapidly restores reflex function.

Suppressor of cytokine signaling (SOCS) proteins They are intracellular molecules that act as a negative feedback system to regulate cytokine and growth factor signaling. They mainly inhibit the JAK/STAT pathway, helping prevent excessive signaling and maintaining proper control of immune responses, cell growth, and differentiation.

Supraoptic nucleus (SON) Hypothalamic nucleus containing magnocellular oxytocin neurons. Acts together with PVN in hormone release. SON neurons show burst firing during MER. It contributes to systemic oxytocin surges.

Synapsids The link between mammals and the amniotes.

T lymphocytes They are a group of lymphocytes that mature in the thymus and play a pivotal role in cell-mediated immune responses. T cells can be classified into helper T cells, suppressor T cells, and cytotoxic or killer T cells. Different types of T cells can be identified by their structural markers. Helper T cells are also called CD4+ due to the presence of CD4 as added co-receptors. Similarly, cytotoxic T cells can be identified through their specific marker CD8, hence called CD8+. T cells can also be classified on the basis of the expression of T-cell receptors (TCR) into two categories, $\alpha\beta$ T-cells and $\gamma\delta$ T-cells. The $\alpha\beta$ T-cells are of two types, namely CD4+ (T-helper) and CD8+ cells. Helper T cells can be subdivided into Th1 and Th2 cells. CD8+ lymphocytes comprise T-cytotoxic and T-suppressor cells.

Teat cannulation It is a procedure in which a thin, hollow tube (cannula) is inserted into the teat canal for the purpose of intra-mammary infusion of medicines, milk drainage, or to maintain the patency of the teat canal after surgery.

Teat cistern (sinus papillaris) The teat cistern is the cavity inside the teat that is connected with the gland cistern. The teat cistern has a storage capacity of 10 to 50 ml. It has a honeycombed appearance due to the presence of multiple overlapping longitudinal and circular folds.

Teat end callosity This is characterized by the appearance of a protruding mass of keratinized tissue around the teat sphincter due to machine milking. It is mostly seen in high-yielding cows during early to mid-lactation and usually disappears during the dry period. Effective milking management practices are the key to its prevention.

Temperature–humidity index (THI) It is used to evaluate the combined effects of air temperature and humidity to gauge heat stress, mainly in livestock like dairy cows. It indicates conditions that may cause discomfort, affect health, reduce milk production, or impair reproduction. THI is calculated using formulas that include dry-bulb temperature and relative humidity, with higher values signaling greater risk—for example, a THI above 74 indicates danger or emergency for cows.

Temporal dynamics Timing characteristics of oxytocin release and milk flow. Includes latency, pulse duration, and clearance. Precise timing ensures efficient milk removal. Disruption alters flow patterns.

Tenascins (TN) They are extracellular matrix glycoproteins that regulate cellular differentiation and morphology.

Terminal ductal-lobular unit (TDLU) This is the primary milk-producing unit of the mammary gland in humans and pigs, comprising a terminal duct and a cluster of ductules. It is also called the terminal ductal unit (TDU) in cows and terminal end buds (TEBs) in rodents.

Tight junctions Tight junctions are narrow, continuous seals between the mammary epithelial cells that facilitate cell–cell communication. They also maintain different internal milieu between ducts and alveoli from the surrounding interstitial space. The shape of the tight junctions is dynamic in nature. There are a number of proteins associated with tight junctions that control the functions of these junctions.

Transcellular transport In this mechanism, water and solutes are transported through the plasma membranes of mammary epithelial cells via transport proteins. The transcellular routes are further classified into the membrane route, Golgi route, milk fat route, and transcytosis. Water, urea, sodium, potassium, and chlorides are carried via the membrane route. Milk proteins, citrate, and calcium are carried through the Golgi route. Milk fats are extruded from mammary epithelial cells by the milk fat route. Immunoglobulins are carried via transcytosis.

Transcytosis In this pathway, the transport cargo is internalized, followed by transport across the cytoplasm and released to the other side of the cell. Proteins such as albumin, immunoglobulins, transferrin, hormones, and growth factors are transported across the mammary epithelial cells through the transcytosis pathway. The major advantage of transcytosis is that the bioactive molecules are carried, avoiding degradation. The process of transcytosis involves three steps: endocytosis of the materials, followed by endosomal trafficking, and finally the exocytosis.

Transferrin (TF) It is an iron-binding protein synthesized locally in the mammary gland (pigs, rodents, and rabbits) or transported from blood (ruminants). TF is a glycoprotein having two lobes, each capable of binding one Fe^{+3}. TF disrupts the microbial membrane potentials by iron sequestration to exert bacteriostatic and bactericidal effects on a variety of pathogens. The concentration of TF is 0.02–0.04 mg/mL in milk. A significantly higher level of TF is reported in the serum of cows suffering from acute mastitis.

Transforming growth factor-α (TGFα) It is a polypeptide under the EGF family and reported to be a potent mitogen for mammary epithelial cells in rats, humans, and cows. It induces lobuloalveolar growth of mammary glands in virgin mice with higher potency than EGF.

Transgenic animal An animal whose genome has been modified to carry and express foreign genes, often to produce special proteins in milk.

Transplacental passage It is the transfer of substances—like nutrients, oxygen, waste, hormones, drugs, alcohol, viruses, or antibodies—from the mother's bloodstream, across the placenta, to the developing fetus. This crucial interface allows for fetal nourishment but also means harmful agents can reach the baby, making it a significant factor in prenatal health, treatment decisions, and understanding congenital conditions.

Udder seborrhea (necrotic dermatitis) It is a kind of moist and foul-smelling superficial dermatitis caused by ischemia in the udder skin, followed by necrosis as a consequence of severe udder edema. It is usually predominant during the first 1–2 weeks after calving.

Udder stimulation Manual or mechanical pre-milking stimulation of teats. It activates afferent pathways and oxytocin release. Optimal stimulation shortens latency. It is essential for efficient dairy management.

Udder The milk-producing organs of ruminants such as cattle, goats, and sheep are usually referred to as an udder. The term udder is analogous to the "breast" in primates. The udder comprises mammary glands that produce milk with teats that drain the milk. In cows, four mammary glands are joined to form an udder.

Vaccination A preventive measure using biological preparations that stimulate the immune system to protect against specific diseases.

Vacuolar H^+-ATPase (V-ATPase) It is a crucial, multi-subunit enzyme complex found in nearly all eukaryotic cells, acting as an ATP-powered proton (H^+) pump that acidifies intracellular compartments like lysosomes and endosomes, regulating pH and facilitating ligand release from receptors. It plays a crucial role in the selective movement of IgG_1.

Vitellogenin A female-specific protein, egg-yolk protein precursor, having lipids, phosphates, and carbohydrates to provide nourishment to the oviparous developing embryos.

Viviparity Development of the embryo inside the mother's body until the young can be metabolically independent.

Wearable sensor A small electronic device attached to an animal to monitor temperature, activity, rumination, or health in real time.

Whole genome sequencing (WGS) It is a technique that determines the complete DNA sequence of an organism, reading all its nucleotides (A, T, C, G) to provide a full genetic blueprint. It is used in medical diagnostics (e.g., rare diseases, cancer), epidemiology (tracking outbreaks), and evolutionary studies, and can detect all types of genetic variations, including SNPs, insertions, deletions, and large structural changes. It has been used to identify genes or specific mutations linked to milk production traits.

Wingless-related integration site (WNT) These are secreted glycoproteins that bind to the Frizzled (Fz) receptor family to regulate crucial developmental aspects and organogenesis in the embryo. The signaling pathway is termed the Wnt signaling pathway. It controls cell migration, determination of cell fate, and neural patterning during embryonic mammary gland development. Wnt ligands such as Wnt3 and Wnt6 are present in the ectoderm, Wnt5a and Wnt11 in the mesenchyme, and Wnt10b in mammary placodes. The Wnt ligands are transcriptional and posttranscriptional regulating proteins that act either canonical (-β-catenin-dependent) or noncanonical (β-catenin-independent) pathways for the appearance of the mammary fate in embryonic ectoderm.

Xanthine oxidase It is an important humoral defense factor that originates from the apical membrane of mammary epithelium and is primarily found in the milk fat globule membrane. The bactericidal activity of xanthine oxidase is mediated by the production of nitric oxide from inorganic nitrite, which is further converted to peroxynitrite. The bacteriostatic action of xanthine oxidase is mediated through the production of hydrogen peroxide in the presence of a reducing substrate.

α-Lactalbumin The protein that regulates the production of lactose in the milk.

β-Casomorphin-7 (BCM-7) It is a bioactive peptide generated during the digestion of β-casein, particularly from the A1 variant. It exhibits opioid-like activity by binding to μ-opioid receptors, thereby interacting with the gut–brain axis and potentially modulating gastrointestinal motility, inflammatory processes, and immune responses.

Index

J. Mukherjee et al., *Veterinary Lactation Physiology*,
https://doi.org/10.1007/978-3-032-21123-1

S

T